Lippincott's Q&A Certification Review

EMERGENCY NURSING

SECOND EDITION

Wolters Kluwer Health | Lippincott Williams & Wilkins
Philadelphia • Baltimore • New York • London
Buenos Aires • Hong Kong • Sydney • Tokyo

Staff

Acquisitions Editor
Bill Lamsback

Clinical Director
Joan M. Robinson, RN, MSN

Clinical Project Manager
Beverly Ann Tscheschlog, RN, MS

Clinical Editor
Leigh Ann Trujillo, RN, BSN

Product Director
David Moreau

Senior Product Manager
Diane Labus

Editor
Shana Harrington

Copy Editor
Heather Ditch

Editorial Assistants
Karen J. Kirk, Jeri O'Shea, Linda K. Ruhf

Art Director
Elaine Kasmer

Design Assistant
Karen Kappe Nugent

Design
Joseph John Clark (design), Scott Rattray (cover)

Vendor Manager
Cynthia Rudy

Senior Manufacturing Coordinator
Beth J. Welsh

Production Services
S4 Carlisle Publishing Services

The clinical treatments described and recommended in this publication are based on research and consultation with nursing, medical, and legal authorities. To the best of our knowledge, these procedures reflect currently accepted practice. Nevertheless, they can't be considered absolute and universal recommendations. For individual applications, all recommendations must be considered in light of the patient's clinical condition and, before administration of new or infrequently used drugs, in light of the latest package-insert information. The authors and publisher disclaim any responsibility for any adverse effects resulting from the suggested procedures, from any undetected errors, or from the reader's misunderstanding of the text.

Printed in China
978-1-4511-7199-0
1-4511-7199-4

LQ&ACRen010912

Library of Congress Cataloging-in-Publication Data

Lippincott's Q & A certification review : emergency nursing. — 2nd ed.
p. ; cm.
Lippincott's Q and A certification review : emergency nursing
Emergency nursing
Includes bibliographical references and index.
ISBN 978-1-4511-7199-0 (alk. paper) — ISBN 1-4511-7199-4 (alk. paper)
I. Lippincott Williams & Wilkins. II. Title: Lippincott's Q and A certification review : emergency nursing. III. Title: Emergency nursing.
[DNLM: 1. Emergencies—nursing—Examination Questions. 2. Emergency Nursing—methods—Examination Questions. WY 18.2]
616.02'5076—dc23
2012022345

CCS0712

Contents

Contributors and consultants

Kelly Allen, RN, MSN, CEN
Clinical Nurse Specialist Emergency/Trauma
Providence Regional Medical Center
Everett, Wash.

Susan Barnason, PhD, APRN-CNS, CEN, CCRN
Professor of Nursing
University of Nebraska Medical Center College of Nursing, Lincoln Division
Lincoln, Neb.

Beth Ann Broering, MSN, RN, CEN, CCRN, CPEN, CCNS, FAEN
Emergency Services Clinical Nurse Specialist
St. Thomas Health Services
Nashville, Tenn.

Cheyenne Brown, RN, BS, CEN
Registered Nurse
Intermountain Healthcare
Salt Lake City, Utah

Laurie Donaghy, BSN, RN, CEN
Staff Nurse
Temple University Hospital
Philadelphia, Pa.

Laura Favand, RN, MS, CEN
Chief of Plans, Training Mobilization, and Security
USA MEDDAC
Fort Knox, Ky.

Andi Foley, MSN, RN, CEN
Emergency Nurse Specialist
University of Washington
Seattle, Wash.

Wm. Bryan Gibboney, MSN, APRN, FNP-C, ACNP-BC, CEN, CPEN, CCRN
Emergency Nurse Practitioner
Biloxi Regional Medical Center
Biloxi, Miss.

Molly Groban, MS, MAEd, RN, CEN, CCRN, LNC, MICN, SANE
Director of Education
JFK Memorial Hospital
Indio, Calif.

Jill Johnson, DNP, APRN, FNP-BC, CCRN, CEN, CFRN
Market Manager Clinical Operation
Take Care Health
PT Emergency Dept.
Team Health Service
Louisville, Ky.

Charles Kunkle, MSN, CEN, CCRN, BC-NA
Director of Emergency/Pediatric Services
St. Mary Medical Center
Langhorne, Pa.

Sharon L. G. Lee, MSN, FNP-C, ARNP, CEN, CCRN
Clinical Educator, Emergency Department
BryanLGH Medical Center
ARNP
Mercy Hospital
Lincoln, Neb.

Charles L. Mandelin, RN, BA, BSN, CEN
Registered Nurse
Duke Hospital
Durham, N.C.

Cheryl Schmitz, MS, RN, BC, CNS-BC, CEN
Clinical Specialist, Emergency Services
Inova Loudoun Hospital
Leesburg, Va.

Dawn M. Specht, MSN, PhD, RN, APRN, CEN, CCRN, CCNS
Clinical Nurse Specialist/Advanced Practice Nurse
AtlantiCare Regional Medical Center
Atlantic City, N.J.

Polly Gerber Zimmermann, RN, MS, MBA, CEN, FAEN
Associate Professor
Harry S. Truman College
Chicago, Ill.

Understanding the CEN examination

According to the National Specialty Nursing Certifying Organization, certification is the process by which a nongovernmental agency or association validates, based on predetermined standards, a registered nurse's qualifications and knowledge for practice in a defined functional or clinical area of nursing. To enhance your performance on the Certified Emergency Nurse (CEN) examination, review the answers to these commonly asked questions.

Who sponsors the CEN examination?

The Board of Certification for Emergency Nurses (BCEN) sponsors the CEN examination. The BCEN evaluates and recognizes nurses who have attained a defined body of emergency nursing knowledge needed to function at a competent level.

Is the CEN examination as difficult as the NCLEX?

Health care professionals who take a certification examination for a specialty area of practice already have the knowledge required by the basic licensure examination. Because the knowledge measured by the CEN examination is specialized for emergency nursing, the CEN examination is more challenging than the National Council Licensure Examination (NCLEX).

If I've been an emergency nurse for years, do I need to study?

As an emergency nurse, you have probably mastered complex technical skills related to the care of emergency clients as well as the theoretical knowledge that underlies these skills. You have also probably developed the ability to make sound nursing judgments in crises that often determine whether a client lives or dies. Despite such advanced knowledge, skill mastery, and decision-making ability, many emergency nurses experience high levels of test-taking anxiety that may prevent them from seeking certification. This book can help alleviate test-taking anxiety by providing a thorough review of the material contained in the CEN examination.

What are the eligibility requirements?

The BCEN establishes criteria for eligibility to take the CEN examination. Current criteria are listed here.

- You must possess a current unrestricted license or nursing certificate as a registered nurse in the United States.
- Nurses from other countries must possess licensure, registration, or certification to practice as a registered nurse in that country. An additional international testing fee will be assessed at the time of application.
- Any restriction, suspension, or probation, or any order arising from a Nursing License Authority that limits your ability to function in an emergency nurse setting and perform those tasks normally associated with emergency nursing practice will disqualify you to sit for the examination unless you're a qualified individual with a disability who can perform the essential functions of emergency nursing with or without reasonable accommodation.
- Although not a requirement, the BCEN recommends that you have 2 years of experience in emergency nursing practice.
- Membership in the Emergency Nurses Association qualifies you for a reduced CEN examination application fee.

How many questions are on the examination?

The CEN examination consists of 175 multiple-choice questions, of which 150 are scored. A candidate is allotted 3 hours to complete the examination.

How is the examination administered?

The CEN examination is administered by computer. Upon special request, a pencil-and-paper test may be available.

What topics does the examination cover?

The content of the CEN examination, based on recognized standards and practices for emergency nursing, is divided into two major areas: clinical practice and professional issues.

Clinical practice

The CEN examination contains, but isn't limited to, the following items. The questions in Chapters 1 to 19 of this book approximate the content areas shown below; the sample test reflects the actual examination.

- Gastrointestinal emergencies (10 items)
- Cardiovascular emergencies (20 items)
- Maxillofacial and ocular emergencies (9 items)
- Medical emergencies and communicable diseases (17 items)
- Neurologic emergencies (15 items)
- Obstetric, genitourinary, and gynecologic emergencies (14 items)
- Orthopedic emergencies and wound management (15 items)
- Psychosocial emergencies (7 items)
- Respiratory emergencies (18 items)
- Shock and multisystem trauma emergencies (9 items)
- Substance abuse, toxicologic, and environmental emergencies (10 items).

When studying for the examination, keep in mind that clinical practice questions also are designed to test your knowledge of the five steps of the nursing process: assessment, analysis, planning, implementation, and evaluation. The outline below shows examples of specific nursing behaviors associated with each step. The CEN examination uses only the NANDA-approved list of nursing diagnoses in test items.

Assessment

These questions test your ability to collect data. They focus on such nursing behaviors as:

- assessing the client's physiologic and psychosocial health as well as safety needs
- collecting information from the client, family, friends, hospital records, and health team members
- recognizing symptoms and findings
- communicating findings to other team members
- challenging orders and decisions by health team members, as appropriate.

Analysis

These questions test your ability to identify real or potential health care needs and problems. They focus on such nursing behaviors as:

- organizing, interpreting, and validating assessment data
- gathering additional data when necessary

- identifying and communicating nursing problems to the health care team
- determining the client's needs and the staff's ability to meet them.

Planning and implementation

These questions test your ability to initiate and complete actions that accomplish defined goals. They focus on such nursing behaviors as:

- including the client, family, friends, and other health team members in setting goals
- mutually establishing goal priorities
- providing a safe, effective care environment for the client
- documenting all information needed to manage the client's needs
- planning for the client's comfort and the maintenance of optimum functioning
- selecting the best nursing measures to deliver effective care
- prioritizing interventions to ensure optimal outcomes
- identifying community resources to assist the client and family
- coordinating the client's care with other health care providers
- delegating care responsibilities to other health care providers
- supervising and validating the activities of other health team members
- formulating outcomes of nursing interventions
- teaching the client and family
- recording all appropriate information, orally and in written reports.

Evaluation

These questions test your ability to measure goal achievement. They focus on such nursing behaviors as:

- comparing actual outcomes with expected outcomes
- evaluating the client's compliance with the prescribed plan of care
- documenting the client's response to care
- revising the plan of care and reordering priorities as needed.

Professional issues

A small percentage of the questions on the CEN examination (11 items) pertain to legal and organizational issues. The focus is on such topics as informed consent, confidentiality, and quality improvement. The questions in Chapters 20 and 21 of this book are examples of these types of questions. The professional issues portion of the examination doesn't include a nursing process dimension.

What's the best way to study?

Although individual study is highly recommended, the "best" way to study is a matter of personal preference. Some test candidates prefer to study alone, whereas others opt for group study, and still others enjoy a combination of the two.

Individual study

No matter what other study strategies you use, individual preparation for the CEN examination is highly recommended. This preparation can take several forms.

- Read review books such as this one to help you pinpoint areas that need improvement. You can then concentrate on reviewing materials in those areas.
- Consult emergency nursing textbooks and study guides. As you read the material, ask yourself multiple-choice questions about the information. Consider how the CEN

examination might test your knowledge of this material.

- Answer practice questions similar to those on the test. Spend about 30 minutes each day answering 10 to 20 questions (don't try to answer 100 questions on your day off). After you answer the questions, compare your answers with the correct answers listed in the review book; also review the rationales provided. If you answer some questions incorrectly and aren't sure why, return to the textbook or review book to find the rationale. By doing this, you'll become more familiar and comfortable with the examination's format while reinforcing the information you've studied.
- If you haven't attended an Advanced Cardiac Life Support course, Pediatric Advanced Life Support course, Trauma Nursing Care course, or an Emergency Nursing Pediatric course, consider attending these courses or review the course provider manuals for these courses. Content that is covered in these courses is often found in the CEN examination.

Group study

Studying with others can effectively prepare you for the CEN examination. To get the most from your sessions, follow these guidelines:

- Be choosy about whom to include in your study group. Limit the number of people (the recommended size is four to six people); larger groups can disrupt study.
- Ask each member to prepare one section of the study topic before the group meets. For example, have one person discuss anatomy and physiology, another review the drugs used for treatments, and a third cover key elements of emergency nursing care.
- Meet regularly (once or twice weekly) to maintain a studious atmosphere.
- Limit each study session to 2 hours. Longer sessions invite participants to wander off the topic and promote a negative attitude toward the examination.
- Avoid turning study sessions into a party. Although snacks and refreshments can help maintain the group's energy, a party atmosphere will render the session ineffective.

How can I master a multiple-choice test?

Multiple-choice questions are one of the most commonly used test formats for such standardized tests as the CEN examination. After you've mastered these test-taking strategies, you'll be able to score better on multiple-choice tests.

- Read the question and all options carefully and completely.
- Treat each question individually. Use only the information provided for that question, and avoid reading into a question information that isn't provided.
- Monitor your time. You'll have approximately 60 seconds per question; because most test-takers average 45 seconds per question, you may finish well before the time limit.
- Narrow your choices by using the process of elimination. If you can identify even one option as incorrect, you can focus your attention on the more plausible answers (and improve your chances of answering correctly).
- Don't change your answer. Studies show that test-takers who change an answer on a multiple-choice examination usually change it from a correct answer to an incorrect one or from one incorrect answer to another

incorrect answer. Rarely do they change to a correct answer.

- Look for qualifying words in the question (such as *first, best, most, better,* and *highest*) that ask you to judge the priority of the options; then select the answer that has the highest priority.
- Look for negative words in the question (such as *not, least, unlikely, inappropriate, unrealistic, lowest, contraindicated, except, inconsistent, all but, atypical,* and *incorrect*). In general, when you're asked a negative question, three of the choices are appropriate actions, and one is inappropriate. You're being asked to select the inappropriate choice as your answer.
- Avoid selecting answers that contain absolute words (including *always, every, only, all, never,* and *none*); these options usually are incorrect.
- Never choose an option that refers the client to a physician. Because the CEN examination is for nurses and includes conditions and problems that nurses should be able to solve independently, an answer that refers a client to the physician usually is incorrect and can be eliminated from consideration.
- Don't look for a pattern (such as C, C, A, B, C, C, A, B) when selecting answers. The questions and answers on the examination are randomly arranged.
- Don't panic if you read a question that you don't understand. Some questions may refer to diseases, drugs, or laboratory tests that you're unfamiliar with. In such cases, remember that nursing care is similar in many situations, even when disease processes differ markedly. Just select the answer that seems logical and involves general nursing care.
- Think positively about the examination. People who have a positive attitude score higher than those who don't.

Are there any other tips I should know?

Proper planning can go a long way toward ensuring your success on the CEN examination. Try these suggestions.

Before examination day

- A week or so before the examination, drive to the test site to familiarize yourself with parking facilities and to locate the test room. Knowing where to go will greatly reduce your anxiety on the day of the examination.
- Follow as normal a schedule as possible on the day before the examination. If you need to travel to the test site and stay away from home overnight, try to follow your usual nightly routine; avoid the urge to do something different.
- The night before the test, avoid drinking alcoholic beverages. Alcohol, a central nervous system (CNS) depressant, interferes with your ability to concentrate. Avoid eating foods you've never eaten before, which may cause adverse GI effects the next day.
- Avoid taking sleep medications you've never taken before. Like alcohol, most sleep aids are CNS depressants; some have a hangover effect, while others produce drowsiness for an extended period.
- Don't stay up late to study; this will make you tired during the test, which will decrease your ability to concentrate. Besides, you're probably as prepared as you can be. Review formulas, charts, and lists for no more than 1 hour. Then relax, perhaps by watching television or reading a magazine or

book. These activities will help decrease your anxiety. Go to bed at your usual time.

Examination day

- On the morning of the examination, don't attempt a major review of the material. The likelihood of learning something new is slim, and intensive study may only increase your anxiety.
- Don't drink excessive amounts of coffee, tea, or caffeine-containing beverages. Caffeine will increase your nervousness and stimulate your renal system. (Rest room visits are permitted, but the allotted test time isn't extended if you leave the room during the test.)
- Eat breakfast, even if you usually don't, and include foods high in glucose and protein to maintain your energy level. Shun greasy, heavy foods, which tend to form an uncomfortable knot in your stomach and may decrease your ability to concentrate.
- Dress in comfortable, layered clothing. Jogging suits are popular. Many rooms are air-conditioned in the summer and may be cool even if it's hot outside. Be prepared by taking a sweater or sweatshirt.
- Arrive at the test site 30 to 45 minutes early, and make sure you have the required papers and documents for admittance to the test room. Latecomers aren't admitted to the examination.
- Do not bring pencils, pens, note paper, calculators, calipers, or other resources. Nothing is permitted to be taken into the testing room.
- At the testing center, you will be given a pencil and a blank piece of paper for notes and calculations. You will be asked to turn in that paper at the completion of the test.
- Think positively about how you'll do. Taking the CEN examination shows confidence in your knowledge of emergency nursing. When you receive your passing results, plan to celebrate your success, a significant achievement in your professional life that deserves to be rewarded.

Who can I contact for more information?

Contact the Board of Certification of Emergency Nursing, 915 Lee Street, Des Plaines Ill. 60016-6569, or phone (800) 900-9659, extension 2630. An online application is available at the BCEN website: *http://www.ena.org/bcen/default.asp.* Other correspondence and requests for information concerning applications for or administration of the CEN examination should be directed to: Applied Measurement Professionals, Inc., Candidate Services – CEN Examination, 8310 Nieman Road, Lenexa, Kans. 66214, USA, or phone (913) 541-0400.

Part I
Clinical practice

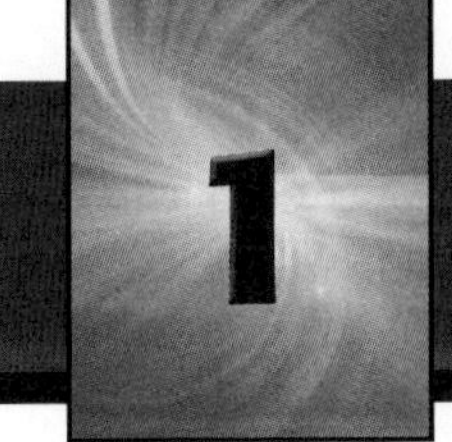

1 Abdominal emergencies

1. A client complains of right lower quadrant abdominal pain, nausea, and vomiting. Which intervention isn't appropriate?
[ ] **A.** Offering clear liquids
[ ] **B.** Obtaining a urine specimen
[ ] **C.** Obtaining a blood specimen for a complete blood count (CBC)
[ ] **D.** Assisting the client to a position of comfort

Correct answer—A. *Rationales:* A client with undiagnosed abdominal pain should receive nothing by mouth in case surgery is required. Obtaining a urine specimen and a CBC can help diagnose the cause of abdominal pain. Repositioning can sometimes diminish the client's pain.
Nursing process step: Intervention

2. A client complains of abdominal pain and distention, fever, tachycardia, and diaphoresis. An abdominal X-ray shows free air under the diaphragm. The emergency department nurse should suspect which condition?
[ ] **A.** Intestinal obstruction
[ ] **B.** Acute appendicitis
[ ] **C.** Intestinal perforation
[ ] **D.** Acute cholelithiasis

Correct answer—C. *Rationales:* Intestinal perforation is associated with free air under the diaphragm. Intestinal obstruction, acute appendicitis, and acute cholelithiasis aren't associated with free air.
Nursing process step: Assessment

3. A client has an intestinal perforation. Which intervention is inappropriate?
[ ] **A.** Inserting a nasogastric (NG) tube
[ ] **B.** Offering clear liquids
[ ] **C.** Administering I.V. antibiotics
[ ] **D.** Preparing the client for surgery

Correct answer—B. *Rationales:* The client with intestinal perforation will require surgery and should receive nothing by mouth. An NG tube should be inserted to decompress the GI tract. Antibiotics should be administered I.V. to prevent sepsis, which can be caused by leakage from the perforation.
Nursing process step: Implementation

4. Which assessment finding is most important for the nurse to act on for a client diagnosed with acute pancreatitis?
[ ] **A.** Sharp, knifelike pain
[ ] **B.** Bluish discoloration around the umbilicus
[ ] **C.** Orthostatic hypotension
[ ] **D.** One episode of emesis

Correct answer—C. *Rationales:* A major complication of pancreatitis is hypovolemia. Because hypovolemia can cause low blood pressure, orthostatic hypotension is associated with hypotension. Sharp, knifelike pain is expected and will be treated, but circulation takes priority. Bluish discoloration around the umbilicus (Cullen's sign) is a result of the exudate from autodigestion of the pancreas in pancreatitis and does not require immediate intervention. One episode of emesis doesn't require intervention.
Nursing process step: Analysis

5. What are three major complications of pancreatitis?
[ ] **A.** Hypervolemia, latent hypocalcemia, and latent hypoxia
[ ] **B.** Hypervolemia, latent hypercalcemia, and latent hypoxia
[ ] **C.** Hypovolemia, latent hypocalcemia, and latent hypoxia
[ ] **D.** Hypovolemia, latent hypercalcemia, and latent hypoxia

Correct answer—C. *Rationales:* The three major complications of pancreatitis include hypovolemia (not hypervolemia), latent hypocalcemia (not hypercalcemia), and latent hypoxia.
Nursing process step: Analysis

6. Peritoneal lavage is a diagnostic tool used in detecting abdominal injuries. Which of the following is a contraindication for peritoneal lavage?
[ ] **A.** An unconscious client
[ ] **B.** A history of abdominal surgery
[ ] **C.** A distended bladder
[ ] **D.** An allergy to radiopaque dye

Correct answer—C. *Rationales:* A distended bladder is an absolute contraindication for peritoneal lavage. Peritoneal lavage involves the instillation and withdrawal of fluid from the abdominal cavity. An indwelling urinary catheter should be inserted before the procedure. Radiopaque dye isn't required. Peritoneal lavage is especially useful for diagnosing abdominal injuries in an unconscious client because he can't report pain. A history of abdominal surgery isn't a contraindication for this procedure.
Nursing process step: Intervention

7. Which organ is most frequently injured in blunt abdominal trauma?
[ ] **A.** Large bowel
[ ] **B.** Spleen
[ ] **C.** Liver
[ ] **D.** Stomach

Correct answer—B. *Rationales:* A highly vascular and encapsulated organ, the spleen is compressed against the vertebral column during blunt abdominal trauma. Injuries to the spleen are commonly seen in clients with left lower rib injuries. Injuries to the liver are common in clients with right lower rib fractures. The large bowel and stomach are seldom injured in blunt abdominal trauma.
Nursing process step: Assessment

8. A 4-year-old child is brought to the emergency department after being hit in the abdomen with a baseball bat. Which of the following isn't a normal finding for this child?
[ ] **A.** High-pitched tympanic sound over the stomach
[ ] **B.** Cylindrical contour of the abdomen
[ ] **C.** Failure of the abdomen to move with respirations
[ ] **D.** Crying during examination

Correct answer—C. *Rationales:* Because children younger than age 9 are abdominal breathers, chest movements are normally synchronized with abdominal movements. Failure of the abdomen to move with respirations could indicate serious abdominal injury. The high-pitched tympanic sounds indicate air in the stomach, a condition common in mouth breathers. Young children have a spinal lordosis that gives the abdomen a cylindrical, prominent contour. They may express their fear by crying during the examination; speaking softly and allowing a caregiver to stay nearby may help ease their fear.
Nursing process step: Assessment

9. Which clinical presentation would be most indicative of a small-bowel obstruction?
[ ] **A.** Dark, tarry stool
[ ] **B.** Bowel sounds occurring at a rate of 5 to 30 per minute
[ ] **C.** Foul-smelling, dark, copious emesis
[ ] **D.** Metallic taste in the mouth

Correct answer—C. *Rationales:* Small-bowel obstructions are higher and tend to lead to reverse peristalsis and emesis of feculent material. Dark, tarry stool is a classic symptom of upper GI bleeding, not obstruction. Normal bowel sounds consist of clicks and gurgles that occur at a rate of 5 to 30 per minute, so this is a normal finding. Bowel sounds are also more indicative of a large-intestine obstruction. The presence of a metallic taste isn't related to a bowel obstruction.
Nursing process step: Analysis

10. A client comes to the emergency department complaining of stomach pain and has several episodes of coffee-ground emesis. What assessment would be most important for the nurse to ask to help determine the cause of this client's symptoms?
[ ] **A.** History of most recent food intake
[ ] **B.** History of nonsteroidal anti-inflammatory drug (NSAID) use
[ ] **C.** History of taking oral iron supplements
[ ] **D.** History of hemorrhoids

Correct answer–B. *Rationales:* Coffee-ground emesis results from upper GI bleeding that has remained in the stomach. Upper GI bleeding is commonly caused by regular intake of NSAIDs. The client's most recent food intake won't help determine the cause of the client's symptoms. Iron supplements could cause abdominal pain from constipation but not coffee-ground emesis. A history of hemorrhoids would cause recent bleeding, not coffee-ground emesis or abdominal pain.
Nursing process step: Analysis

11. The client with liver failure will have which of the following laboratory values?
[ ] **A.** Increased platelets, increased magnesium
[ ] **B.** Increased lipase, increased amylase PT
[ ] **C.** Decreased ALT, decreased AST PT
[ ] **D.** Decreased albumin, increased PT

Correct answer–D. *Rationales:* Albumin decreases because the liver can't synthesize blood proteins. PT increases because the diseased liver can't make clotting factors in sufficient amounts. These clients are prone to bleeding.
Nursing process step: Assessment

12. A mother brings her 2-month-old infant to the emergency department (ED). His abdomen is distended, and he has been vomiting forcefully and with increasing frequency over the past 2 weeks. On examination, the ED nurse notes signs of dehydration and a palpable mass to the right of the umbilicus. Peristaltic waves are visible, moving from left to right. The nurse should suspect which condition?
[ ] **A.** Colic
[ ] **B.** Failure to thrive
[ ] **C.** Intussusception
[ ] **D.** Pyloric stenosis

Correct answer–D. *Rationales:* These are classic symptoms of pyloric stenosis caused by hypertrophy of the circular pylorus muscle. Surgery is the standard treatment for this disorder. Abdominal masses and abnormal peristalsis aren't necessarily related to colic or failure to thrive. Intussusception is usually characterized by acute onset and severe abdominal pain.
Nursing process step: Assessment

13. What is the FAST examination used for in clients with primarily blunt abdominal trauma?
[ ] **A.** As a fecal assay screening test
[ ] **B.** To determine the presence of hemoperitoneum
[ ] **C.** To determine the presence of free air from perforation
[ ] **D.** To determine whether bladder injury has occurred

Correct answer–B. *Rationales:* The FAST test is a focused assessment sonography for trauma ultrasonography. It is a bedside, rapid, accurate diagnostic tool to detect the presence of hemoperitoneum. Four areas are examined: the hepatorenal fossa, the splenorenal fossa, the pericardial sac, and the pelvis. It isn't a fecal assay screening test, nor does it determine whether free air is present or whether a bladder injury has occurred.
Nursing process step: Analysis

14. Acute abdominal pain in the geriatric client may be related to which of the following?
[ ] **A.** Inflammatory bowel disease
[ ] **B.** Diverticulitis
[ ] **C.** Bowel obstruction with intussusception
[ ] **D.** Ulcerative colitis

Correct answer–B. *Rationales:* Diverticulitis is one of the most common causes of acute abdominal pain in the geriatric population. About 50% of all Americans from ages 60 to 80 have diverticulitis, as do most Americans over age 80. Inflammatory bowel disease is more common in clients aged 10 to 30. Bowel obstructions are commonly caused by adhesions from previous surgeries, fecal impaction, or tumors—not intussusception—in this population. Ulcerative colitis is more prevalent in clients aged 30 to 50.
Nursing process step: Assessment

15. A client in the emergency department has severe nausea and has been vomiting every 30 to 45 minutes for the past 8 hours. This client is at risk for developing which condition?
[ ] **A.** Metabolic acidosis and hyperkalemia
[ ] **B.** Metabolic acidosis and hypokalemia
[ ] **C.** Metabolic alkalosis and hyperkalemia
[ ] **D.** Metabolic alkalosis and hypokalemia

Correct answer—D. *Rationales:* Excessive vomiting, which reduces hydrochloric acid in the stomach, causes metabolic alkalosis. It also leads to hypokalemia. Clients with the above symptoms would not be prone to acidosis or hyperkalemia.
Nursing process step: Assessment

16. The client presents to the emergency department with vomiting and diarrhea and is diagnosed with gastroenteritis. Which of the following is most important prior to allowing the client to be discharged home?
[ ] **A.** Administration of antidiarrheal medication
[ ] **B.** Ability to repeat back the BRAT diet requirements
[ ] **C.** Ability to tolerate oral fluids
[ ] **D.** Bowel sounds within normal limits

Correct answer—C. *Rationales:* Before a client goes home, the client must be able to take and keep oral fluids so no dehydration occurs at home. Antidiarrheal medications aren't routinely used for gastroenteritis. Repeating the BRAT diet requirements or hearing normal bowel sounds isn't as important as the ability to tolerate oral fluids.
Nursing process step: Intervention

17. Which of the following isn't indicative of a stomach injury?
[ ] **A.** Blood in the nasogastric (NG) aspirate
[ ] **B.** Bowel sounds in the chest
[ ] **C.** Epigastric pain and tenderness
[ ] **D.** Decreased or absent bowel sounds

Correct answer—B. *Rationales:* The client with a stomach injury may have blood in the NG aspirate as well as epigastric pain and tenderness. Bowel sounds may be decreased or absent. Signs of peritonitis may be present if acidic gastric contents have been released. Bowel sounds in the chest are indicative of diaphragmatic rupture, not stomach injury.
Nursing process step: Evaluation

18. Which of the following is the most distinguishing factor of a pancreatic injury?
[ ] **A.** Flank ecchymosis
[ ] **B.** Dullness in flank area
[ ] **C.** Right upper quadrant tenderness
[ ] **D.** Rectal bleeding

Correct answer—A. *Rationales:* Ecchymosis in the flank area (known as Turner's sign) suggests retroperitoneal bleeding and is commonly associated with pancreatic injury. Dullness in the flank area (Ballance's sign) is characterized by two types of dullness: a fixed dullness to percussion in the left flank and a dullness in the right flank that disappears with a change in position. Ballance's sign is usually associated with splenic injuries. Option C is associated with liver injuries; option D is associated with colon injuries. A client with pancreatic injury may also demonstrate ileus, epigastric pain radiating to the back or left upper quadrant, a positive Kehr's sign (pain in the left shoulder secondary to diaphragmatic irritation by blood), and pain, nausea, and vomiting.
Nursing process step: Assessment

19. Decreased or absent bowel sounds may result from which condition?
[ ] **A.** Irritants inside the bowel
[ ] **B.** Irritants outside the bowel
[ ] **C.** Hypovolemia
[ ] **D.** Anxiety

Correct answer—B. *Rationales:* Decreased or absent bowel sounds may be caused by an irritant, such as blood or intestinal contents, outside the bowel. Irritants inside the bowel usually cause hyperactive bowel sounds. Hypovolemia and anxiety don't cause decreased or absent bowel sounds.
Nursing process step: Evaluation

20. Which statement about a penetrating abdominal trauma is true?
[ ] **A.** The outside appearance of the wound reflects the extent of internal injury.
[ ] **B.** The outside appearance of the wound doesn't reflect the extent of internal injury.
[ ] **C.** Death occurs more commonly after penetrating trauma than after blunt trauma.
[ ] **D.** Objects impaled in the abdomen should be removed soon after the client arrives in the emergency department.

Correct answer—B. *Rationales:* The appearance of entrance and exit wounds doesn't reflect the extent of internal injury; for example, a bullet may fragment and change direction once inside the body. Death occurs more commonly after blunt abdominal trauma, in which case external signs of injury aren't obvious; therefore, detection and treatment may be delayed. Impaled objects shouldn't be removed—instead, these objects should be stabilized with a dressing to prevent further injury to the client.
Nursing process step: Evaluation

21. A client with upper GI bleeding and a history of liver disease arrives at the emergency department (ED). The ED nurse may need to administer which drug by way of a nasogastric (NG) tube?
[ ] **A.** Vasopressin (Pitressin)
[ ] **B.** Heparin
[ ] **C.** Magnesium citrate
[ ] **D.** Propylthiouracil (PTU)

Correct answer—C. *Rationales:* Magnesium citrate helps rid the bowel of blood and fecal matter; digested blood releases ammonia and other toxins into the bloodstream, increasing the risk of hepatic encephalopathy. Vasopressin is administered I.V. to control bleeding. Heparin is contraindicated because the client may have coagulation defects from the liver disease. PTU is given via an NG tube but is used to treat thyroid storm.
Nursing process step: Intervention

22. For which of the following clients is it most important to receive I.V. hydration?
[ ] **A.** A 30-year-old who has vomited several times today
[ ] **B.** A 6-month-old who had two wet diapers today
[ ] **C.** An 80-year-old with skin tenting noted on the forearm
[ ] **D.** A 15-year-old with 450 mL output in 8 hours

Correct answer—B. *Rationales:* An infant is at highest risk for decompensation from dehydration and has fewer diapers than usual. An elderly client will have forearm skin tenting that is related to the loss of collagen, not dehydration. A 30-year-old who has vomited several times will more than likely be able to compensate for the fluid loss. A 15-year-old who has a urinary output of 450 mL in 8 hours isn't in danger of dehydration.
Nursing process step: Evaluation

23. For a client with upper GI bleeding, gastric lavage is used to achieve the following with which exception?
[ ] **A.** Removing blood from the stomach
[ ] **B.** Reducing acid-peptide activity in the stomach
[ ] **C.** Reducing gastric mucosal blood flow
[ ] **D.** Sclerosing bleeding varices

Correct answer—D. *Rationales:* Gastric lavage with room temperature saline solution or water removes blood from the stomach. (The absorption of this blood may increase the client's ammonia levels.) Lavage also reduces acid-peptide activity in the stomach, reduces gastric mucosal blood flow, and prepares the client for diagnostic procedures such as endoscopy. Gastric lavage isn't effective in sclerosing bleeding varices.
Nursing process step: Intervention

24. Assessment of the abdomen should be performed in what sequence?
[ ] **A.** Percussion, palpation, auscultation, inspection
[ ] **B.** Inspection, percussion, auscultation, palpation
[ ] **C.** Inspection, auscultation, percussion, palpation
[ ] **D.** Auscultation, percussion, palpation, inspection

Correct answer—C. *Rationales:* Inspection, followed by auscultation, should be the first part of an abdominal assessment. Percussion and palpation may alter bowel sounds, so they should be done after auscultation. Palpation should be the last step in the examination because it may cause client discomfort and guarding.
Nursing process step: Assessment

25. A common finding during the evaluation of a client with cholecystitis is:
[ ] **A.** increased right lower quadrant pain.
[ ] **B.** pain during liver palpation.
[ ] **C.** periumbilical bruising.
[ ] **D.** shocklike pain with neck flexion.

Correct answer—B. *Rationales:* Pain during liver palpation when the client inhales and the inflammed gallbladder slides over the examiner's fingers (called Murphy's sign) is a positive finding for cholecystitis. In appendicitis, increased right lower quadrant pain can be elicited by hyperextension of the right hip and elevation of the right leg (Psoas sign); Periumbilical bruising (Cullen's sign), may be found in intraperitoneal bleeding. Pain resembling a sudden electric shock throughout the body produced by flexing the neck (Lhermitte's sign) is caused by cervical spine trauma, multiple sclerosis, cervical cord tumor, or cervical spondylosis.
Nursing process step: Assessment

26. A client with upper GI bleeding may require medications to reduce the acidity of gastric secretions, which can irritate the bleeding site. Which drug doesn't reduce gastric secretion acidity?
[ ] **A.** Cimetidine (Tagamet)
[ ] **B.** Vasopressin
[ ] **C.** Famotidine (Pepcid)
[ ] **D.** Ranitidine (Zantac)

Correct answer—B. *Rationales:* Vasopressin decreases blood flow to the site. The other drugs are histamine antagonists and reduce gastric acidity.
Nursing process step: Intervention

27. The difference between ulcerative colitis and Crohn's disease is that ulcerative colitis:
[ ] **A.** reveals patchy areas of full-thickness inflammation anywhere along the GI tract from the mouth to the anus.
[ ] **B.** recurs despite surgical intervention.
[ ] **C.** is an inflammatory disorder affecting the mucosal lining of the colon and rectum.
[ ] **D.** is more common among females.

Correct answer—C. *Rationales:* Ulcerative colitis begins as an inflammatory intestinal disorder affecting the mucosal lining of the colon and the rectum. The chronic inflammatory process can cause diffuse mucosal bleeding. A total colectomy offers complete cure and remission of peripheral symptoms. Crohn's disease involves recurrent inflammation of the entire GI tract and involves the mucosa as well as the surrounding musculature. More commonly found in females, the goals of treatment and management of Crohn's disease include improving symptoms and controlling the disease process.
Nursing process step: Assessment

28. A client has a history of liver failure and elevated ammonia levels. The client reports having had two soft, formed bowel movements yesterday. What action should the nurse take?
[ ] **A.** Administer the laxative lactulose.
[ ] **B.** Force oral fluids.
[ ] **C.** Encourage protein intake.
[ ] **D.** Administer activated charcoal.

Correct answer—A. *Rationales:* Lactulose is used to excrete ammonia. It should be held only if the client has constant diarrheal stools, in which case the colon is sterilized with neomycin. Forcing oral fluids or administering activated charcoal isn't indicated in the treatment of elevated ammonia levels in liver failure. Protein intake wouldn't be encouraged because the liver can't metabolize the byproducts of protein.
Nursing process step: Evaluation

29. Peritoneal lavage is appropriate for which of the following?
[ ] **A.** Rapidly increasing abdominal distention
[ ] **B.** An impaled object in the abdomen
[ ] **C.** A blood alcohol level of 0.240 mg/dl and a tender abdomen
[ ] **D.** Hypotension unresponsive to fluid bolus

Correct answer–C. *Rationales:* Peritoneal lavage is commonly used when a client can't participate in the abdominal examination (because of injuries or intoxication) or when the examination doesn't rule out the possibility of abdominal injury. A client with rapidly increasing abdominal distention or with an impaled object in the abdomen has abdominal injuries, and peritoneal lavage would serve no diagnostic purpose. A client with hypotension that's unresponsive to fluid boluses needs immediate treatment; peritoneal lavage would waste time.
Nursing process step: Intervention

30. A client with peritonitis will most likely show which symptom?
[ ] **A.** Guarding
[ ] **B.** Left lower quadrant abdominal pain
[ ] **C.** Increased bowel sounds
[ ] **D.** Hyperactive bowel sounds

Correct answer–A. *Rationales:* Peritoneal irritation causes guarding, generalized abdominal pain, and hypoactive bowel sounds. In addition, this client may experience nausea, vomiting, low-grade fever, and shallow respirations secondary to the abdominal pain.
Nursing process step: Assessment

31. Which intervention is inappropriate for a client with acute rectal bleeding?
[ ] **A.** Insertion of a nasogastric (NG) tube
[ ] **B.** Administration of enemas until clear
[ ] **C.** Insertion of an indwelling urinary catheter
[ ] **D.** Initiation of large-bore I.V. lines

Correct answer–B. *Rationales:* Enemas aren't appropriate for a client with lower GI bleeding because they may increase bleeding. Even though rectal bleeding seems to indicate lower GI bleeding, the blood could be coming from a rapid upper GI bleed; therefore, an NG tube is appropriate. An indwelling urinary catheter is helpful in maintaining accurate intake and output. Because this client may need fluid resuscitation, large-bore I.V. lines are indicated.
Nursing process step: Intervention

32. Which of the following is characteristic of a small-bowel obstruction?
[ ] **A.** Hyperactive bowel sounds
[ ] **B.** Copious vomiting
[ ] **C.** Gradual onset
[ ] **D.** Metabolic acidosis

Correct answer–B. *Rationales:* Obstruction of the small intestine is characterized by frequent and copious vomiting, a rapid (not gradual) onset, and colicky, intermittent, cramplike abdominal pain. Bowel sounds are present but not hyperactive in the large intestines. Small-bowel obstructions place the client at risk for metabolic alkalosis (not metabolic acidosis) because of fluid and electrolyte deficiencies due to loss of gastric acid.
Nursing process step: Analysis

33. A child has swallowed a quarter. What's the nurse's primary concern?
[ ] **A.** Corrosion of the stomach's mucosal lining
[ ] **B.** Bowel obstruction
[ ] **C.** Bowel perforation
[ ] **D.** Airway obstruction

Correct answer–D. *Rationales:* First, the child should be assessed to determine whether the quarter has obstructed his airway. Next, he should be observed for signs of mucosal lining corrosion and bowel obstruction or perforation.
Nursing process step: Evaluation

34. What are the most common causes of acute pancreatitis?
[ ] **A.** Trauma and postoperative syndrome
[ ] **B.** Alcohol abuse and biliary tract disease
[ ] **C.** Hypercalcemia and drug use
[ ] **D.** Trauma and alcohol abuse

Correct answer—B. *Rationales:* Alcoholism and biliary tract disease cause 80% of all cases of pancreatitis. The other options are less common.
Nursing process step: Evaluation

35. What treatment does the nurse anticipate for a client with upper-bowel obstruction?
[ ] **A.** Soapsuds enema
[ ] **B.** Warm, moist compresses
[ ] **C.** Oral fluids
[ ] **D.** Nasogastric (NG) tube

Correct answer—D. *Rationales:* A client with bowel obstruction will usually need the GI tract to be decompressed by insertion of an NG tube. A soapsuds enema or the use of warm, moist compresses isn't indicated as treatment for an upper-bowel obstruction. Oral fluids can be given only if the GI tract is functional.
Nursing process step: Intervention

36. Which statement about GI bleeding isn't true?
[ ] **A.** The color of passed blood is a product of GI transit time.
[ ] **B.** Melena is a chemical interaction of gastric acid with blood over several hours.
[ ] **C.** Bright red rectal bleeding rules out upper GI bleeding.
[ ] **D.** As little as 50 mL of blood can cause clinical melena.

Correct answer—C. *Rationales:* Brisk upper GI bleeding with a quick passage of blood through the GI tract can result in bright red rectal bleeding. The other options are accurate.
Nursing process step: Evaluation

37. A client has corrosive injury to the esophagus from ingesting a liquid alkali substance. What should be included in the treatment?
[ ] **A.** Induce vomiting.
[ ] **B.** Insert a nasogastric (NG) tube.
[ ] **C.** Manage the airway.
[ ] **D.** Administer steroids.

Correct answer—C. *Rationales:* Airway management is important in a client with corrosive injury to the esophagus because aspiration of the alkali substance may have occurred. Esophageal perforation may be present. Vomiting shouldn't be induced because this will further expose tissue to the alkali. Insertion of an NG tube should be avoided except with endoscopy or fluoroscopy. The administration of steroids probably isn't beneficial to this client. If the client is seen within 1 hour of ingestion, water may be given.
Nursing process step: Intervention

38. The nurse would expect to hear which sound during percussion of the stomach?
[ ] **A.** Resonance
[ ] **B.** Dullness
[ ] **C.** Hyperresonance
[ ] **D.** Tympany

Correct answer—D. *Rationales:* Tympany is normally heard over air-filled viscera such as the stomach. Hyperresonance and resonance are more commonly heard over lung tissue. Dullness is heard over solid organs.
Nursing process step: Assessment

39. The client with pancreatitis has signs of hypovolemia. What would the nurse anticipate administering?
[ ] **A.** D_5W and half-normal saline solution at 125 mL/hour
[ ] **B.** Normal saline at 80 mL/hour
[ ] **C.** Lactated Ringer's solution at 150 mL/hour
[ ] **D.** Clear oral liquids

Correct answer—C. *Rationales:* Replacement fluids should be isotonic normal saline or lactated Ringer's solution. Dextrose wouldn't be used because dextrose is metabolized readily and then the solution infused becomes hypotonic rather than isotonic. Normal saline could be given, but the replacement rate is 125 to 150 mL/hour; the maintenance rate is 60 to 80 mL/hour. Clear liquids administered orally aren't an option treating hypovolemia because the client can't take in enough to replace what has been lost.
Nursing process step: Analysis

40. Ascites may be caused by which condition?
[ ] **A.** Cirrhosis
[ ] **B.** Ectopic pregnancy
[ ] **C.** Chronic obstructive pulmonary disease (COPD)
[ ] **D.** Crohn's disease

Correct answer—A. *Rationales:* Ascites is an accumulation of fluid in the peritoneal cavity that may be caused by various factors, such as cirrhosis and peritonitis. Ascites isn't caused by an ectopic pregnancy, COPD, or Crohn's disease.
Nursing process step: Assessment

41. The pain of mesenteric vascular infarction is commonly associated with which condition?
[ ] **A.** Abdominal distention and bloody diarrhea
[ ] **B.** Constipation
[ ] **C.** Abdominal distention and abdominal free air
[ ] **D.** Vomiting

Correct answer—A. *Rationales:* Mesenteric vascular infarction is usually associated with vomiting, bloody diarrhea, abdominal distention and tenderness, and hypotension. Constipation and vomiting are more commonly associated with intestinal obstruction. Abdominal distention and abdominal free air are associated with perforated viscous.
Nursing process step: Assessment

42. A client arrives at the emergency department (ED) complaining of a burning, gnawing epigastric pain that occurs 1 to 2 hours after meals. Symptoms have been present for 2 weeks. The ED nurse recognizes these symptoms as indicative of which condition?
[ ] **A.** Pancreatitis
[ ] **B.** Irritable bowel syndrome
[ ] **C.** Peptic ulcer disease
[ ] **D.** Cholecystitis

Correct answer—C. *Rationales:* These are common symptoms of peptic ulcer disease. Symptoms of pancreatitis include epigastric pain that radiates to the back with nausea and vomiting. Clients with irritable bowel syndrome complain of left lower quadrant pain and constipation or diarrhea. The pain of cholecystitis is epigastric or, more commonly, located in the right upper quadrant.
Nursing process step: Assessment

43. A client is complaining of dark stools. The nurse should assess for which of the following?
[ ] **A.** Ingestion of beets
[ ] **B.** Ingestion of bismuth-containing compounds
[ ] **C.** Ingestion of red meat
[ ] **D.** Ingestion of green vegetables

Correct answer—B. *Rationales:* Ingestion of bismuth-containing compounds, such as Pepto-Bismol, may result in black stools. Iron and charcoal may also cause dark stools. Ingestion of beets may cause red stools. Red meat shouldn't alter the color of stools. Green vegetables can cause green stools.
Nursing process step: Assessment

44. For a client with gastroesophageal reflux disease (GERD), discharge instructions should include which of the following?
[ ] **A.** "Lie down and rest after each meal."
[ ] **B.** "Avoid fried and fatty foods."
[ ] **C.** "Drink 16 ounces of water with each meal."
[ ] **D.** "Wine with your dinner is okay."

Correct answer—B. *Rationales:* Foods that irritate the esophagus should be avoided. They include fried and fatty foods, alcoholic beverages, and chocolate. A client with GERD should be instructed not to lie down for 3 hours after a meal. Overeating and drinking excessively should be avoided; both contribute to lower esophageal sphincter relaxation.
Nursing process step: Evaluation

45. Which of the following findings would make the nurse suspect intussusception in a child?
[ ] **A.** Dark, tarry stool
[ ] **B.** Delayed growth and development
[ ] **C.** Sharp, intermittent abdominal pain
[ ] **D.** Daily episodes of bright red rectal bleeding

Correct answer—C. *Rationales:* Obstruction in the small intestine is characterized classically by sharp, intermittent abdominal pain. Dark, tarry stools are a classic sign of upper GI bleeding. Delayed growth and development is primarily due to inadequate nutritional intake or absorption problems, not an obstruction. Episodes of bright red rectal bleeding indicate a lower GI bleed caused by hemorrhoids, not an obstruction.
Nursing process step: Analysis

46. The client with inflammatory bowel disease (IBD) comes to the emergency department with an exacerbation of his disease. What finding is most important for the nurse to follow up related to potential peritonitis?

[ ] **A.** White blood cell count (WBC) of 11,000mm³
[ ] **B.** Oral temperature of 100.4° F (38° C)
[ ] **C.** Positive rebound tenderness
[ ] **D.** Abdominal cramping

Correct answer—C. *Rationales:* Positive rebound tenderness is not associated with IBD and would indicate the client is developing peritonitis. Clients developing peritonitis will exhibit sharp pain with voluntary and involuntary abdominal muscle rigidity, not abdominal cramping or irritation, which is more likely to be present with gastroenteritis. An elevated white blood cell count and an elevated temperature are most likely due to an infectious process.
Nursing process step: Analysis

47. A client with a history of alcohol abuse and cirrhosis is vomiting large amounts of bright red blood. The client's responses are poor. Vital signs include blood pressure, 80/50 mm Hg; pulse, 140 beats/minute; respirations, 36 breaths/minute; and temperature, 99.8° F (37.7° C). What should the emergency department nurse do first?

[ ] **A.** Suction blood from the airway.
[ ] **B.** Insert two large-bore I.V. lines.
[ ] **C.** Insert a nasogastric tube.
[ ] **D.** Administer I.V. vitamin K.

Correct answer—A. *Rationales:* Establishing a clear airway is the first priority. Airway, breathing, and circulation are always included in the primary assessment. The other interventions are important but shouldn't precede the establishment of an airway.
Nursing process step: Intervention

48. Risk factors for Crohn's disease include:

[ ] **A.** smoking.
[ ] **B.** hypertension.
[ ] **C.** hispanic ancestry.
[ ] **D.** eating hot, spicy foods.

Correct answer—A. *Rationales:* Smokers are twice as likely to develop the disease than nonsmokers. Those of Jewish ancestry—not Hispanic—are at five times greater risk than the general population. Hypertension or the ingestion of hot, spicy foods has no effect on the tendency to develop Crohn's disease.
Nursing process step: Assessment

49. The diagnostic test of choice for the client with cholecystitis is:

[ ] **A.** abdominal X-ray.
[ ] **B.** upper GI barium swallow.
[ ] **C.** right upper quadrant (RUQ) abdominal ultrasound.
[ ] **D.** oral cholecystogram.

Correct answer—C. *Rationales:* RUQ abdominal ultrasound is more sensitive and less invasive for diagnosing gallbladder disease than an oral cholecystogram. The oral cholecystogram requires oral preparation the evening before the examination, which may not be an option for the emergency client. The ultrasound can reveal the thickened gallbladder wall, gallbladder distention, fluid around the gallbladder, and gallstones. An upper GI barium swallow is used to examine the upper GI digestive tract.
Nursing process step: Intervention

50. Most hiatal hernias are asymptomatic. Though rare, complications include the following *except*:

[ ] **A.** gastric volvulus or strangulation.
[ ] **B.** aortic aneurysm.
[ ] **C.** esophagitis.
[ ] **D.** gastric reflux.

Correct answer—B. *Rationales:* Hiatal hernias result from muscle weakening and loss of elasticity. Some people with a hiatal hernia will experience heartburn with reflux. In certain people, this reflux damages the esophageal lining, resulting in esophagitis. Aortic aneurysm is an arterial-wall weakening that can occur anywhere along the aorta; however, 80% occur in the abdominal aorta.
Nursing process step: Assessment

51. Which of the following isn't a physical indication of a potential liver injury?
[ ] **A.** Trauma to the right upper quadrant (RUQ) or right lower chest wall
[ ] **B.** Right-sided rib fractures
[ ] **C.** Referred pain to right shoulder
[ ] **D.** Kehr's sign

Correct answer—D. *Rationales:* The liver is located in the RUQ. It's the second most commonly injured solid organ in blunt trauma. Kehr's sign is left shoulder pain caused by diaphragmatic irritation, usually as a result of splenic bleeding. Both rib fractures and referred pain to the right shoulder may be physical indicators of liver injury.
Nursing process step: Assessment

52. A 30-year-old female complains of sharp right lower quadrant pain. Which finding would be indicative of appendicitis rather than of an ectopic pregnancy?
[ ] **A.** Negative pregnancy test
[ ] **B.** Right lower quadrant (RLQ) tenderness
[ ] **C.** Low-grade fever
[ ] **D.** Last menstrual period 14 days ago

Correct answer—A. *Rationales:* A key distinction between appendicitis and ectopic pregnancy is that appendicitis doesn't have a positive pregnancy test. Both appendicitis and an ectopic pregnancy could exhibit RLQ tenderness and a low-grade fever, especially if there was a perforation. The timing of the last menstrual period could indicate an ectopic pregnancy.
Nursing process step: Analysis

53. Which medication should be avoided in the client with biliary colic?
[ ] **A.** Ampicillin/sulbactam (Unasyn)
[ ] **B.** Morphine
[ ] **C.** Demerol (Meperidine)
[ ] **D.** Ketorolac tromethamine

Correct answer—B. *Rationales:* Morphine should be avoided because it can cause spasm of the sphincter of Oddi at the common bile duct, worsening the pain. Demerol and Toradol may be used for short-term pain control. Secondary infection of the gallbladder can occur as a result of cystic duct obstruction and bile stasis. The most frequent organisms are *Escherichia coli* (41%), *Enterococcus* (12%), *Klebsiella* (11%), and *Enterobacter* (9%). A third-generation cephalosporin and metronidazole or Unasyn will cover most common organisms.
Nursing process step: Intervention

54. The client comes to the emergency department complaining of upper abdominal pain that he describes as 7 on a scale of 0 to 10. What laboratory findings would specifically indicate the pancreas is involved?
[ ] **A.** Elevated amylase and lipase
[ ] **B.** Decreased hemoglobin and hematocrit
[ ] **C.** Elevated white blood cells
[ ] **D.** Decreased platelets

Correct answer—A. *Rationales:* Amylase and lipase are enzymes released when pancreatic tissue is destroyed. Pancreatitis involves autodigestion of the pancreas, and elevated pancreatic enzymes that are two to three times the normal value are indicative of pancreatic injury. Decreased hemoglobin and hematocrit, elevated white blood cells, and decreased platelets are not indicative of pancreatic involvement.
Nursing process step: Analysis

55. What is important to teach a client with chronic gastritis?
[ ] **A.** Consume milk with meals.
[ ] **B.** Remain upright 1 hour after eating.
[ ] **C.** Avoid foods with gluten.
[ ] **C.** Do not smoke.

Correct answer—D. *Rationales:* Smoking is contraindicated in all forms of gastritis. Milk is not an essential part of the diet. Option B shows basic instructions for gastroesophageal reflux, or GERD. Gluten is avoided with gluten-sensitive enteropathy.
Nursing process step: Implementation

56. A client comes to the emergency department with a two-day history of abdominal cramping and watery diarrhea that has become bloody. Which assessment question should the nurse ask related to the possibility of *Escherichia coli* etiology?
[ ] **A.** "Did anyone else eat the same food, and are they ill?"
[ ] **B.** "Did you eat any improperly cooked eggs in the last 24 hours?"
[ ] **C.** "Have you taken any over-the-counter medications in the last week?"
[ ] **D.** "Do you have a family history of inflammatory bowel disease (IBD)?"

Correct answer—A. *Rationales: E. coli* 0157:H7 is obtained from contaminated beef, pork, milk, cheese, fish, and cookie dough. The clinical manifestation typically includes abdominal cramping for 2 to 8 days and diarrhea (often bloody). Determining if others ate the food and had a similar reaction would help pinpoint the cause to a foodborne illness. Improperly cooked eggs are usually related to *Salmonella*. Over-the-counter medication use and a family history of IBD aren't related to an *E. coli* etiology.
Nursing process step: Assessment

57. The nurse is providing discharge instructions to a client with gastroenteritis. Which of the following is an example of initial intake the nurse should encourage?
[ ] **A.** Milkshake
[ ] **B.** Banana
[ ] **C.** Gatorade
[ ] **D.** Oatmeal

Correct answer—C. *Rationales:* Most gastroenteritis is self-limiting. Initially, oral hydration is done with clear liquids, such as cola, ginger ale, apple juice, tea, broth, and electrolyte replacement drinks like Gatorade (Pedialyte). After the diarrhea subsides, the BRAT diet (bananas, rice, applesauce, and toast) can be started. A milkshake and oatmeal are too irritating to the GI system and difficult to digest at this point; they shouldn't be offered.
Nursing process step: Implementation

58. A client is diagnosed with Hepatitis B. What question would help determine how the disease was contracted?
[ ] **A.** "Did you eat any raw shellfish?"
[ ] **B.** "How much alcohol do you drink?"
[ ] **C.** "Do you use I.V. drugs?"
[ ] **D.** "Have you donated blood recently?"

Correct answer—C. *Rationales:* Hepatitis B is mainly contracted by blood and by sexual activity. Hepatitis B is neither transmitted through the oral or fecal route nor contracted by contaminated food. Alcohol consumption isn't relevant to hepatitis B transmission. Receiving blood—not donating it—would be relevant to this client's diagnosis.
Nursing process step: Analysis

59. What instructions should the nurse give to a client diagnosed with hepatitis A?
[ ] **A.** Wear a condom during sexual relationships.
[ ] **B.** Avoid alcohol as long as jaundice is present.
[ ] **C.** Avoid acetaminophen (Tylenol) for at least a year.
[ ] **D.** Consume a low-residue diet.

Correct answer—C. *Rationales:* Acetaminophen should be avoided for at least a year. Alcohol should be avoided regardless of whether jaundice is present. Hepatitis B is contracted mainly through blood or sex. A low-residue diet is used with inflammatory bowel disease.
Nursing process step: Intervention

60. A client has been diagnosed with Crohn's disease. Which assessment finding is most important for the nurse to follow up on immediately?
[ ] **A.** Rigid abdomen
[ ] **B.** Elevated white blood cells (WBCs)
[ ] **C.** Temperature of 100.4° F (38° C)
[ ] **D.** Four diarrheal stools in one day

Correct answer—A. *Rationales:* A rigid, or boardlike, abdomen is indicative of GI perforation, which is a complication of Crohn's disease. Elevated WBCs, temperature of 100.4° F, and four diarrheal stools in one day are symptoms of an exacerbation of irritable bowel disease, not Crohn's disease.
Nursing process step: Analysis

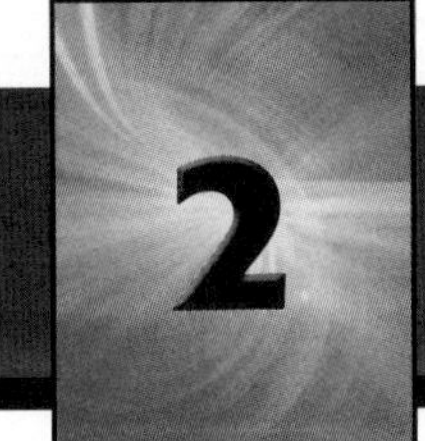

2 Cardiovascular emergencies

1. Which drug shouldn't be given by way of an endotracheal (ET) tube?
[ ] **A.** Atropine
[ ] **B.** Sodium bicarbonate
[ ] **C.** Epinephrine
[ ] **D.** Lidocaine (Xylocaine)

Correct answer—B. *Rationales:* Sodium bicarbonate shouldn't be given by way of an ET tube because of its alkalinity and because the large amounts required shouldn't be administered by this route. Atropine, epinephrine, and lidocaine are absorbed rapidly by the lungs and may be given safely by way of an ET tube.
Nursing process step: Intervention

2. A client has the following symptoms: dyspnea, dependent edema, hepatomegaly, crackles, and distended jugular veins. The nurse should suspect which condition?
[ ] **A.** Pulmonary embolism
[ ] **B.** Heart failure
[ ] **C.** Cardiac tamponade
[ ] **D.** Tension pneumothorax

Correct answer—B. *Rationales:* A client with heart failure has reduced cardiac output because of the heart's decreased pumping ability. Therefore, fluid builds up and causes dyspnea, edema, hepatomegaly, crackles, and dis tended jugular veins. A client with pulmonary embolism has acute shortness of breath, pleuritic chest pain, hemoptysis, and fever. A client with cardiac tamponade has muffled heart sounds, hypotension, and elevated venous pressure. A client with tension pneumothorax has a deviated trachea and no breath sounds on the affected side as well as dyspnea and distended jugular veins.
Nursing process step: Assessment

3. A client arrives in the emergency department complaining of nausea, diaphoresis, shortness of breath, and squeezing substernal pain that radiates to the left shoulder and teeth. The nurse should perform which intervention?
[ ] **A.** Complete registration, order an electrocardiogram, establish I.V. access, and record vital signs.
[ ] **B.** Alert the catheter laboratory team, administer oxygen, apply a cardiac monitor, and notify the physician.
[ ] **C.** Take the client to the examination room, establish I.V. access, give sublingual nitroglycerin, and alert the catheter laboratory team.
[ ] **D.** Administer oxygen, apply a cardiac monitor, record the client's vital signs, and give sublingual nitroglycerin.

Correct answer—D. *Rationales:* The client's pain is caused by myocardial ischemia. Oxygen increases the myo cardial oxygen supply. Cardiac monitoring reveals life-threatening arrhythmias. The nurse should ensure that the client isn't hypotensive before giving sublingual nitroglycerin for chest pain. Registration may be delayed until the client is stabilized. Alerting the catheter laboratory team before completing an initial assessment is premature.
Nursing process step: Intervention

4. The cardiac monitor reveals the following rhythm on a client who's complaining of substernal chest pains.

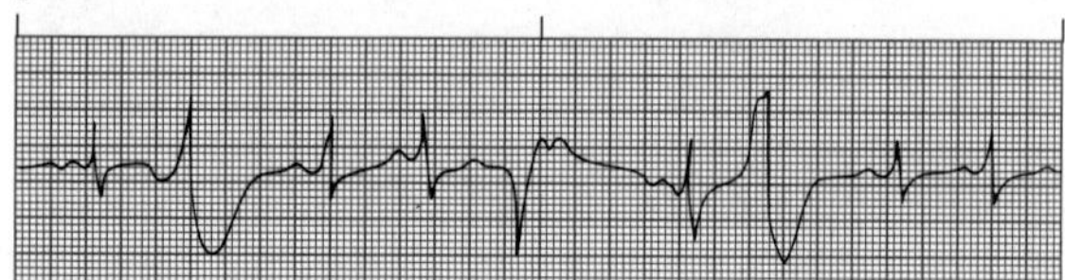

After administering oxygen by nasal cannula, what medication would be the initial treatment for this arrhythmia?

[ ] **A.** Magnesium sulfate
[ ] **B.** Amiodarone
[ ] **C.** Lidocaine (Xylocaine)
[ ] **D.** Atropine

Correct answer—C. *Rationales:* The client is experiencing premature ventricular contractions (PVCs). Lidocaine is the drug of choice for PVCs associated with chest pain and a normal heart rate. Magnesium sulfate is used in torsades de pointes. Amiodarone is used only for life-threatening ventricular arrhythmias. Atropine is used to increase heart rate, which is not necessary in this situation.
Nursing process step: Intervention

5. The nurse is asked to begin a lidocaine infusion. The premixed bag contains 2 g of lidocaine in 500 mL of dextrose 5% in water. What's the drip rate for 2 mg/minute to be delivered by infusion pump?

[ ] **A.** 15 mL/hour
[ ] **B.** 30 mL/hour
[ ] **C.** 45 mL/hour
[ ] **D.** 60 mL/hour

Correct answer—B. *Rationales:* First determine the concentration:

2 g = 2,000 mg

$$\frac{2{,}000 \text{ mg}}{500 \text{ mL}} = 4 \text{ mg/mL}$$

Then determine the drip rate:

2 mg/minute × 60 = 120 mg/hour

$$\frac{120 \text{ mg/hour}}{4 \text{ mg/mL}} = 30 \text{ mL/hour}$$

Nursing process step: Intervention

6. Which of the following is an absolute contraindication for thrombolytic therapy?

[ ] **A.** Active bleeding
[ ] **B.** Current anticoagulant therapy
[ ] **C.** Over age 75
[ ] **D.** Severe hepatic disease

Correct answer—A. *Rationales:* Active bleeding is an absolute contraindication for thrombolytic therapy. The other options are considered relative risks and should be evaluated before administering thrombolytics.
Nursing process step: Assessment

7. Which of the following are complications of thrombolytic (reperfusion) therapy?

[ ] **A.** Puncture site oozing and GI bleeding
[ ] **B.** Tachycardia
[ ] **C.** Chest pain
[ ] **D.** Headache

Correct answer—A. *Rationales:* Bleeding is a com plication of thrombolytic therapy. Bradycardia—not tachy cardia—is a common reperfusion arrhythmia (others are accelerated idioventricular and ventricular ectopy). The client should also have less chest pain. Headache isn't as sociated with thrombolytic therapy.
Nursing process step: Assessment

8. Diuretic therapy is deemed effective in a client with heart failure if:

[ ] **A.** dyspnea decreases and jugular vein distention (JVD) increases.
[ ] **B.** JVD decreases and urine output increases.
[ ] **C.** dyspnea decreases, urine output increases, and JVD decreases.
[ ] **D.** dyspnea decreases and JVD decreases.

Correct answer—C. *Rationales:* Diuretics decrease preload by eliminating sodium and water from the body and decrease dyspnea, increase urine output, and decrease JVD.
Nursing process step: Evaluation

9. A client with acute heart failure exhibits these hemodynamic parameters: central venous pressure, 15 mm Hg; blood pressure, 90/50 mm Hg; pulse, 132 beats/minute; and respirations, 36 breaths/minute. What are the therapy goals for this client?

[ ] **A.** To decrease myocardial workload, decrease volume, and increase myocardial contractility

[ ] **B.** To decrease volume, decrease cardiac output, and increase myocardial contractility

[ ] **C.** To increase volume, decrease cardiac output, and increase myocardial contractility

[ ] **D.** To decrease myocardial workload, increase volume, and increase myocardial contractility

Correct answer—A. *Rationales:* Therapy goals for a client with acute heart failure are to reduce myocardial workload in order to increase cardiac output; decrease volume, which causes dyspnea and edema; and increase myocardial contractility to increase cardiac output. Heart failure is a low cardiac output state.

Nursing process step: Evaluation

10. A 34-year-old client is brought to the emergency department with a stab wound to the right lower chest. His vital signs are as follows: blood pressure, 80/50 mm Hg; pulse, 130 beats/minute; and respirations, 24 breaths/minute. Breath sounds are present bilaterally, and heart sounds are muffled. Based on these assessment findings, what should the nurse anticipate happening next?

[ ] **A.** Computed tomography (CT) of the chest

[ ] **B.** Pericardiocentesis

[ ] **C.** Central venous catheter insertion

[ ] **D.** Chest tube insertion

Correct answer—B. *Rationales:* Based on the assessment findings of both hypotension and muffled heart sounds, the client is experiencing cardiac tamponade. Immediate intervention by way of pericardiocentesis is necessary to correct the problem in order to prevent the client from experiencing cardiac arrest. CT of the chest will confirm fluid accumulation around the pericardium but will delay treatment. Insertion of the central venous catheter may be needed for fluid replacement in the absence of I.V. access. Insertion of a chest tube isn't necessary at this time because the client has equal breath sounds bilaterally.

Nursing process step: Analysis

11. A 75-year-old male is brought to the emergency department. He's complaining of chest pain, headaches, and blurred vision. He states he has a history of hypertension but hasn't been taking his medication because he ran out. Vital signs are as follows: blood pressure, 210/130 mm Hg; pulse, 110 beats/minute, and regular and respiratory rate of 18 breaths/minute. Breath sounds are clear bilaterally, and pulse oximetry is 98% on room air. Based on the above assessment findings, what might this client be experiencing?

[ ] **A.** Acute myocardial infarction (MI)

[ ] **B.** Heart failure

[ ] **C.** Hypertensive crisis

[ ] **D.** Pericarditis

Correct answer—C. *Rationales:* The client presents with a blood pressure of 210/130 mm Hg, blurred vision, headaches, and chest pain, which are all consistent findings of a client experiencing a hypertensive crisis. The findings listed here aren't consistent with acute MI, heart failure, or pericarditis.

Nursing process step: Analysis

12. In order to control a hypertensive crisis and prevent further damage, the physician orders labetalol I.V. push. To ensure safe medication administration, what should the nurse keep in mind?

[ ] **A.** Dilute the medication and hang as a piggyback.

[ ] **B.** Administer the medication over 10 seconds.

[ ] **C.** Place the client on a cardiac monitor and noninvasive blood pressure monitoring.

[ ] **D.** Divide into 4 equal doses for administration.

Correct answer—C. *Rationales:* Labetalol administration can cause hypotension, bradycardia, and heart blocks, so monitoring of both the blood pressure and the heart rate and rhythm is essential for safe administration. It isn't necessary to dilute the medication and hang as a piggyback. Labetalol can be administered I.V. push over 2 minutes—not 10 seconds. Labetalol doesn't need to be divided into 4 equal doses for administration.

Nursing process step: Intervention

13. The emergency department nurse should prepare a client with a ruptured aorta for:
[ ] **A.** emergency surgery.
[ ] **B.** chest tube insertion.
[ ] **C.** chest computed tomography (CT) scan.
[ ] **D.** immediate intubation.

Correct answer—A. *Rationales:* A client with a ruptured aorta requires immediate surgery. Chest tubes shouldn't be inserted. Diagnosis can be made with chest X-ray. A CT scan would delay definitive treatment. Intubation is done at the time of surgery, unless otherwise indicated.
Nursing process step: Intervention

14. A client with hypotension and dyspnea has the following rhythm:

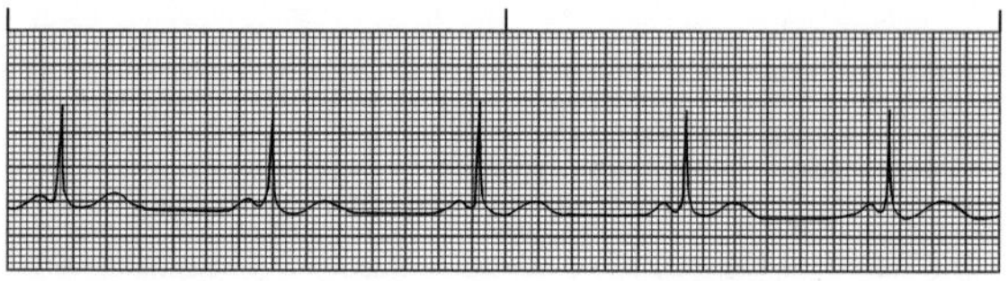

The emergency nurse should immediately do which of the following?
[ ] **A.** Administer lidocaine (Xylocaine) 1 mg/kg I.V. push.
[ ] **B.** Prepare for external pacing.
[ ] **C.** Administer atropine 0.5 mg I.V. push.
[ ] **D.** Begin a dopamine infusion at 5 g/kg per minute.

Correct answer—C. *Rationales:* The client's ECG strip shows bradycardia, and atropine is the drug of choice for treating symptomatic bradycardia. The 2010 American Heart Association guidelines recommend repeating the 0.5-mg dose at 3- to 5-minute intervals until 3 mg has been given. Pacing may be indicated if atropine is ineffective. Dopamine isn't a first-line drug for treating bradycardia. However, it's used to treat hypotension. In this case, bradycardia is the cause of hypotension and should be addressed first. Lidocaine shouldn't be given for bradycardia because it may suppress the escape rhythm and lead to further hypotension and, possibly, asystole.
Nursing process step: Intervention

15. The nurse has delivered synchronized cardioversion to a symptomatic client with supraventricular tachycardia. The client then develops pulseless ventricular tachycardia. What should the nurse do immediately?
[ ] **A.** Deliver a precordial thump.
[ ] **B.** Administer lidocaine (Xylocaine) 1 mg/kg I.V. push.
[ ] **C.** Defibrillate at 200 joules.
[ ] **D.** Administer adenosine (Adenocard) 6 mg I.V. push.

Correct answer—C. *Rationales:* Immediately defib rillate at 200 joules according to advanced cardiac life support protocol. A precordial thump isn't part of the 2010 American Heart Association guidelines. Lidocaine can be administered as an alternative to amiodarone for persistent pulseless ventricular tachycardia if defibrillation and epinephrine are ineffective. Adenosine isn't effective for ventricular tachycardias.
Nursing process step: Intervention

16. An 80-year-old client has received a lidocaine bolus and infusion after suffering nonsustained ventricular tachycardia. For which symptom of lidocaine toxicity should the nurse monitor?
[ ] **A.** Hypertension
[ ] **B.** Tachycardia
[ ] **C.** Increased intracranial pressure
[ ] **D.** Seizures

Correct answer—D. *Rationales:* Seizures are a symptom of lidocaine toxicity. Hypertension, tachycardia, and increased intracranial pressure aren't commonly associated with lidocaine toxicity.
Nursing process step: Evaluation

17. Which of the following best demonstrates the effectiveness of thrombolytic therapy?
[ ] **A.** Greater than 2-mm elevation in the ST segment
[ ] **B.** Oozing from I.V. sites
[ ] **C.** Relief of chest pain
[ ] **D.** Absence of arrhythmias

Correct answer—C. *Rationales:* Thrombolytic therapy effectiveness is measured by the relief of chest pain, presence of reperfusion arrhythmias, and normalization of the ST segment. Oozing of blood from I.V. sites may occur because thrombolytic therapy may increase bleeding time, but bleeding doesn't demonstrate its effectiveness.
Nursing process step: Assessment

18. Which intervention is inappropriate for a client with acute arterial occlusion?
[ ] **A.** Maintain the affected extremity in a dependent position.
[ ] **B.** Apply a heating pad to the affected extremity.
[ ] **C.** Use a Doppler ultrasound device to auscultate pulses.
[ ] **D.** Prepare the client for possible surgery.

Correct answer—B. *Rationales:* Increased tempera ture increases oxygen demands on the extremity. Maintain ing the extremity in a dependent position promotes blood flow. Using Doppler ultrasound aids in assessing for wor sening of the occlusion. The client may need surgery.
Nursing process step: Intervention

19. A client who has been kicked in the chest by a bull arrives in the emergency department. Vital signs are blood pressure, 80/50 mm Hg; pulse, 144 beats/minute; respirations, 36 breaths/minute; and temperature, 98.5° F (36.9° C). Heart sounds are muffled and facial cyanosis is present. A bolus of 1,000 mL of fluid is infused. Blood pressure remains 82/50 mm Hg and pulse increases to 150 beats/minute. The client is most likely to have:
[ ] **A.** myocardial contusion.
[ ] **B.** tension pneumothorax.
[ ] **C.** cardiac tamponade.
[ ] **D.** aortic injury.

Correct answer—C. *Rationales:* Muffled heart sounds are associated with cardiac tamponade. A volume-depleted client with cardiac tamponade may not respond to volume infusion. Myocardial contusion presents with chest pain and electrocardiogram changes. Tension pneumothorax presents with acute increases in respiratory rate and heart rate, chest pain, tracheal deviation to the unaffected side, and an absence of breath sounds on the affected side. Aortic injury presents with a widened mediastinum by chest X-ray, hypotension, respiratory distress, and chest pain.
Nursing process step: Assessment

20. The aorta is most commonly injured during which type of trauma?
[ ] **A.** Deceleration trauma that causes shearing
[ ] **B.** Penetrating trauma
[ ] **C.** Blunt chest trauma
[ ] **D.** Chest injuries that cause rib fractures

Correct answer—A. *Rationales:* Deceleration may cause laceration to the aorta by shearing forces. The other options may cause aortic injuries but aren't the primary mechanisms of injury.
Nursing process step: Assessment

21. A client is undergoing pericardiocentesis. The rhythm previously showed sinus tachycardia. Premature ventricular contractions (PVCs) are now noted on the monitor. This condition indicates which of the following?
[ ] **A.** It's time for the physician to begin aspirating the syringe.
[ ] **B.** The pericardial sac has been entered, and it's time to attach a clamp to the needle at the skin level to prevent further insertion.
[ ] **C.** The needle has entered the heart.
[ ] **D.** The needle is touching the myocardium.

Correct answer—D. *Rationales:* If the needle touches the myocardium, PVCs or ST-segment elevation may be observed. The needle hasn't necessarily entered the heart. At this time, the needle should be withdrawn slightly. The physician should aspirate the syringe while advancing the needle and should stop as soon as blood is obtained.
Nursing process step: Intervention

22. Cardiac tamponade may result from which condition?
[ ] **A.** Myasthenia gravis
[ ] **B.** Endocarditis
[ ] **C.** Systemic lupus erythematosus
[ ] **D.** Guillain-Barré syndrome

Correct answer—C. *Rationales:* Systemic lupus erythematosus as well as chest trauma and pericarditis may cause an accumulation of fluid in the pericardial sac, leading to cardiac tamponade. The other options don't result in cardiac tamponade.
Nursing process step: Evaluation

23. A client with a ruptured descending aorta may exhibit which of the following?
[ ] **A.** Greater pulse amplitude in the arms than in the legs
[ ] **B.** Greater pulse amplitude in the legs than in the arms
[ ] **C.** Blood pressure differences in right and left arms
[ ] **D.** Distended jugular veins and muffled heart sounds

Correct answer—A. *Rationales:* A client with a ruptured descending aorta may have a greater pulse amplitude in the arms than in the legs because of decreased perfusion to the legs. Blood pressure differences in arms are indicative of ruptured subclavian arteries. Distended jugular veins and muffled heart sounds aren't likely to be present in this client.
Nursing process step: Assessment

24. A client with electrocardiogram (ECG) changes in leads V1, V2, and V3 may be suffering from which injury?
[ ] **A.** Inferior wall injury
[ ] **B.** Anterior wall injury
[ ] **C.** Lateral wall injury
[ ] **D.** Posterior wall injury

Correct answer—B. *Rationales:* Anterior wall injury is associated with ECG changes in leads V1, V2, and V3. Inferior wall injury is associated with ECG changes in leads II, III, and aVF. Lateral wall injury is associated with ECG changes in leads I, aVL, V5, and V6. Posterior wall injury is associated with ECG changes in leads V1 and V2.
Nursing process step: Assessment

25. A client with a history of hypertension and coronary artery disease (CAD) presents with substernal chest pain and shortness of breath. The pain is unrelieved with multiple doses of nitroglycerin and the administration of oxygen, but it responds to morphine. This may indicate that the pain is caused by:
[ ] **A.** angina pectoris because this type of pain is usually unresponsive to nitroglycerin and oxygen administration.
[ ] **B.** acute myocardial infarction (MI) because the pain of acute MI isn't usually relieved by nitroglycerin and oxygen administration.
[ ] **C.** heart failure because this may cause chest pain that's unrelieved by nitroglycerin and oxygen administration.
[ ] **D.** pericarditis because this disorder is commonly seen in a hypertensive client with CAD and won't respond to nitroglycerin or oxygen administration.

Correct answer—B. *Rationales:* The pain of acute MI won't be relieved by the administration of nitroglycerin. This differentiates it from anginal pain, which should respond to nitroglycerin administration and oxygen. Heart failure isn't commonly associated with substernal chest pain, and pericarditis isn't common in a hypertensive client with CAD.
Nursing process step: Assessment

26. A client in ventricular fibrillation hasn't responded to standard treatment—defibrillation, epinephrine, and lidocaine (Xylocaine). Which of the following is a potentially reversible cause of ventricular fibrillation?

[ ] **A.** Hypothermia
[ ] **B.** Hypervolemia
[ ] **C.** Hyperthermia
[ ] **D.** Digoxin toxicity

Correct answer—A. *Rationales:* Hypothermia, hypovolemia, and electrolyte imbalances can potentially cause ventricular fibrillation and may need to be treated before standard measures are effective. Digoxin toxicity can cause atrial tachycardia—not ventricular fibrillation.
Nursing process step: Evaluation

27. What's the maximum number of times a client can be defibrillated safely?

[ ] **A.** 10
[ ] **B.** 15
[ ] **C.** 18
[ ] **D.** There's no limit

Correct answer—D. *Rationales:* There's no maximum number of times a client can be defibrillated. However, if the client remains in ventricular fibrillation for more than 30 minutes, the chances of survival are low. Exceptions would be resuscitation of children, hypothermic individuals, drowning victims, and clients who go in and out of ventricular fibrillation multiple times. These clients may benefit from longer resuscitation.
Nursing process step: Evaluation

28. An elderly client arrives in the emergency department complaining of diarrhea, weakness, headache, and "yellowish" vision. The client has a history of hypertension and "heart" problems. Home medications aren't available. Vital signs are blood pressure, 90/68 mm Hg; pulse, 52 beats/minute; respirations, 22 breaths/minute; and temperature, 98.4° F (36.9° C). The nurse should suspect which condition?

[ ] **A.** Gastroenteritis
[ ] **B.** Viral syndrome
[ ] **C.** Digoxin (Lanoxin) toxicity
[ ] **D.** Overdose of antihypertensive medication

Correct answer—C. *Rationales:* The client's complaints along with vital signs suggest digoxin toxicity. The nurse should attempt to obtain a list of home medications from the client's family, physician, or medical records. Obtaining a serum digoxin level would be appropriate. The therapeutic digoxin level is 0.8 to 2.0 ng/mL. A client with gastroenteritis would complain of abdominal cramps, diarrhea, and vomiting. Viral syndrome includes symptoms of malaise and, possibly, fever. A client with an antihypertensive overdose would exhibit hypotension and weakness but wouldn't have "yellowish" vision.
Nursing process step: Analysis

29. Which of the following isn't generally associated with pulseless electrical activity (PEA)?

[ ] **A.** Hypovolemia
[ ] **B.** Alkalosis
[ ] **C.** Massive pulmonary embolism
[ ] **D.** Acidosis

Correct answer—B. *Rationales:* These rhythms aren't associated with alkalosis. The other options may all be causes of PEA. Other possible causes include hypoxia, cardiac tamponade, tension pneumothorax, hypothermia, drug overdose, hyperkalemia, and massive myocardial infarction.
Nursing process step: Assessment

30. A client complaining of severe chest pain is brought to the emergency department and suddenly becomes unresponsive. The monitor shows the following rhythm:

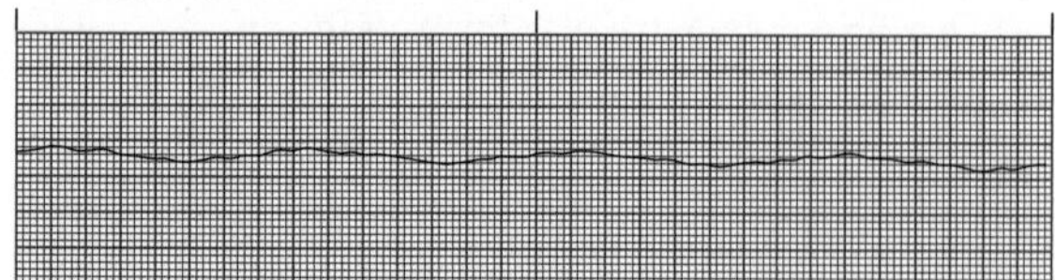

What should the nurse do immediately?

[ ] **A.** Check for pulse and check monitor leads.
[ ] **B.** Begin cardiopulmonary resuscitation (CPR).
[ ] **C.** Administer atropine 1 mg I.V.
[ ] **D.** Defibrillate at 200 joules.

Correct answer—A. *Rationales:* Check the client and monitor leads before initiating treatment. The monitor strip shows asystole; therefore, CPR should then be initiated. The client should be intubated at once and I.V. access obtained. Epinephrine 1 mg I.V. or vasopressin 40 units I.V. is given. Defibrillation isn't indicated for a client in asystole.
Nursing process step: Intervention

31. Nitrates have which effects?

[ ] **A.** Increase preload, increase afterload
[ ] **B.** Increase preload, decrease afterload
[ ] **C.** Decrease preload, decrease afterload
[ ] **D.** Decrease preload, increase afterload

Correct answer—C. *Rationales:* Nitrates decrease preload and afterload, thereby decreasing myocardial oxygen demand and increasing myocardial oxygen supply.
Nursing process step: Evaluation

32. What's the primary effect of vagal stimulation on the heart?

[ ] **A.** Increases parasympathetic tone
[ ] **B.** Increases sympathetic tone
[ ] **C.** Decreases parasympathetic tone
[ ] **D.** Decreases sympathetic tone

Correct answer—A. *Rationales:* Vagal stimulation increases parasympathetic tone, which decreases the heart rate and may slow atrioventricular conduction. An increase in sympathetic tone results in increased heart rate and cardiac output. A decrease in sympathetic tone would have the opposite effect.
Nursing process step: Analysis

33. How much pressure should be applied to the paddles during defibrillation?

[ ] **A.** 10 lb
[ ] **B.** 15 lb
[ ] **C.** 20 lb
[ ] **D.** 25 lb

Correct answer—D. *Rationales:* Apply 25 lb of pressure to both paddles. Applying less pressure increases the risk of burns and makes defibrillation less effective. Conductor pads or gel should be used to ensure good contact.
Nursing process step: Intervention

34. A client in ventricular fibrillation has received initial defibrillation at 200 joules. The monitor continues to show ventricular fibrillation. What's the next action?

[ ] **A.** Charge the defibrillator and deliver 300 joules.
[ ] **B.** Check for a pulse.
[ ] **C.** Resume cardiopulmonary resuscitation (CPR).
[ ] **D.** Deliver synchronized cardioversion at 200 joules.

Correct answer—C. *Rationales:* According to the 2010 American Heart Association advanced cardiac life support guidelines, CPR should be resumed immediately and continued for 2 minutes or 5 cycles before rechecking the rhythm. Pulse check, defibrillation, and cardioversion are not indicated treatments according to AHA.
Nursing process step: Intervention

35. What's the purpose of defibrillation?

[ ] **A.** To produce temporary asystole
[ ] **B.** To "jump-start" the heart
[ ] **C.** To produce a sinus rhythm
[ ] **D.** To synchronize the rhythm

Correct answer—A. *Rationales:* The purpose of defibrillation is to produce temporary asystole to completely depolarize the myocardium. Depolarizing allows the heart's natural pacemakers to resume normal activity. Other choices are not the correct purpose of defibrillation.
Nursing process step: Evaluation

36. Which drug is inappropriate for a client with a wide-complex tachycardia?
[ ] **A.** Lidocaine (Xylocaine)
[ ] **B.** Amiodarone
[ ] **C.** Procainamide
[ ] **D.** Verapamil

Correct answer—D. *Rationales:* Administering verapamil to a client with ventricular tachycardia can be lethal. Verapamil may accelerate the heart rate and decrease blood pressure, particularly in clients with atrial fibrillation and Wolff-Parkinson-White syndrome. The other options would be appropriate for a client with wide-complex tachycardia.
Nursing process step: Intervention

37. What's the role of beta-adrenergic blockers in a client with acute myocardial infarction?
[ ] **A.** To reduce myocardial oxygen consumption
[ ] **B.** To increase blood pressure
[ ] **C.** To increase catecholamine levels
[ ] **D.** To increase oxygen demand

Correct answer—A. *Rationales:* Beta-adrenergic blockers decrease myocardial oxygen consumption and demands of the ischemic areas of the heart. They're used to reduce infarct size by decreasing sympathetic tone, thereby decreasing afterload. They also lower blood pressure and decrease arrhythmias by decreasing catecholamine levels.
Nursing process step: Analysis

38. A client with a serum potassium level of 7.8 mEq/L may manifest which electrocardiogram changes?
[ ] **A.** Peaked T waves, tachycardia, and widened QRS complex
[ ] **B.** Bradycardia, peaked T waves, and widened QRS complex
[ ] **C.** Tachycardia and widened QRS complex
[ ] **D.** Bradycardia and widened QRS complex

Correct answer—B. *Rationales:* A client with hyperkalemia may exhibit peaked T waves, a widened QRS complex with bradycardia, disappearance of P waves and, eventually, idioventricular rhythm and asystole.
Nursing process step: Analysis

39. Which drug is considered a negative inotrope?
[ ] **A.** Epinephrine
[ ] **B.** Dobutamine
[ ] **C.** Propranolol (Inderal)
[ ] **D.** Digoxin (Lanoxin)

Correct answer—C. *Rationales:* Propranolol is a negative inotrope; it decreases the contractile state of the myocardium. The other options are all positive inotropes; that is, they increase the contractile state of the myocardium.
Nursing process step: Evaluation

40. A client complaining of severe "tearing" chest pain that radiates to the back is probably experiencing:
[ ] **A.** pericarditis.
[ ] **B.** endocarditis.
[ ] **C.** myocardial infarction (MI).
[ ] **D.** dissecting abdominal aneurysm.

Correct answer—D. *Rationales:* Sudden onset of severe chest pain that radiates to the back with a tearing sensation is the classic presentation of dissecting abdominal aneurysm. A client with pericarditis may complain of chest pain that's relieved by sitting forward. A client with endocarditis has a fever, a heart murmur, weight loss, and fatigue but no chest pain. A client with an MI presents with chest pain or pressure radiating to the left arm, neck, or jaw; the pain is unrelieved by rest or change in position.
Nursing process step: Assessment

41. Occlusion of the left coronary artery will probably result in damage to which of the following?
[ ] **A.** Inferior wall of the myocardium
[ ] **B.** Anterior wall of the myocardium
[ ] **C.** Posterior wall of the myocardium
[ ] **D.** Right ventricle

Correct answer—B. *Rationales:* The left coronary artery supplies the anterior and lateral walls of the myocardium. The inferior wall is usually supplied by the right coronary artery. The posterior wall is supplied by a branch of the posterior descending artery. The right ventricle is supplied by the right coronary artery.
Nursing process step: Analysis

42. Percutaneous coronary intervention (PCI) is preferred over thrombolytic therapy for ST-segment elevation myocardial infarction (MI) in all of the following cases except when:

[ ] **A.** the presentation from the time of symptom onset is less than 3 hours.

[ ] **B.** the presentation from the time of symptom onset is more than 3 hours.

[ ] **C.** the client has increased risk of bleeding.

[ ] **D.** the client presents in shock or heart failure.

Correct answer—A. *Rationales:* If presentation from the time of symptom onset is less than 3 hours, there's no preference for either PCI or thrombolytic therapy. PCI is preferred for late presentation (more than 3 hours from symptom onset), with increased risk of bleeding, and when the client is at high risk, presenting in shock or heart failure.
Nursing process step: Intervention

43. Low-molecular-weight heparin is indicated for non-ST elevation myocardial infarctions for which of the following reasons?

[ ] **A.** Reduction of afterload

[ ] **B.** Inhibition of thrombin generation or formation

[ ] **C.** Exhibiting of lytic-action on thrombus or area of infarct

[ ] **D.** Inhibition of platelet formation

Correct answer—B. *Rationales:* Low-molecular-weight heparin inhibits thrombin generation by factor Xa inhibition and indirectly inhibits thrombin by formation of a complex with antithrombin III. Low-molecular-weight heparin doesn't reduce afterload, exhibit a lytic action on the thrombus or the area of infarct, or inhibit platelet formation.
Nursing process step: Intervention

44. Which of the following is the term for the force against which a cardiac chamber must eject blood during systole?

[ ] **A.** Systemic vascular resistance

[ ] **B.** Preload

[ ] **C.** Afterload

[ ] **D.** Stroke volume

Correct answer—C. *Rationales:* Afterload is the force against which a cardiac chamber must eject blood during systole. Systemic vascular resistance is this force. Preload is the amount of stretch on the myocardium before systole. Stroke volume is the amount of blood ejected by the left ventricle during systole.
Nursing process step: Assessment

45. Which of the following best describes a pericardial friction rub?

[ ] **A.** Classified as systolic

[ ] **B.** Best heard at the apex with the bell of the stethoscope

[ ] **C.** Varies in intensity with respiration

[ ] **D.** May be accentuated by having the client lean forward and exhale

Correct answer—D. *Rationales:* A pericardial friction rub may be heard when the pericardial surfaces are inflamed. The sound can be heard over the entire pericardium by using the diaphragm of the stethoscope. Unlike a pleural friction rub, it doesn't vary in intensity during respiration. It may be accentuated if the client leans forward and exhales.
Nursing process step: Assessment

46. Which blood test is most indicative of cardiac damage?

[ ] **A.** Lactate dehydrogenase (LD)

[ ] **B.** Complete blood count (CBC)

[ ] **C.** Troponin I

[ ] **D.** Creatine kinase (CK)

Correct answer—C. *Rationales:* Troponin I levels rise rapidly and are detectable within 1 hour after myocardial injury. Troponin I levels aren't detectable in people without cardiac injury. LD is present in almost all body tissue and isn't specific to heart muscle. LD isoenzymes are useful in diagnosing cardiac injury. CBC is used to review blood counts, and a complete chemistry is obtained to review electrolytes. Because CK levels may rise with skeletal muscle injury, CK isoenzymes are required to detect cardiac injury.
Nursing process step: Analysis

47. Which of the following is an important sign of left-sided heart failure in adults?
[ ] **A.** Systolic murmur
[ ] **B.** S3 or ventricular gallop
[ ] **C.** Diastolic murmur
[ ] **D.** S1 heart sound

Correct answer—B. *Rationales:* S3 is a sign of left-sided heart failure in adults and warrants treatment. It may be heard in early diastole. A systolic murmur is heard with mitral insufficiency; a diastolic murmur is heard with mitral stenosis. An S1 heart sound is the normal simultaneous closing of the mitral and tricuspid valves.
Nursing process step: Assessment

48. A client is in the emergency department receiving treatment for chest pain. The nurse has applied oxygen via nasal cannula and administered sublingual nitroglycerin and aspirin. What is the primary goal for this client?
[ ] **A.** Alleviate acute pain.
[ ] **B.** Reverse hypoxia.
[ ] **C.** Decrease myocardial oxygen demand.
[ ] **D.** Increase cardiac output.

Correct answer—C. *Rationales:* Chest pain, or angina, is caused by myocardial ischemia, and interventions should be aimed at decreasing myocardial oxygen demands. Making the client comfortable by alleviating his acute pain is a priority, but the pain will decrease as the cardiac tissue is better perfused. It isn't necessary to reverse hypoxia because generalized hypoxia isn't the cause of the myocardial ischemia. Increasing the cardiac output isn't necessary because the cardiac output may not be altered for the client experiencing angina.
Nursing process step: Intervention

49. Why are diuretics used in the treatment of heart failure?
[ ] **A.** To increase cardiac output
[ ] **B.** To decrease myocardial oxygen consumption
[ ] **C.** To decrease fluid volume
[ ] **D.** To decrease cardiac output

Correct answer—C. *Rationales:* Diuretics reduce total fluid volume and relieve the symptoms of congestion. They don't affect cardiac output or myocardial oxygen consumption.
Nursing process step: Analysis

50. Which drug may be used to reduce afterload in a client with heart failure?
[ ] **A.** Morphine
[ ] **B.** Digoxin (Lanoxin)
[ ] **C.** Dobutamine
[ ] **D.** Metoprolol (Lopressor)

Correct answer—A. *Rationales:* Morphine reduces afterload and decreases myocardial oxygen demand. It also decreases anxiety and dyspnea. Digoxin and dobutamine are positive inotropes and increase cardiac contractility. Meto prolol is a beta-adrenergic blocker that decreases myocar dial contractility, heart rate, and cardiac output.
Nursing process step: Evaluation

51. Which thrombolytic agent is most likely to cause an allergic reaction?
[ ] **A.** Streptokinase (Streptase)
[ ] **B.** Reteplase (Retavase)
[ ] **C.** Tenecteplase (TNKase)
[ ] **D.** Alteplase (Activase)

Correct answer—A. *Rationales:* Allergic reactions, most commonly manifested by fever and rash, occur in about 5% of clients who receive streptokinase. To help prevent allergic reactions, clients are usually given steroids and antihistamines before streptokinase is administered.
Nursing process step: Evaluation

52. Which is the most common cause of cardiac arrest in an adult?
[ ] **A.** Electrolyte disturbances
[ ] **B.** Respiratory arrest
[ ] **C.** Ventricular fibrillation
[ ] **D.** Drug toxicity

Correct answer—C. *Rationales:* Ventricular fibrillation is the most common cause of cardiopulmonary arrest. The other options may result in cardiac arrest but aren't the most common causes.
Nursing process step: Evaluation

53. A client with acute shortness of breath and frothy pink-tinged sputum arrives at the emergency department. Crackles and wheezes are present. Vital signs are blood pressure, 90/50 mm Hg; pulse, 120 beats/minute; respirations, 34 breaths/minute; and temperature, 98.6° F (37° C). The client has a history of diabetes, hypertension, and heart failure. Which of the following should the nurse suspect?
[ ] **A.** Cardiac tamponade
[ ] **B.** Pneumothorax
[ ] **C.** Pulmonary embolus
[ ] **D.** Pulmonary edema

Correct answer—D. *Rationales:* These symptoms are typical of acute pulmonary edema related to heart failure. A client with cardiac tamponade has muffled heart sounds and elevated venous pressure. A client with a pneumothorax has shortness of breath and chest pain. Breath sounds are decreased on the affected side. Clients with pulmonary embolus commonly report chest pain.
Nursing process step: Assessment

54. Which drugs are used to treat acute pulmonary edema associated with heart failure?
[ ] **A.** Digoxin (Lanoxin), morphine, and furosemide (Lasix)
[ ] **B.** Furosemide (Lasix), morphine, and nitroglycerin
[ ] **C.** Amrinone, digoxin (Lanoxin), and dopamine (Intropin)
[ ] **D.** Norepinephrine (Levophed), amrinone (Inocor), and propranolol (Inderal)

Correct answer—B. *Rationales:* Drug therapy in acute pulmonary edema is aimed at reducing preload. Furosemide, morphine, and nitroglycerin are first-line drugs used to reduce preload. Digoxin has little role in the treatment of acute pulmonary edema. Amrinone may be used in cardiogenic shock after other drugs have failed. Norepinephrine has no role in the treatment of acute pulmonary edema.
Nursing process step: Intervention

55. Which of the following is the most common cause of acute cardiac tamponade?
[ ] **A.** Pericarditis
[ ] **B.** Penetrating chest trauma
[ ] **C.** Blunt chest trauma
[ ] **D.** Myocardial infarction (MI)

Correct answer—B. *Rationales:* Although pericarditis, blunt chest trauma, and MI can cause cardiac tamponade, penetrating chest trauma is the most common cause of acute cardiac tamponade.
Nursing process step: Assessment

56. A client who has had shaking chills and fever for 3 days comes to the emergency department. Assessment reveals splinter hemorrhaging of the nail beds and a systolic murmur. The nurse should suspect which condition?
[ ] **A.** Pericarditis
[ ] **B.** Endocarditis
[ ] **C.** Myocarditis
[ ] **D.** Rheumatic endocarditis

Correct answer—B. *Rationales:* These are the hallmark symptoms of endocarditis. A client with pericarditis complains of chest pain that's relieved by leaning forward. A precordial friction rub may be heard on auscultation. A client with myocarditis may complain of fatigue, dyspnea, palpitations, and mild discomfort. Auscultation may reveal an S3 and a systolic murmur. Rheumatic endocarditis usually produces symptoms of left-sided heart failure: shortness of breath, crackles, and wheezing.
Nursing process step: Assessment

57. Cardiopulmonary resuscitation is being performed on an intubated client. Gastric distention is present. What should the nurse do first?
[ ] **A.** Insert a nasogastric (NG) tube.
[ ] **B.** Retract the endotracheal (ET) tube ¾″ (2 cm).
[ ] **C.** Perform 5-point auscultation
[ ] **D.** Apply direct abdominal pressure.

Correct answer—C. *Rationales:* First, the nurse should make sure the ET tube is correctly positioned by auscultating the left and right anterior chest, the left and right midaxillary line, and over the epigastrium (5-point auscultation). The nurse should then insert an NG tube to relieve gastric distention. The nurse shouldn't apply abdominal pressure after ET tube placement is confirmed. Gastric distention should be relieved because it can interfere with adequate lung inflation.
Nursing process step: Implementation

58. The pathophysiology involved in myocardial contusion is related to which of the following?
[ ] **A.** Penetrating injuries of the myocardium
[ ] **B.** Bleeding into and direct injury to the myocardium
[ ] **C.** Occlusion of coronary vessels
[ ] **D.** Stab wound to the chest

Correct answer—B. *Rationales:* Myocardial contusion is caused by blunt trauma to the myocardium—not by penetrating injuries. The pathophysiology relates to bleeding into the myocardium as well as direct injury to the muscle, not to occlusion of coronary vessels.
Nursing process step: Analysis

59. Cardiac output is a product of what?
[ ] **A.** Heart rate times central venous pressure
[ ] **B.** Heart rate times systemic vascular resistance
[ ] **C.** Heart rate times stroke volume
[ ] **D.** Heart rate times cardiac index

Correct answer—C. *Rationales:* Cardiac output is a product of heart rate times stroke volume. It's measured in liters per minute. The normal value is 4 to 6 L/minute. The other options are incorrect.
Nursing process step: Assessment

60. Which statement concerning unstable angina isn't true?
[ ] **A.** It occurs more frequently at rest.
[ ] **B.** It's relieved with doses of sublingual nitroglycerin.
[ ] **C.** The chest pain is of increasing duration.
[ ] **D.** It's associated with reversible depression of ST segments.

Correct answer—B. *Rationales:* Unstable angina isn't usually relieved with sublingual nitroglycerin. The other statements are true. A client with unstable angina requires hospitalization.
Nursing process step: Assessment

61. Which of the following isn't an action of lidocaine (Xylocaine)?
[ ] **A.** Decreases automaticity
[ ] **B.** Increases fibrillation threshold
[ ] **C.** Decreases fibrillation threshold
[ ] **D.** Suppresses ischemic tissue conduction

Correct answer—C. *Rationales:* Lidocaine increases the fibrillation threshold and makes the myocardium less susceptible to fibrillation, which is why it's used to treat ventricular ectopy. The fibrillation threshold shouldn't be decreased.
Nursing process step: Evaluation

62. For the nurse to hear S3 and S4, what's the best position for the client?
[ ] **A.** Left lateral
[ ] **B.** Supine
[ ] **C.** High Fowler's
[ ] **D.** Right lateral

Correct answer—A. *Rationales:* S3 and S4 are best heard when the client is in the left lateral position. The bell of the stethoscope should be placed at the point of maximal impulse. S3 is known as a ventricular gallop, and S4 is known as an *atrial gallop*. All other positions would make it difficult to ascultate S_3 and S_4.
Nursing process step: Assessment

63. A client comes to the emergency department after a syncopal episode and responds to questions but is difficult to arouse. The client's 12-lead ECG shows a superventricular (SVT) with a regular rhythm and a narrow QRS complex; heart rate, 190 beats/minute; blood pressure, 80/50 mm Hg; and a respiratory rate of 30 breaths/minute. Which of the following would be the most appropriate electrical intervention for this client?
[ ] **A.** Monophasic defibrillation using 200 joules
[ ] **B.** Monophasic synchronized cardioversion using 200 joules
[ ] **C.** Biphasic synchronized cardioversion using 120 joules.
[ ] **D.** Biphasic synchronized cardioversion using 50 joules

Correct answer—D. *Rationales:* This client is unstable with a high-rate, regular SVT, which requires immediate biphasic synchronized cardioversion using 50 to 100 joules. Defibrillation is only to be used for ventricular fibrillation and wide-irregular complex pulseless ventricular tachycardia. Monophasic synchronized cardioversion using 200 joules or biphasic synchronized cardioversion using 120 joules is appropriate for a client with a high-rate, irregular rhythm with a narrow QRS complex, such as atrial fibrillation.
Nursing process step: Intervention

64. A 74-year-old male arrives in the emergency department complaining of a sudden onset of abdominal pain that radiates to his back. His heart rate is 140 beats/minute, and his blood pressure is 80/50 mm Hg. What condition should the nurse suspect?

[ ] **A.** Ruptured abdominal aortic aneurysm (AAA)
[ ] **B.** ST elevation myocardial infarction
[ ] **C.** Ruptured appendix
[ ] **D.** Ruptured spleen

Correct answer—A. *Rationales:* Sudden onset of abdominal or back pain with tachycardia and hypotension are characteristic signs of a ruptured AAA. The unstable vital signs are indicative of hemorrhagic shock from the rupture of a large vessel. These aren't typical signs and symptoms for an MI or a ruptured appendix or spleen.
Nursing process step: Analysis

65. Appropriate interventions for a client complaining of syncope include which of the following?

[ ] **A.** Obtaining orthostatic vital signs
[ ] **B.** Obtaining hearing test
[ ] **C.** Magnetic resonance imaging (MRI)
[ ] **D.** Computed tomography (CT) scan

Correct answer—A. *Rationales:* Orthostatic vital signs reveal orthostatic hypotension, which may be the result of medications or hypovolemia. Syncope may also be related to cardiac arrhythmias—not hearing difficulties. An MRI or CT scan may be ordered if the other options don't reveal the cause of the syncope.
Nursing process step: Intervention

66. A client in ventricular tachycardia arrives at the emergency department. What should the nurse do first?

[ ] **A.** Administer amiodarone.
[ ] **B.** Defibrillate at 200 joules.
[ ] **C.** Assess the client.
[ ] **D.** Administer lidocaine (Xylocaine).

Correct answer—C. *Rationales:* The nurse should first assess the client. A client in ventricular tachycardia may be hemodynamically stable for hours to days. Performing defibrillation isn't appropriate for a client with a pulse. Amiodarone and lidocaine may be appropriate if the client is hemodynamically stable.
Nursing process step: Intervention

67. What drug should the nurse anticipate giving to a client suffering from acute myocardial infarction (MI)?

[ ] **A.** Morphine
[ ] **B.** Sodium bicarbonate
[ ] **C.** Atropine
[ ] **D.** Adenosine (Adenocard)

Correct answer—A. *Rationales:* A client with acute MI may receive morphine to decrease pain, anxiety, and myocardial oxygen consumption. Sodium bicarbonate isn't indicated for this client. Atropine is given only for sympto matic bradycardias. Adenosine is given to a client with supraventricular tachycardia.
Nursing process step: Intervention

68. Which of the following characterizes complete atrioventricular (AV) block?

[ ] **A.** The atria and ventricles beat independently of one another.
[ ] **B.** The PR interval is greater than 0.20 second.
[ ] **C.** There's a cyclical prolongation of the PR interval.
[ ] **D.** The PR interval is greater than 0.20 second and consistent with periodic failure of the ventricle to respond.

Correct answer—A. *Rationales:* In complete AV block, there's no association between the atria and the ventricles. Option B describes a first-degree AV block. Option C describes a Mobitz Type I or Wenckebach AV block. Option D describes a Mobitz Type II block.
Nursing process step: Assessment

69. A 22-year-old unrestrained driver arrives in the emergency department after being involved in a high-speed single vehicle rollover crash in which he was partially ejected through the windshield. He's unconscious and has no spontaneous respiratory efforts, and his abdomen is markedly distended. Based on the history, what's the most likely cause of this client's pulseless electrical activity (PEA)?

[ ] **A.** Cardiac tamponade due to undiagnosed chest trauma

[ ] **B.** Hypovolemia due to blood loss

[ ] **C.** Acidosis

[ ] **D.** Electrolyte imbalances due to massive volume infusion

Correct answer—B. *Rationales:* Hypovolemia is the most common cause of shock in an injured client. This client had a significant mechanism of injury. His possible abdominal injury could be the source of massive blood loss. There may be undiagnosed chest trauma as well, but there's no indication of that in the scenario. Acidosis is a complication of inadequate perfusion and may be complicating the resuscitation of this client. Massive volume infusions aren't likely to result in PEA in the acutely injured client in the resuscitation phase.

Nursing process step: Assessment

70. Which intervention is most likely to resolve the pulseless electrical activity (PEA) in a client who sustained massive internal injuries in a motor vehicle accident?

[ ] **A.** Administration of a dopamine infusion

[ ] **B.** Administration of crystalloid and blood products

[ ] **C.** Surgical repair of his bilateral femur fractures

[ ] **D.** Antibiotic administration to prevent infection

Correct answer—B. *Rationales:* The most likely cause of this client's PEA is massive volume loss, so the best approach to correcting the problem is to administer volume, including crystalloids and blood products. Dopamine might increase the client's blood pressure, but at the cost of worsening tissue perfusion. Antibiotic administration and surgical repair are important goals after the client has been initially stabilized.

Nursing process step: Intervention

71. A 66-year-old man presents complaining of a sudden onset of abdominal pain radiating to the flank. He has a history of poorly controlled hypertension, coronary artery disease (CAD), and heart failure. Which condition may be associated with his presentation and history?

[ ] **A.** Angina pectoris

[ ] **B.** Gastroesophageal reflux disease

[ ] **C.** Pulmonary embolus

[ ] **D.** Abdominal aortic aneurysm dissection

Correct answer—D. *Rationales:* Abdominal pain radiating to the flank area in a 66-year-old male with a history of hypertension and CAD should be assumed to be related to abdominal aortic aneurysm dissection until this cause can be ruled out. Abdominal pain with a sudden onset isn't a common presentation of the other disorders listed.

Nursing process step: Assessment

72. Appropriate interventions for a client with a possible abdominal aortic aneurysm would include:

[ ] **A.** immediate electrocardiogram, upright chest X-ray, and administration of an oral antacid.

[ ] **B.** placing the client in bed, assessing vital signs, and notifying the physician of the client's arrival and assessment findings.

[ ] **C.** initiating I.V. sodium nitroprusside infusion, titrated until the pain is relieved.

[ ] **D.** administering oxygen and preparing the client for the cardiac catheterization laboratory.

Correct answer—B. *Rationales:* Placing the client in bed, assessing vital signs, and notifying the physician of the client's arrival will assist in a more rapid diagnosis. The other actions aren't indicated.

Nursing process step: Intervention

73. When performing cardiopulmonary resuscitation on an adult client, how far should the sternum be depressed to obtain adequate cardiac compression?
[ ] **A.** At least ½″ (1 cm)
[ ] **B.** At least 1″ (2.5 cm)
[ ] **C.** At least 1½″ (3.5 cm)
[ ] **D.** At least 2″ (5 cm)

Correct answer—D. *Rationales:* In adults, the sternum must be depressed at least 2″ to adequately compress the heart between the sternum and spine. Less cardiac compression may result in inadequate generation of cardiac output.
Nursing process step: Intervention

74. A 79-year-old man presents complaining of numbness in his lower leg and foot. He states that the affected foot feels cooler than his other foot and that the numbness began while he was at rest. He also relates that he has a history of atrial fibrillation and that he was taking warfarin (Coumadin) until 2 weeks ago, when his prescription ran out. The nurse's assessment will include:
[ ] **A.** 12-lead electrocardiograph (ECG).
[ ] **B.** palpation of pulses in bilateral lower extremities.
[ ] **C.** auscultation of bowel tones.
[ ] **D.** percussion of the abdomen.

Correct answer—B. *Rationales:* Palpation of the pulses in both lower extremities will determine whether the pulses are equal or whether the pulse is decreased in the affected extremity. The client's history of atrial fibrillation and abrupt cessation of anticoagulant therapy places him at risk for embolization, which may cause the symptoms he reported. Auscultation of bowel tones and percussion of the abdomen won't assist in determining this client's problem. A 12-lead ECG will likely be performed, but immediate assessment of the extremity takes precedence.
Nursing process step: Assessment

75. Which condition would be a contraindication to the administration of tPA?
[ ] **A.** Recent head injury with subdural hematoma
[ ] **B.** History of coronary artery bypass surgery 10 months ago
[ ] **C.** History of receiving streptokinase in the past 3 months
[ ] **D.** Elevated serum cholesterol

Correct answer—A. *Rationales:* A recent head injury with subdural hematoma contraindicates the administration of any thrombolytic agent. A history of surgery 10 months ago isn't a contraindication, but recent surgery would be a contraindication. Clients who have recently received streptokinase shouldn't receive it again but may receive tPA. Elevated serum cholesterol is common in clients with coronary artery disease and isn't a contraindication to the administration of thrombolytic agents.
Nursing process step: Assessment

76. During the administration of the thrombolytic agent, the client states that his pain has resolved, and the nurse notes an accelerated idioventricular rhythm. The client remains alert, and his blood pressure is 100/64 mm Hg. His respirations are regular at 16 breaths/minute. These signs may indicate:
[ ] **A.** worsening ischemia and growing infarction.
[ ] **B.** immediate transfer to a facility with cardiac surgical capability.
[ ] **C.** emergency I.V. pacemaker placement.
[ ] **D.** reperfusion symptoms.

Correct answer—D. *Rationales:* Cessation of pain and observation of an accelerated idioventricular rhythm may be associated with reperfusion and aren't signs of deterioration. Worsening ischemia would be indicated by continuing pain and unstable vital signs. Idioventricular rhythm associated with reperfusion is usually transient and likely won't require pacemaker placement unless the arrhythmia persists and is associated with unstable vital signs.
Nursing process step: Assessment

77. After the administration of thrombolytic agents, which procedure shouldn't be performed?
[ ] **A.** Arterial puncture, due to increased risk of bleeding
[ ] **B.** Administration of contrast, due to increased risk of renal failure
[ ] **C.** I.V. fluid infusion, due to increased risk of heart failure
[ ] **D.** Incentive spirometry, due to increased risk of atelectasis

Correct answer—A. *Rationales:* Arterial and venous punctures during and after the administration of thrombo lytic agents increase the risk of bleeding. Administration of contrast, I.V. fluids, and incentive spirometry may be contraindicated in some clients for reasons unrelated to thrombolytic therapy.
Nursing process step: Intervention

78. A client's electrocardiogram shows a prolonged QT interval. Which arrhythmia is associated with a prolonged QT interval?
[ ] **A.** Atrial fibrillation
[ ] **B.** First-degree atrioventricular block
[ ] **C.** Torsades de pointes
[ ] **D.** Junctional rhythm

Correct answer—C. *Rationales:* Torsades de pointes is associated with a prolonged QT interval. Atrial fibrillation, first-degree atrioventricular block, and a junctional rhythm aren't associated with a prolonged QT interval.
Nursing process step: Analysis

79. A client's lab work indicates hypokalemia and hypomagnesemia. Which arrhythmia is the client at greatest risk for developing?
[ ] **A.** Bradycardia
[ ] **B.** Torsades de pointes
[ ] **C.** Atrial fibrillation
[ ] **D.** Supraventricular tachycardia

Correct answer—B. *Rationales:* A low magnesium level can induce torsades de pointes. Bradycardia, atrial fibrillation, and supraventricular tachycardia aren't associated with hypokalemia and hypomagnesemia.
Nursing process step: Analysis

80. An overdose of which medication would put a client at highest risk for torsades de pointes?
[ ] **A.** Sotalol (Betapace)
[ ] **B.** Acetaminophen
[ ] **C.** Alprazolam (Xanax)
[ ] **D.** Hydromorphone

Correct answer—A. *Rationales:* Sotalol is a beta blocker as well as an antiarrhythmic and is associated with prolongation of the PR and QT interval, which places a client at risk for developing torsades de pointes. Acetaminophen, alprazolam, and hydromorphone aren't associated with a prolonged QT interval.
Nursing process step: Analysis

81. Which diagnostic tool would be the most important when endocarditis is suspected?
[ ] **A.** Troponin I
[ ] **B.** Blood cultures
[ ] **C.** Electrocardiogram
[ ] **D.** Chest X-ray

Correct answer—B. *Rationales:* Blood cultures would show systemic bacteremia, which is the standard test for diagnosing endocarditis. Troponin I measures myocardial injury and would be used to diagnose a myocardial infarction. Electrocardiograms and chest X-rays wouldn't indicate specific abnormalities associated with endocarditis.
Nursing process step: Evaluation

82. A client comes to the emergency department with a low-grade fever, general malaise, and nontender maculae (Janeway lesions) on the palms of both hands and the soles of both feet. What disorder should the nurse suspect?
[ ] **A.** Meningitis
[ ] **B.** Infective endocarditis
[ ] **C.** Hand-foot-and-mouth disease
[ ] **D.** Splenic abscess

Correct answer—B. *Rationales:* Janeway lesions are most common with infective endocarditis. Janeway lesions aren't a dermatologic manifestation of meningitis, hand-foot-and-mouth disease, or splenic abscess.
Nursing process step: Assessment

83. What history assessment finding would alert the nurse to the possibility of bacterial endocarditis in a client with fever, cough, malaise, and shortness of breath?

[ ] **A.** History of Lyme disease
[ ] **B.** History of I.V. drug abuse
[ ] **C.** History of heart failure
[ ] **D.** History of myocardial infarction (MI)

Correct answer–B. *Rationales:* Endocarditis is a common infection caused by I.V. drug use and should be suspected for all clients with an infection from an unknown source and a history of I.V. drug use. A history of Lyme disease, heart failure, and MI aren't associated with endocarditis.

Nursing process step: Analysis

84. Which drug would be most appropriate to control blood pressure immediately for a client with hypertensive emergency?

[ ] **A.** Intravenous labetalol
[ ] **B.** Oral metoprolol (Lopressor)
[ ] **C.** Intravenous furosemide (Lasix)
[ ] **D.** Oral furosemide (Lasix)

Correct answer–A. *Rationales:* Labetalol, an alpha- and beta-blocking medication, is beneficial in lowering blood pressure. Oral metoprolol and oral furosemide would be ineffective because of the time needed for full effect due to the route given. I.V. furosemide may lower the blood pressure but is not the first medication indicated for hypertensive emergency.

Nursing process step: Intervention

85. Which of the following is not a risk of hypertension?

[ ] **A.** Renal failure
[ ] **B.** Cerebral infarct
[ ] **C.** Deep vein thrombosis
[ ] **D.** Retinal hemorrhage

Correct answer–C. *Rationales:* Deep vein thrombosis isn't a common risk of hypertension; arterial infarcts are more common. Renal failure, cerebral infarct, and retinal hemorrhage are all common examples of end-organ damage from hypertension.

Nursing process step: Analysis

3 Disaster management

1. What's an event that involves fewer than 100 victims called?

[ ] **A.** Multiple-client incident
[ ] **B.** Multiple-casualty incident
[ ] **C.** Mass-casualty incident
[ ] **D.** Mass-client incident

Correct answer–B. *Rationales:* The triage classification of disasters occurs in three tiers. The first is a multiple-client incident, which is a common occurrence involving fewer than 10 casualties. The next is a multiple-casualty incident, which involves fires, natural occurrences (hurricanes and tornadoes), radiation or biochemical accidents, and air, train, and bus crashes. Casualties number 100 or fewer.
A multiple-casualty incident strains the existing emergency medical system but doesn't overwhelm the components.
A mass-casualty incident is the least common. It occurs with major earthquakes, explosions, structural failures, and large-scale fires. Casualties number more than 100. There are many deaths and injuries; property damage is extensive as well. The emergency medical system and health care facilities are overwhelmed. Mass-client incidents are not part of the triage classification of disasters.
Nursing process step: Assessment

2. Which of the following is one of the four key components of an emergency preparedness program?

[ ] **A.** Mitigation and prevention
[ ] **B.** Analysis
[ ] **C.** Intervention
[ ] **D.** Reassimilation

Correct answer–A. *Rationales:* Analysis, intervention, and reassimilation aren't part of the four key components of an emergency preparedness program. The four components include:

◆ Mitigation and prevention: These components are crucial in helping to curtail or severely limit a disaster's severity.
◆ Planning: It's essential to have emergency preparedness plans that have been practiced, critiqued, and periodically updated. Such plans help ensure that emergency medical systems and health care facilities can respond to a disaster.
◆ Response: The ability to respond to disasters with adequate staff, a mix of personnel, sufficient supplies, and a clear chain of command is paramount to the implementation of an emergency preparedness plan.
◆ Recovery: This phase assesses the number of casualties, types of treatment, utilization of resources, and disposition of the incident. Overall response is evaluated, and recommendations are made. The economic impact of the disaster is assessed, and all workers should receive critical incident stress debriefing.

Nursing process step: Analysis

3. Which hospital department provides the crucial interface during a disaster?
[ ] **A.** Administration
[ ] **B.** Emergency department
[ ] **C.** Morgue
[ ] **D.** Operating room

Correct answer—B. *Rationales:* The Emergency department is the interface between the hospital and the disaster scene and is the institution's first "clinical domino" to sustain the burden of client care. The staff's performance during the initial disaster response affects the entire hospital. Administration's role is to support the emergency department by setting up command operations and securing adequate staff to care for incoming casualties. The morgue's role is to hold casualties triaged as mortally injured or dead on arrival. The operating room is the second most critical area for handling incoming casualties; many of the victims may need surgical intervention.
Nursing process step: Analysis

4. What organization is intended to provide a nationwide template to enable federal, state, local, and tribal governments to work together for a range of domestic incidents?
[ ] **A.** National Incident Management System (NIMS)
[ ] **B.** Federal Response Plan (FRP)
[ ] **C.** Federal Bureau of Investigation (FBI)
[ ] **D.** Disaster Relief and Emergency Assistance Act

Correct answer—A. *Rationales:* NIMS integrates emergency preparedness and response into a national framework for incident management. Incident Command Structures are based on a three-organization system: incident command, multiagency coordination, and public information. The Federal Response Plan was created as a guide for an all-hazards approach to domestic incidents and how to group them. The Disaster Relief and Emergency Assistance Act was enacted as statutory author for most federal disaster response activities and created the Federal Response Plan.
Nursing process step: Analysis

5. The Joint Commission has explicit requirements for hospital disaster preparedness. Which of the following is part of those requirements?
[ ] **A.** A description of the hospital's role in community-wide emergency preparedness planning
[ ] **B.** Classification system used in triage
[ ] **C.** Evidence of annual disaster plan implementation either through drills or in actual disaster situations
[ ] **D.** To assess the need for additional personnel in a disaster area

Correct answer—A. *Rationales:* The Joint Commission requires each hospital to describe its role in the community-wide emergency preparedness plan. Each hospital must also be able to show evidence of staff education and training and of semiannual disaster plan implementation. The classification system used in triage is the job of the hospital Incident Command System, not The Joint Commission. The National Disaster Management System, not The Joint Commission, assesses the need for additional personnel in a disaster area.
Nursing process step: Evaluation

6. After a disaster, the nurse caring for survivors may experience stress reactions that are both expected and normal. Which of the following isn't an example of immediate stress?
[ ] **A.** Anxiety
[ ] **B.** Frustration and anger
[ ] **C.** Physical symptoms
[ ] **D.** Alcohol and drug use

Correct answer—D. *Rationales:* The use of alcohol and drugs is considered a delayed reaction to the stress of a disaster. Anxiety manifests itself almost immediately after the staff learns of a disaster. Frustration and anger occur as the victims arrive and the staff deals with the pain and suffering of innocent casualties. This emotion is intensified if the disaster was caused deliberately.
Nursing process step: Evaluation

7. The Homeland security all-hazards taxonomy lists the four mission stages as prevent, protect, respond, and recover. Which is an example of prevention?

[ ] **A.** Controlling access
[ ] **B.** Guarding cyber assets
[ ] **C.** Donning protective garments
[ ] **D.** Disposing of materials

Correct answer–A. *Rationales:* Prevention migrates the effect of a disaster; controlling access will prevent or minimize a disaster from occurring. Guarding cyber assets involves protection of physical and cyber assets and systems. Donning protective garments involves responding to the incident and dealing with it. Disposing of materials involves recovery that includes a restoration of the environment.

Nursing process step: Analysis

8. Which statement is true concerning immediate mass evacuation?

[ ] **A.** Immediate mass evacuation involves the evacuation of people from a geographical area in response to a potential disaster.
[ ] **B.** A sudden, unexpected event has occurred that immediately threatens the health and safety of a population.
[ ] **C.** Residents living in a disaster area need to evacuate but may have a few hours to retrieve personal property.
[ ] **D.** This type of evacuation is orderly and allows time for warning the population of potential disaster; the population is given updated information if the situation worsens as well as instructions for evacuating.

Correct answer–B. *Rationales:* Immediate evacuation occurs without advance warning and requires the population to leave belongings and property behind. A potential mass evacuation involves the evacuation of people from a geographical area when the threat of disaster exists. Those living in the area may have a few hours to gather personal belongings. Evacuation is orderly and allows time for warning the population of potential disaster; the population is given updated information if the situation worsens as well as instructions for evacuating.

Nursing process step: Intervention

9. Which of the following isn't considered when developing an emergency department disaster plan?

[ ] **A.** How the plan will be activated?
[ ] **B.** Who will be in charge of managing incoming casualties?
[ ] **C.** Which client classification system will be used to triage casualties?
[ ] **D.** How injured, but ambulatory, clients will be transported to hospitals from the disaster scene?

Correct answer–D. *Rationales:* How the plan will be activated, who will be in charge of the incoming casualties, and which classification system will be used to triage casualties should be considered when developing an emergency department disaster plan. Casualty transportation is handled by the community disaster plan and emergency medical services.

Nursing process step: Intervention

10. Under the Homeland Security all-hazards taxonomy, which of the following is included in the response stage?

[ ] **A.** Devaluing physical assets and defending systems
[ ] **B.** Identifying terrorist capabilities
[ ] **C.** Screening and restricting people
[ ] **D.** Providing medical care and distributing prophylaxis

Correct answer–D. *Rationales:* Providing medical care and distributing prophylaxis are actions related to the incident itself. Devaluing physical assets and defending systems is in the protection stage. Identifying terrorist capabilities and screening and restricting people are both under the prevention stage.

Nursing process step: Intervention

11. Which of the following is an example of a natural disaster?
[ ] **A.** Hurricane Katrina in 2005
[ ] **B.** The attack on the World Trade Center of 2001
[ ] **C.** The Bhopal, India, gas leak of 1984
[ ] **D.** The Kansas City Hyatt Regency skywalk collapse of 1981

Correct answer—A. *Rationales:* Natural disasters arise from forces of nature, such as earthquakes, hurricanes, floods, and tornadoes. Natural disasters create a heavy death toll, suffering, and destruction. The attack on the World Trade Center, the gas leak in India, and the collapse in Kansas City were all human-made disasters.
Nursing process step: Assessment

12. Which statement about disaster committee organization is true?
[ ] **A.** The selection of committee members must be based on the individuals' seniority.
[ ] **B.** The committee should have a statement of accountability.
[ ] **C.** Each committee member should have defined roles and responsibilities.
[ ] **D.** The selection of committee members must be based on their role in the facility.

Correct answer—C. *Rationales:* Each member should have defined roles and responsibilities. Members of a disaster committee must be chosen for their ability to take action and produce results, not based on their personality or role in the facility. The committee should have a statement of philosophy that all members can uphold.
Nursing process step: Analysis

13. Which of the following is essential in the development of a disaster plan?
[ ] **A.** Organizing a disaster committee
[ ] **B.** Having only verbal authority for the initiation of the disaster plan
[ ] **C.** Eliminating the command center for the hospital disaster plan
[ ] **D.** Holding biannual disaster drills

Correct answer—A. *Rationales:* Essential elements for disaster plan development include having an organized disaster committee, authority to develop and initiate the plan, and a disaster control (or command) center in the hospital. On-scene medical teams, although integrated effectively into some plans, aren't essential elements of the hospital disaster plan.
Nursing process step: Analysis

14. Which statement about disaster drills isn't true?
[ ] **A.** They provide excellent feedback about how staff will perform in an actual disaster.
[ ] **B.** They provide an opportunity to educate the staff about emergency preparedness.
[ ] **C.** They allow the disaster committee to evaluate the disaster plan.
[ ] **D.** They provide a valuable mechanism for disaster plan feedback.

Correct answer—A. *Rationales:* There's no way to know how staff will perform in an actual disaster. Drills are best suited to educating staff, evaluating the plan, critiquing the drill and making modifications, and developing interagency relationships. All these elements prepare the committee and hospital staff for an actual disaster.
Nursing process step: Assessment

15. Which of the following isn't a disaster drill?
[ ] **A.** Tabletop exercise
[ ] **B.** Functional exercise
[ ] **C.** Full-scale exercise
[ ] **D.** Participatory exercise

Correct answer—D. *Rationales:* A participatory exercise isn't a disaster drill. Tabletop exercises, which are done on paper, provide a simulated disaster without time constraints. Key disaster-response personnel have an opportunity to evaluate the plan and resolve issues in a nonthreatening manner. A functional exercise evaluates one or more complex activities in the plan. These scaled-down simulated disasters focus on a few aspects of the plan. A full-scale exercise evaluates all major aspects of the preparedness program. This type of drill involves the use of personnel, supplies, and equipment to simulate as closely as possible an actual disaster.
Nursing process step: Assessment

16. Several victims have arrived from a chemical plant after a bomb exploded. The victims are covered with a strong-smelling liquid and have labored respirations. What action should the nurse responding take *first?*
[ ] **A.** Apply oxygen per nasal cannula.
[ ] **B.** Assess what chemicals the victims were exposed to.
[ ] **C.** Don personal protective garments.
[ ] **D.** Remove the victims' clothes.

Correct answer–C. *Rationales:* The first thing the nurse should do is protect herself by donning personal protective garments. Then decontamination of the victims can occur prior to treatment, which includes removal of the victims' clothes and dilution of the chemical. The next action would be to apply oxygen to the victims followed by additional assessments, such as what chemicals the victims were exposed to.
Nursing process step: Intervention

17. The hospital Incident Command System (ICS) was developed and is used for the following reasons:
[ ] **A.** To use the same terminology for Emergency Medical Services and Fire personnel
[ ] **B.** Communication within a specific department
[ ] **C.** Satisfy Health Insurance Portability and Accountability Act (HIPAA) regulations
[ ] **D.** Satisfy Joint Commission (TJC) requirements

Correct answer–A. *Rationales:* The ICS was developed in California in the 1970s after a large fire. During the incident, it was discovered that none of the agencies were using the same terminology or system to manage the situation. This led to confusion and inefficiencies. After the ICS was developed, hospitals began to adopt it because of communications issues with outside agencies during a major incident. HIPAA and TJC didn't develop the ICS.
Nursing process step: Analysis

18. Several clients present to the emergency department triage desk complaining of excessive salivation, rhinorrhea, vomiting, watery eyes, and diarrhea. The nurse also notices that all of the clients have miosis. What does the nurse suspect is the problem?
[ ] **A.** These clients were exposed to pepper spray.
[ ] **B.** They have experienced carbon monoxide poisoning.
[ ] **C.** They were all using drugs.
[ ] **D.** A nerve agent was used on passengers on the bus.

Correct answer–D. *Rationales:* The symptoms are typical of an exposure to a nerve agent. Pepper spray wouldn't cause vomiting and diarrhea. Most drugs may cause one of the listed symptoms but not all of them. Carbon monoxide poisoning wouldn't cause diarrhea, vomiting, or rhinorrhea.
Nursing process step: Assessment

19. A client who has been exposed to a nerve agent will need all of the following *except:*
[ ] **A.** antinausea medications.
[ ] **B.** decontamination.
[ ] **C.** pralidoxime.
[ ] **D.** atropine in large doses.

Correct answer–A. *Rationales:* Antinausea medications and decontamination won't break the cycle. An anticholinesterase agent, such as pralidoxime, will break the agent enzyme bond and restore normal activity. Atropine should also be given in large doses.
Nursing process step: Analysis

20. Why does a client who was exposed to a nerve agent require decontamination if the agent was a gas?
[ ] **A.** Decontamination will prevent the client's further exposure to the agent.
[ ] **B.** Decontamination will prevent exposure to the nurse and to others.
[ ] **C.** Decontamination isn't necessary because the agent was a gas and it has dissipated.
[ ] **D.** A and B.

Correct answer–D. *Rationales:* A gas can be absorbed into clothing and continue to expose others. Never assume that the client isn't contaminated because he was exposed to a gas.
Nursing process step: Intervention

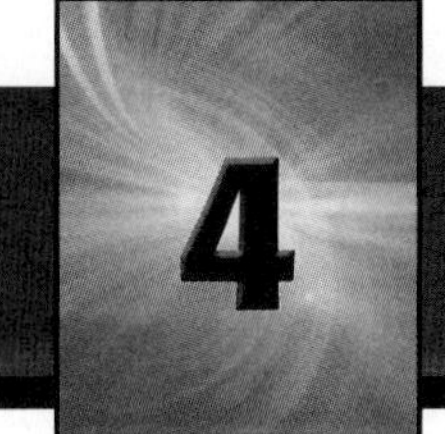

4 Environmental emergencies

1. Which intervention is inappropriate for a client with partial-thickness burns over 20% of his body surface area?

[ ] **A.** Remove restrictive clothing and jewelry.

[ ] **B.** Assess for tetanus prophylaxis.

[ ] **C.** Debride all blisters.

[ ] **D.** Don't shave the eyebrows if the burn involves the face.

Correct answer—C. *Rationales:* Blisters should be left intact because they're a natural barrier to infection. (Some believe that blisters should be removed for proper assessment only if they impede joint movement. If the blisters require aspiration, the outer layer should be left intact for protection.) Restrictive clothing and jewelry should be removed before edema develops. A client with a burn should receive appropriate tetanus prophylaxis. Eyebrows shouldn't be shaved because they may not grow back.

Nursing process step: Intervention

2. Which statement about frostbite is true?

[ ] **A.** Frostbite is reversible.

[ ] **B.** The nurse should vigorously rub the affected area.

[ ] **C.** Frostbite is usually accompanied by hypothermia.

[ ] **D.** The emergency department nurse should immerse the affected area in hot (120° to 130° F [48.9° to 54.4° C]) water.

Correct answer—C. *Rationales:* Frostbite occurs from overexposure to cold. It's usually accompanied by hypothermia, which may need to be addressed first. After frostbite has occurred, it isn't reversible; however, surrounding tissues should be protected from injury. The affected area shouldn't be rubbed; ice crystals have formed within the tissues, and rubbing would damage the tissue further. The affected area should be immersed in warm water (100° to 110° F [37.8° to 43.3° C]).

Nursing process step: Assessment

3. Which of the following are the initial signs and symptoms consistent with a Portuguese man o' war jellyfish sting?

[ ] **A.** Severe incapacitating localized pain with wide erythematous bands on the skin

[ ] **B.** Pain at the site with central radiation of discomfort

[ ] **C.** Painful lesions having a "string of beads" appearance

[ ] **D.** Initial sting barely felt and pain without skin signs developing slowly beginning in the sacral area and progressing to the entire body

Correct answer—C. *Rationales:* The sting of the Portuguese man o' war is painful and leaves a lesion having a "string of beads" appearance on the skin. The deadliest of the jellyfish is the box jellyfish. Its sting is severe and immediately incapacitating, with wide erythematous banded lesions on the skin. Pain at the site of a lesion with a central radiation of discomfort is a hallmark of the sting of a scorpion fish. The initial sting of the Irukandji jellyfish is barely felt, and a progressive painful syndrome develops rapidly about 30 to 60 minutes after envenomation.

Nursing process step: Assessment

4. A client has a core temperature of 90° F (32.2° C). The emergency department nurse should expect this client to have which reaction?

[ ] **A.** Shivering

[ ] **B.** Apnea

[ ] **C.** Muscle rigidity, no shivering

[ ] **D.** Cold, pale skin

Correct answer—C. *Rationales:* A client with a core body temperature of 90° F usually doesn't shiver. Shivering is present at higher temperatures. Clients generally don't become apneic or have cold, pale skin until their core body temperature reaches 77° F (25° C).

Nursing process step: Assessment

5. Which intervention is inappropriate for a client with severe burns?
[ ] **A.** Administration of subcutaneous heparin
[ ] **B.** Administration of humidified oxygen
[ ] **C.** Aggressive fluid resuscitation
[ ] **D.** Administration of tetanus prophylaxis

Correct answer–A. *Rationales:* A burn client shouldn't receive I.M. or subcutaneous injections because of erratic drug uptake related to decreased peripheral circulation and fluid volume changes. Administration of humidified oxygen is appropriate for a trauma client but is particularly important in the severely burned client if upper airway damage is suspected. Aggressive fluid resuscitation is essential to prevent hypovolemic shock. Burns are especially prone to tetanus, and clients should receive tetanus toxoid and tetanus immune globulin on the basis of their immunization status.
Nursing process step: Intervention

6. A 2-year-old child is brought to the emergency department after being found submerged in a neighborhood pool. The child is unconscious with a pulse of 60 beats/minute and respirations of 4 breaths/minute. Breathing is being assisted with a bag-valve-mask device. What should be the first action of the nurse?
[ ] **A.** Administer epinephrine (Adrenalin).
[ ] **B.** Assist with intubation.
[ ] **C.** Begin an intraosseous infusion.
[ ] **D.** Obtain a cervical spine X-ray.

Correct answer–B. *Rationales:* Airway, breathing, and circulation are always first priority actions. Therefore, the nurse should first assist with intubation. After the airway is stabilized, I.V. access can be attempted; if unsuccessful, the intraosseous route can be established. Epinephrine is used to treat circulation problems, but this would be addressed after the client's airway was established. After the client is stabilized, a cervical spine X-ray can be obtained.
Nursing process step: Intervention

7. Which client should be referred to a burn center?
[ ] **A.** A 54-year-old with full-thickness burns over 10% of the body surface area (BSA)
[ ] **B.** A 30-year-old with partial-thickness burns over 15% of the BSA
[ ] **C.** A 40-year-old with partial- and full-thickness burns over 15% of the BSA
[ ] **D.** An 8-year-old with partial- and full-thickness burns over 5% of the BSA

Correct answer–A. *Rationales:* The American Burn Association and the American College of Surgeons have issued guidelines outlining the categories of burn victims who should be referred to a burn center.
- Partial- and full-thickness burns greater than 10% of the BSA in clients under age 10 or over age 50
- Partial- and full-thickness burns greater than 20% of the BSA in all age-groups
- Deep partial- and full-thickness burns that involve the face, hands, feet, genitalia, perineum, and overlying major joints in all age-groups
- Full-thickness burns greater than 5% of the BSA in all age-groups

Nursing process step: Assessment

8. A client arrives in the emergency department after suffering chemical burns to his body while at work. What's the first priority of care for this client?
[ ] **A.** Remove his clothes and irrigate the burns with lots of water.
[ ] **B.** Establish two large-bore I.V. lines and infuse lactated Ringer's solution.
[ ] **C.** Contact the poison control center for specific instructions.
[ ] **D.** Determine the type of chemical involved.

Correct answer–A. *Rationales:* The most important intervention is to wash off the chemical with lots of water to prevent further tissue damage. Most chemicals are safely removed in this manner. The nurse shouldn't attempt to neutralize the chemical; neutralizing may generate heat and cause further tissue damage. After the burn has been irrigated, determine the type of chemical involved and contact the poison control center for additional instructions. I.V. line placement and infusion of lactated Ringer's solution may also be helpful.
Nursing process step: Intervention

9. Fluid resuscitation in a burn victim may be deemed effective if what happens?
[ ] **A.** Central venous pressure (CVP) is decreased.
[ ] **B.** Urine output is 0.5 to 1.0 mL/kg/hour.
[ ] **C.** Electrolyte balance is achieved.
[ ] **D.** Level of consciousness (LOC) is improved.

Correct answer–B. *Rationales:* The goal of therapy is to maintain a urine output of 0.5 to 1.0 mL/kg/hour; for electrical burns, increase intake to maintain a urine output of 1.5 to 2.0 mL/kg/hour. Adequate fluid volume should result in a normal—not decreased—CVP. Electrolyte balance is important but may not be achieved early in the resuscitation phase. LOC in the burn client may be affected by many things, including concomitant injuries and opioid administration.
Nursing process step: Evaluation

10. A client is diagnosed with heat exhaustion. The nurse should expect the client to exhibit which symptoms?
[ ] **A.** Tachycardia, hypotension, and hot, dry skin
[ ] **B.** Core body temperature of 105.6° F (40.9° C)
[ ] **C.** Headache, nausea, and dizziness
[ ] **D.** Profuse sweating, tachycardia, and hypotension

Correct answer–C. *Rationales:* A client with heat exhaustion exhibits profuse sweating, headache, nausea, and dizziness. Blood pressure, heart rate, and respirations are usually normal, and body temperature is only mildly elevated. A client with tachycardia, hypotension, and hot, dry skin with a temperature of 105.6° F is suffering from heatstroke.
Nursing process step: Assessment

11. Which statement regarding decompression sickness (the "bends") isn't true?
[ ] **A.** A diver at great depths for long periods may experience decompression sickness if he ascends rapidly.
[ ] **B.** The gas that's the problem in decompression sickness is oxygen.
[ ] **C.** Extremes of water temperature and poor physical condition are factors that increase the severity of this condition.
[ ] **D.** The treatment of choice for decompression sickness is recompression.

Correct answer–B. *Rationales:* Nitrogen is dissolved in solution because a diver at great depths for long periods breathes nitrogen at greater pressures than normal. However, the "bends" can occur at depths less than 33 feet. Ascending rapidly doesn't allow time for the nitrogen to reabsorb, and bubbles form, causing decompression sickness. The other options are correct.
Nursing process step: Evaluation

12. A client arrives at the emergency department after suffering a burn injury. The burned area is white and leathery, with no blisters. What's the best classification for this burn?
[ ] **A.** First-degree burn
[ ] **B.** Second-degree burn (superficial partial thickness)
[ ] **C.** Second-degree burn (deep partial thickness)
[ ] **D.** Third-degree burn (full thickness)

Correct answer–D. *Rationales:* Third-degree, full-thickness burns may appear white, red, or black. These burns are dry and leathery, with no blisters. Hair can be pulled out easily. The client may experience little or no pain because nerve endings have been destroyed. First-degree burns are superficial, involving only the epidermis. These burns are accompanied by local pain and redness but no blistering. Second-degree, superficial partial-thickness burns appear red and moist with blister formation; these burns are painful. Second-degree, deep partial-thickness burns may convert to full thickness in the presence of trauma, decreased blood supply, or infection.
Nursing process step: Assessment

13. A client with suspected burn inhalation injury is tested for carboxyhemoglobin. What's the normal carboxyhemoglobin level?
[ ] **A.** Less than 5%
[ ] **B.** 5% to 10%
[ ] **C.** 10% to 20%
[ ] **D.** 20% to 40%

Correct answer–A. *Rationales:* In nonsmokers, less than 5% is a normal carboxyhemoglobin level. Smokers may have carboxyhemoglobin levels of 5% to 10%. Higher levels are considered abnormal. At levels of 20%, a client may experience mild headache. As levels approach 40%, the client may exhibit dizziness, confusion, nausea, vomiting, and loss of consciousness. Levels of 60% to 80% may result in death.
Nursing process step: Assessment

14. Which of the following is the primary cause of hypovolemia in a burn client?
[ ] **A.** Increased capillary permeability
[ ] **B.** Blood loss
[ ] **C.** Neurogenic shock
[ ] **D.** Nausea and vomiting

Correct answer–A. *Rationales:* Capillary damage leads to increased capillary permeability. Fluid shifts into the interstitial spaces, leading to hypovolemia. Aggressive fluid resuscitation should be implemented. Options B and C may occur if there are concurrent injuries, but they aren't the primary causes of hypovolemia. A burn client doesn't usually experience nausea and vomiting unless there are underlying conditions.
Nursing process step: Evaluation

15. A 34-year-old male presents to the emergency department with the following vital signs: blood pressure, 85/50 mm Hg; temperature, 101.8° F (38.8° C); pulse, 132 beats/minute; respirations, 22 breaths/minute; and oxygen saturation, 100%. He reports he was bitten by an unknown type of snake while canoeing on the river. What type of snakebite should be suspected?
[ ] **A.** Nonpoisonous snakebite
[ ] **B.** Crotalid or pit viper envenomation (most rattlesnakes)
[ ] **C.** Sea snake envenomation
[ ] **D.** Elapid envenomation (coral snakes and cobras)

Correct answer–B. *Rationales:* Symptoms of the crotalid envenomation include nausea, weakness, hypotension, fever, vomiting, and sweating. Sea snake envenomation usually manifests as rapid paralysis of the affected limb and respiratory muscles. Elapid envenomation symptoms are neurologic, resulting in parasthesias, fasciculations, slurred speech, drowsiness, and vertigo. Nonpoisonous snakes don't produce systemic signs and symptoms after a bite.
Nursing process step: Analysis

16. Why are alkali burns more serious than acid burns?
[ ] **A.** They're generally full thickness.
[ ] **B.** They produce liquefaction necrosis.
[ ] **C.** They produce coagulation necrosis.
[ ] **D.** They cause extensive damage to fascia and muscle.

Correct answer–B. *Rationales:* Alkali burns cause liquefaction necrosis, deeper penetration, less pain, and loosening of tissues, all of which increase the spread of the offending agent. Treatment includes irrigation with lots of water for at least 30 minutes to prevent further tissue damage. Acid burns cause coagulation necrosis. Extensive damage to fascia and muscle is likely to occur with electrical burns.
Nursing process step: Analysis

17. Which of the following isn't a reason children have a better survival rate than adults in drowning accidents?
[ ] **A.** Children experience a higher incidence of laryngospasm.
[ ] **B.** Children become hypothermic more rapidly than adults.
[ ] **C.** Children are more susceptible to the diving reflex.
[ ] **D.** Children have a relatively larger surface area.

Correct answer–A. *Rationales:* Children become hypothermic more rapidly than adults because of their relatively larger surface area and smaller amount of subcutaneous fat. They're also more susceptible to the diving reflex, which induces bradycardia and redistributes blood flow to the heart and brain.
Nursing process step: Evaluation

18. An adult weighing 194 lb (88 kg) is brought to the emergency department after sustaining a thermal injury. Burns are partial and full thickness over 38% of the body surface area. According to the Parkland formula, what would this client's fluid requirements be for the first 24 hours after injury?

[ ] **A.** 3,344 mL
[ ] **B.** 13,376 mL
[ ] **C.** 6,688 mL
[ ] **D.** 18,796 mL

Correct answer–B. *Rationales:* The Parkland formula is as follows: 4 mL of lactated Ringer's solution × kg of body weight × % of total body surface burned. In this example, 4 mL × 88 kg × 38% = 13,376 mL of lactated Ringer's solution. One-half the total volume should be administered in the first 8 hours after injury, one-quarter in the second 8 hours, and one-quarter in the remaining 8 hours. The nurse should remember to calculate the time from the time of injury.

Nursing process step: Intervention

19. At what core body temperature should aggressive internal rewarming be initiated in a hypothermic client?

[ ] **A.** 95° F (35° C)
[ ] **B.** 78° F (25.6° C)
[ ] **C.** 86° F (30° C)
[ ] **D.** 90° F (32.2° C)

Correct answer–C. *Rationales:* It's recommended by the American Heart Association that internal rewarming begin at 86° F. Below this point, the client may develop rewarming shock. Below 78° F, death usually occurs.

Nursing process step: Intervention

20. A client arrives at the emergency department after collapsing while running a 5K race. His core body temperature is 105° F (40.6° C), and his urine is tea-colored. What does this mean?

[ ] **A.** He's dehydrated and needs fluids.
[ ] **B.** His urine contains myoglobin, and he's in danger of renal failure.
[ ] **C.** There are red blood cells present in his urine.
[ ] **D.** Urine is normally concentrated when a client is hyperthermic.

Correct answer–B. *Rationales:* Myoglobin is produced when there's a breakdown of muscle tissue, which is then filtered out through the kidneys, causing renal failure. When a client is dehydrated, his urine is normally dark orange-yellow, not tea-colored. The presence of blood in the urine will cause it to look red, not brown.

Nursing process step: Assessment

21. A 54-year-old male was out shoveling snow for several hours. The wind was blowing at about 30 miles per hour; with a temperature of 25° F (−3.9° C), the windchill was −25° F (−31.7° C). He didn't wear a hat and took his gloves off after the first hour because they were wet. When he finally went into the house to "warm up," he complained to his wife that his hands were itching, but not painful. Based on the above description, what type of cold-related injury does he have?

[ ] **A.** Frostbite
[ ] **B.** Chilblains
[ ] **C.** Superficial frostbite
[ ] **D.** Hypothermia

Correct answer–B. *Rationales:* Chilblains, which is considered a mild form of frostbite. The symptoms are normally mild and don't cause pain. Frostbite is usually very painful when the area is rewarming, and swelling of the area usually occurs as the frozen part thaws. Hypothermia is a systematic illness as a result of prolonged exposure to extreme cold temperatures.

Nursing process step: Assessment

5 Maxillofacial emergencies

1. Which of the following isn't indicated for a client with a nasal fracture?
[ ] **A.** Pain medication
[ ] **B.** Tetanus prophylaxis
[ ] **C.** Antibiotic therapy
[ ] **D.** Topical vasoconstriction

Correct answer—D. *Rationales:* The administration of pain medication, tetanus prophylaxis, and antibiotics are all appropriate interventions because nasal fractures should be treated like open fractures. A topical vasoconstriction is used for the treatment of epistaxis or foreign-body extraction.
Nursing process step: Implementation

2. A client who has recently been involved in an altercation arrives in the emergency department. A zygomatic fracture is suspected. The nurse should check for anesthesia or hyperesthesia from infraorbital nerve damage on the affected side in all the following areas *except:*
[ ] **A.** mandible.
[ ] **B.** cheek.
[ ] **C.** nose.
[ ] **D.** upper lip.

Correct answer—A. *Rationales:* The cheek, nose, and upper lip are all supplied by the infraorbital nerve as it exits through the zygoma. The mandible is supplied by a branch of the facial nerve.
Nursing process step: Assessment

3. A client with multiple traumas—a right fractured femur, right clavicle fracture, and right-sided pneumothorax—is suspected of having a zygomatic fracture. The physician orders a Waters' view X-ray to obtain a definitive diagnosis of the zygomatic fracture. Why should the nurse question this X-ray view?
[ ] **A.** It requires a supine position with forward flexion of the neck.
[ ] **B.** It requires a right lateral position with hyperextension of the neck.
[ ] **C.** It requires a prone position with hyperextension of the neck.
[ ] **D.** It requires a left lateral position with flexion of the neck.

Correct answer—C. *Rationales:* The Waters' view requires the client to lie in a prone position with hyperextension of the neck. This client wouldn't be able to safely assume this position because of the multiple injuries. Supine position with forward flexion of the neck represents a submentovertex view that could be used if cervical spine injury were ruled out. A right lateral position with hyperextension of the neck and a left lateral position with flexion of the neck aren't positions of either view.
Nursing process step: Assessment

4. When considering a client's medical history and general appearance, what predisposing factor may be significant to a diagnosis of sinusitis?
[ ] **A.** Dental abscesses
[ ] **B.** Presence of dentures
[ ] **C.** Deviated septum repair
[ ] **D.** Asthma

Correct answer—A. *Rationales:* Dental abscesses, cocaine use, and smoking are all significant predisposing factors to a diagnosis of sinusitis. Other factors include foreign bodies in the nose, allergic rhinitis, use of nasogastric tubes, and air pollution. Dentures, rhinoplasty, and asthma don't contribute to sinusitis.
Nursing process step: Assessment

5. Other evidence that supports a diagnosis of sinusitis includes all of the following *except:*
[ ] **A.** conjunctivitis.
[ ] **B.** periorbital edema.
[ ] **C.** paresthesia of the cheek.
[ ] **D.** opacification to transillumination.

Correct answer—C. *Rationales:* Conjunctivitis, periorbital edema, and opacification to transillumination all indicate sinusitis. Paresthesia of the cheek is present with a zygomatic fracture.
Nursing process step: Assessment

6. Which statement expresses a clear understanding of the client's discharge instructions for use of a decongestant medication?
[ ] **A.** "I need to spray one time in each nostril with the decongestant."
[ ] **B.** "I'll buy an ice pack to use."
[ ] **C.** "I'll use this spray (decongestant) for only 3 days."
[ ] **D.** "When I feel better, I can stop the antibiotics."

Correct answer—C. *Rationales:* Decongestants should be used for only about 3 days. If used for an extended period, a rebound occurs and may cause severe nasal congestion when the drug is discontinued. Two sprays are recommended: one to shrink the mucosa so the second spray (dose) can reach the upper turbinate and sinus ostia. Heat treatment is preferred to cold applications. Antibiotics should be taken for the full course of therapy; discontinuing early may cause the infection to return.
Nursing process step: Evaluation

7. Neosynephrine is used in the treatment of epistaxis to:
[ ] **A.** reduce vomiting.
[ ] **B.** reduce anxiety.
[ ] **C.** constrict vessels.
[ ] **D.** dilate vessels.

Correct answer—C. *Rationales:* Neosynephrine on a saturated pledget that's inserted into the nares assists in epistaxis treatment by constricting blood vessels, thereby decreasing bleeding and improving visualization of the area. Reducing vomiting and anxiety and dilating vessels aren't effects of neosynephrine.
Nursing process step: Analysis

8. All of the following infectious processes can cause significant airway obstruction, necessitating incision and drainage and, possibly, acute airway intervention *except:*
[ ] **A.** epiglottiditis.
[ ] **B.** peritonsillar abscess.
[ ] **C.** retropharyngeal abscess.
[ ] **D.** Ludwig's angina.

Correct answer—A. *Rationales:* Epiglottiditis, an acute bacterial infection, causes swelling of the epiglottis and subsequent airway obstruction. It's treated with antibiotics, humidified oxygen, intubation, or cricothyrotomy; incision and drainage are unnecessary. Peritonsillar abscess and retropharyngeal abscess are complications of acute suppurative tonsillitis. Symptoms include a septic appearance, fever, drooling, foul breath, and a muffled voice. Clients with these abscesses require close airway monitoring, incisions, and drainage. Ludwig's angina presents with high fever, dyspnea, and elevation of the tongue and floor of the mouth. It's caused by streptococcal bacilli and results in a bilateral boardlike swelling of the neck. Sudden airway obstruction can occur; incision and drainage may be required.
Nursing process step: Analysis

9. What element of medical history information wouldn't be important in the assessment of a client with epistaxis?
[ ] **A.** Hypertension
[ ] **B.** Arteriosclerotic heart disease
[ ] **C.** Arthritis
[ ] **D.** Chronic obstructive pulmonary disease (COPD)

Correct answer—D. *Rationales:* COPD wouldn't be of concern regarding a nosebleed. Hypertension may be a cause of epistaxis. Arteriosclerotic heart disease may predispose a client to hypertension secondary to decreased compliance of the arterial walls or decreased arterial vessel lumen. Medications used to treat arthritis may increase a client's hemostatic abnormalities.
Nursing process step: Assessment

10. A client arrives in the emergency department with obvious facial injuries. The client has a laceration and swelling over the left eye as well as pain and ecchymosis on the left side of the face. He can close his eyes tightly, wrinkle his forehead, and elevate his upper lip. Sensation to touch on the left side is absent. Which cranial nerve may be damaged?

[ ] **A.** Oculomotor
[ ] **B.** Trochlear
[ ] **C.** Trigeminal
[ ] **D.** Facial

Correct answer—C. *Rationales:* The trigeminal nerve provides facial sensation and jaw movements. These tests assess trigeminal nerve injury: pain, touch, hot and cold sensations, biting, and the ability to open the mouth against resistance. The facial nerve has three branches that deal with facial expression and taste. The zygomatic branch provides the ability to close the eyes tightly; the temporal branch provides the ability to elevate the brows and wrinkle the forehead; and the buccal branch provides the ability to wrinkle the nose, whistle, and elevate the upper lip. The oculomotor and trochlear nerves elicit eyeball movement as well as pupillary response.
Nursing process step: Assessment

11. Which discharge instruction is inappropriate for a client with a diagnosis of trigeminal neuralgia?

[ ] **A.** Avoid cold drinks.
[ ] **B.** Wash the face gently.
[ ] **C.** Instill artificial tears.
[ ] **D.** Use analgesics as ordered.

Correct answer—C. *Rationales:* Instilling artificial tears is an appropriate intervention for Bell's palsy, in which the eyelid can't close and injury and damage to the eye are potential problems. Trigeminal neuralgia causes severe, intermittent facial pain that can be elicited by stimulating a trigger zone on the face; these clients should avoid cold drinks, cold wind, and swimming in cold water. Gentle washing of the face assists in decreased stimulation of the trigger zone. The client needs to understand that analgesic medications are indicated until the problem resolves.
Nursing process step: Intervention

12. A 50-year-old client comes to the emergency department after being found in a local park confused, weak, and complaining of a "sore mouth." The client appears unkempt, has poor dentition, an edematous tongue, and a foul odor coming from her mouth. She is confused and febrile and is unable to close her mouth completely. She is noted to have firm edema tracking from the left lower mandible into the neck. Palpation produces pain in the neck, and the client is unable to turn her head from side to side. The nurse should be concerned that the client has symptoms of:

[ ] **A.** stroke.
[ ] **B.** Ludwig's angina.
[ ] **C.** epiglottiditis.
[ ] **D.** anaphylactic reaction.

Correct answer—B. *Rationales:* Ludwig's angina refers to cellulitis involving the floor of the mouth. This infection is usually due to *Streptococcus* or *Staphylococcus* species in adults. Clients usually present with pain, tenderness, and swelling of the mouth floor. Stroke symptoms don't include edema of the mouth. Epiglottiditis symptoms are located in the posterior pharynx. An anaphylactic reaction wouldn't cause fever and would be generalized versus specific to left side of the face.
Nursing process step: Analysis

13. Which of the following best describes the proper application of a dressing after incision and drainage of an auricular hematoma?
[ ] **A.** Provide support for the pinna with gauze in, around, and behind it. Place a slit 4″ × 4″ behind the ear, cover the ear with fluffed gauze, and apply a fluff roll bandage or a conforming gauze bandage circumferentially.
[ ] **B.** No dressing is required; simply apply antibiotic ointment and instruct the client to keep the area clean and dry.
[ ] **C.** Place Vaseline gauze over the incision area. Cover the gauze with several 4″ × 4″ gauze pads, and tape them in place.
[ ] **D.** Fill the ear canal and pinna with gauze. Cover the area with 4″ × 4″ gauze pads, wrap with a conforming gauze bandage, then apply a fairly tight elastic bandage.

Correct answer—A. *Rationales:* To reduce pain and cartilage necrosis, the nurse should support the pinna with gauze in, around, and behind it, thereby decreasing and preventing pressure. Cover the ear with fluffed gauze, and apply a fluff roll bandage or conforming gauze bandage circumferentially. The ear should be protected and well-padded with a bulky dressing. A constrictive dressing causes more damage, and no dressing will leave the ear itself unprotected and increase the risk of bacterial invasion. Taping a dressing won't keep it in place or provide the needed bulkiness.
Nursing process step: Intervention

14. Fourteen days after an altercation, a client complains of outer ear pain. The nurse notes necrotic areas of auricular cartilage, and a diagnosis of "cauliflower ear" is made. Evaluation shows that initial treatment of the client's wounds should have included:
[ ] **A.** instillation of antibiotic eardrops for 5 days.
[ ] **B.** incision and drainage or aspiration of auricular hematoma.
[ ] **C.** omission of tetanus toxoid prophylaxis regimen.
[ ] **D.** application of ice packs to the affected ear.

Correct answer—B. *Rationales:* A hematoma to the pinna must be drained by either aspiration or incision. The outer ear cartilage is avascular and receives its nutrients from the perichondrial vessels. Disruption of this supply by a hematoma between the perichondrium and cartilage can cause necrosis and the resultant "cauliflower ear." The use of antibiotic drops is unnecessary for this injury because it is an external injury. Tetanus prophylaxis relates to the prevention of tetanus and is indicated in open or contaminated wounds. Cold packs may reduce swelling, but if they're used inappropriately, they may further decrease blood supply. Cold packs alone aren't sufficient to reduce the hematoma and its subsequent complications.
Nursing process step: Evaluation

15. A client with gingival pain, fever, chills, fatigue, bleeding gums, and foul breath odor is admitted to the emergency department. The diagnosis is trench mouth, or necrotizing ulcerative gingivitis. What's another term for this disease?
[ ] **A.** Vincent's angina
[ ] **B.** Ludwig's angina
[ ] **C.** Prinzmetal's angina
[ ] **D.** Variant angina

Correct answer—A. *Rationales:* Vincent's angina is another name for necrotizing ulcerative gingivitis, caused by infectious organisms. Ludwig's angina is a generalized septic cellulitis surrounding the submandibular gland, beneath the jaw, and around the floor of the mouth. Prinzmetal's angina and variant angina relate to coronary artery spasm.
Nursing process step: Assessment

16. A client with a fractured larynx as a result of being hit in the upper chest by a thrown ball arrives at the emergency department. Which of the following isn't likely to be the cause of airway obstruction?
[ ] **A.** Edema
[ ] **B.** Foreign body
[ ] **C.** Hemorrhage
[ ] **D.** Fracture

Correct answer—B. *Rationales:* The airway obstruction is caused by edema, hemorrhage, or the fracture itself. No indication was given that the presence of a foreign body is suspected.
Nursing process step: Analysis

17. The client with neck trauma continues to worsen, and an emergency needle cricothyroidotomy is performed. Which statement regarding cricothyroidotomy is true?
[ ] **A.** Aspiration of sanguineous fluid confirms placement of the cannula in the trachea.
[ ] **B.** A 20G I.V. catheter should be used for insertion.
[ ] **C.** This method of ventilation can be used for up to 6 hours.
[ ] **D.** A #3 French endotracheal (ET) tube adaptor fits on the end of the cannula for use with a bag-valve-mask device.

Correct answer—D. *Rationales:* An adaptor can be removed from a #3 French ET tube and fits snugly into the hub of the cannula for use with a bag-valve-mask device. Aspiration of air—not sanguineous fluid—as the trachea is entered confirms that the cannula is in the correct place. A large-gauge needle (12G or 14G) should be used for cricothyroidotomy to assist respirations effectively. This is an emergency procedure and can only be used short term until ET intubation or a tracheostomy can be accomplished emergently.
Nursing process step: Intervention

18. Children are more prone to acute otitis media because the eustachian tube in children has which of these properties?
[ ] **A.** More tortuous
[ ] **B.** Vertical lying
[ ] **C.** Shorter
[ ] **D.** Contains positive pressure

Correct answer—C. *Rationales:* The eustachian tube in children is short and lies in a horizontal plane that prevents secretions from draining into the nasopharynx. It also has a negative pressure from the middle ear that allows aspiration of nasopharyngeal secretions into the middle ear. The tube isn't tortuous.
Nursing process step: Analysis

19. Treatment for a client with external otitis media should include:
[ ] **A.** instructions for decongestant.
[ ] **B.** insertion of an antibiotic-soaked wick.
[ ] **C.** performance of myringotomy.
[ ] **D.** ear canal irrigation.

Correct answer—B. *Rationales:* The usual treatment for acute external otitis is the insertion of a wick soaked in antibiotic solution or ointment. Other treatments may include culture of purulent drainage, analgesics, abscess incision and drainage, and application of hot compresses. Decongestants and myringotomy (incision of tympanic membrane) are possible treatments for acute otitis media. Do not irrigate; doing so may spread debris, drainage, and infection to the inner ear.
Nursing process step: Intervention

20. A 35-year-old male presents to the emergency department with complaints of bloody drainage from his left ear canal. He denies pain, fever, cough, chills, dysphagia, or recent illness but complains of decreased hearing sensation in the left ear. Recently, he had participated in a scuba diving class while on vacation. He denies previous hearing or ear problems. The most likely cause of the client's symptoms is:
[ ] **A.** ruptured tympanic membrane.
[ ] **B.** pharyngitis.
[ ] **C.** cerumen impaction.
[ ] **D.** otitis externa.

Correct answer—A. *Rationales:* The client probably has a ruptured tympanic membrane related to pressure changes while diving. Upon membrane rupture, pressure is relieved and drainage—but not necessarily pain—will be present in the ear canal. The client has denied any other symptoms that may indicate pharyngitis. Cerumen impaction wouldn't result in bloody drainage in the ear canal, and otitis externa would produce both bloody drainage and ear pain.
Nursing process step: Analysis

21. All of the following may be appropriate treatments for postextraction bleeding *except:*
[ ] **A.** using oil of cloves at the area of injury.
[ ] **B.** administering Surgicel to the site.
[ ] **C.** using a wet tea bag over the socket.
[ ] **D.** applying a pressure pack to the hemorrhagic area.

Correct answer—A. *Rationales:* Possible treatment regimens for postextraction bleeding include the application of a pressure pack, the use of a wet tea bag (because tannic acid may produce hemostasis), and the administration of Surgicel, Gelfoam, or thrombin. Oil of cloves, another home remedy, is used for analgesia.
Nursing process step: Intervetion

22. A client is brought to the emergency department after a motorcycle accident. He has a fractured right humerus, a large laceration to the right lower leg and, possibly, a head injury. At present, the Glasgow Coma Scale is 8. Two avulsed teeth are located in the client's mouth. All of the following are appropriate placements for the avulsed teeth to protect them for reimplantation *except:*

[ ] **A.** in saline solution.
[ ] **B.** in between the client's gum and lip.
[ ] **C.** in Hank's solution.
[ ] **D.** in a container of milk.

Correct answer—B. *Rationales:* Avulsed teeth can be protected for reimplantation in saline solution, Hank's solution, or milk. A tooth placed in Hank's balanced salt solution can remain viable for up to 24 hours. This solution rehydrates the periodontal ligament cells and renourishes cellular nutrients. When placed in milk, a tooth can be maintained for 3 hours. If the client is awake and aware, the teeth shouldn't be saved by placing them between his gum and lip (due to incompatible osmolarity, pH, and presence of bacteria). However, the client described isn't fully conscious (Glasgow of 8); therefore, this wouldn't be an appropriate action.
Nursing process step: Intervention

23. All of the following statements indicate an understanding of Ménière's disease *except:*

[ ] **A.** "I need to remove excess furniture in my home."
[ ] **B.** "I'll be glad when this is over so it never happens again."
[ ] **C.** "I need to stand up slowly when I get up from a chair."
[ ] **D.** "I may need to have someone with me whenever I go out."

Correct answer—B. *Rationales:* Ménière's disease is a dysfunction of the labyrinth and causes vertigo, tinnitus, and unilateral hearing loss. These symptoms occur suddenly and last from a few minutes to several hours with recurrences over several weeks or months. Therefore, removing excess furniture from the home, standing up slowly when getting out of a chair, and having someone accompany the client outside the house would help him with safety related to the disease. The belief that it won't occur again is incorrect.
Nursing process step: Evaluation

24. A client is admitted to the emergency department complaining of swelling to the neck and shortness of breath. Vital signs are as follows: blood pressure, 140/88 mm Hg; pulse, 98 beats/minute; respirations, 32 breaths/minute; temperature, 102° F (38.9° C); and pulse oximetry, 95% (on room air). When examining the client, the nurse notices that the client's tongue is elevated. After ensuring the airway is patent, what would the next nursing intervention include?

[ ] **A.** Giving oral acetaminophen to treat the fever
[ ] **B.** Initiating an I.V. line and starting antibiotics
[ ] **C.** Preparing the client for emergency surgery
[ ] **D.** Consulting a dentist

Correct answer—B. *Rationales:* The client's presentation is suspicious for Ludwig's angina, which is caused by a spreading infection. Airway management is a priority followed by antibiotics. The client shouldn't be given oral medications; thus the acetaminophen should be given rectally. The client doesn't need to be prepared for emergency surgery. An oral surgeon or an ear, nose, and throat specialist—not a dentist—would be an appropriate consult.
Nursing process step: Intervention

25. Which of the following areas should be avoided when using lidocaine with epinephrine for local anesthetic purposes?

[ ] **A.** Pinna
[ ] **B.** Eyebrow
[ ] **C.** Scalp
[ ] **D.** Vermilion border

Correct answer—A. *Rationales:* Lidocaine with epinephrine shouldn't be used on the tip of the nose and the ears because those areas lack good peripheral circulation and epinephrine has a constricting effect. All other facial areas are considered appropriate for use with epinephrine.
Nursing process step: Intervention

26. Which of the following indicates the proper position for a client during reduction of a dislocated temporomandibular joint?
[ ] **A.** Fowler's
[ ] **B.** Prone
[ ] **C.** Reverse Trendelenburg's
[ ] **D.** Flat supine

Correct answer—A. *Rationales:* For reduction of a temporomandibular joint, the physician should be above the client and the client should be in Fowler's position (upright position) with good back support. Constant downward pressure enables the mandible to slide backward into proper alignment. The other positions don't allow for the proper movement and pressure needed to reduce the joint.
Nursing process step: Analysis

27. All of the following are likely to have airway management problems *except:*
[ ] **A.** mandibular fracture.
[ ] **B.** LeFort II fracture.
[ ] **C.** Ludwig's angina.
[ ] **D.** zygomatic fracture.

Correct answer—D. *Rationales:* A zygomatic fracture doesn't normally cause an edematous or hemorrhagic airway problem. It's also anatomically farther away from the airway. A mandibular fracture and a LeFort II maxillary fracture can cause airway obstruction from hemorrhage or edema formation and bony disturbance. Ludwig's angina causes edema related to the inflammatory process.
Nursing process step: Analysis

28. A 22-year-old client is brought to the emergency department after being struck in the face with a baseball bat. He denies loss of consciousness, vision loss, or bleeding but complains of numbness in the cheek area below his eye and increasing swelling around the eye. During the examination, the nurse notes the client is unable to look up or down with the affected eye. The nurse would be most concerned that this client has:
[ ] **A.** an orbital floor fracture with entrapment.
[ ] **B.** a global rupture.
[ ] **C.** a basal skull fracture.
[ ] **D.** a nasal fracture.

Correct answer—A. *Rationales:* Trauma to the orbital area and inability to move the eye in a vertical motion are common symptoms of an orbital floor fracture. An eye global rupture would include vision loss. A basal skull fracture doesn't cause inability to move the eye. A nasal fracture is possible with this type of injury, but the client didn't complain of bleeding or pain, which would be symptoms of a nasal fracture.
Nursing process step: Assessment

29. After reduction of a dislocated temporomandibular joint, the client will have what response?
[ ] **A.** Spasms of the masseter muscle
[ ] **B.** Full range of motion (ROM) of the temporomandibular joint
[ ] **C.** Severe pain for a period of time
[ ] **D.** Numbness from the injection of lidocaine (Xylocaine)

Correct answer—B. *Rationales:* After reduction, a client with a dislocated temporomandibular joint will have pain relief and full ROM. Spasms of the masseter muscle occur before reduction. Lidocaine isn't used in reduction.
Nursing process step: Evaluation

30. Cerebrospinal fluid leak *isn't* normally objective data for:
[ ] **A.** LeFort I.
[ ] **B.** LeFort II.
[ ] **C.** LeFort III.
[ ] **D.** mandible fracture.

Correct answer—A. *Rationales:* A LeFort I fracture involves the area immediately inferior to the nose and above the lip. LeFort II and LeFort III fractures involve more facial structures and are prone to cerebrospinal fluid leaks. A mandibular fracture can cause cerebrospinal fluid otorrhea, especially if the condyles are fractured.
Nursing process step: Assessment

31. A client with a LeFort II fracture is transferred to the emergency department. The nurse will look for free-floating movement in:
[ ] **A.** the unilateral periorbital area.
[ ] **B.** the nose and dental arch.
[ ] **C.** the teeth and lower maxilla.
[ ] **D.** all facial bones.

Correct answer—B. *Rationales:* A LeFort II fracture is a pyramidal fracture involving the central portion of the maxilla across the superior nasal area; it may also involve the orbit. This produces a free-floating nose and dental arch. Free-floating movement of the unilateral periorbital area doesn't describe a clinical situation. The free-floating movement of the teeth and maxilla describes a LeFort I fracture, and the free-floating movement of all the facial bones describes a LeFort III fracture.
Nursing process step: Assessment

32. Which statement from a client discharged after postextraction bleeding indicates an understanding of instructions?
[ ] **A.** "I need to rinse my mouth three times a day with hydrogen peroxide until the bleeding stops completely."
[ ] **B.** "I need to drink warm tea and coffee several times a day while bleeding is present."
[ ] **C.** "I can have foods like ice cream, macaroni, and cooked oatmeal for the next several days."
[ ] **D.** "I can have any type of liquids, especially those with which I can use a straw."

Correct answer—C. *Rationales:* After postextraction bleeding, a client should be instructed to eat only soft foods for several days. The client also needs to understand that the oral cavity shouldn't be rinsed until bleeding has stopped. The client should avoid warm or hot liquids and shouldn't drink through a straw as this can increase circulation and pressure, which causes more bleeding. The client should use ice packs intermittently.
Nursing process step: Evaluation

33. Which product is indicated for posterior epistaxis?
[ ] **A.** Merocel nasal tampon
[ ] **B.** 16 French indwelling urinary catheter
[ ] **C.** Nasostat nasal balloon
[ ] **D.** Gelfoam hemostatic agent

Correct answer—B. *Rationales:* A 16 French indwelling urinary catheter can be used to control bleeding and provide hemostasis for a posterior nosebleed. It's inserted into the nares and the posterior nasal passage, inflated, and pulled against the nasopharynx. Other choices include gauze packs connected to a string, the Merocel posterior pack, and the Epistat (a double-ballooned catheter). The Merocel nasal tampon is inserted into the anterior nares and swells with blood and nasal secretions, then it exerts gentle pressure on the inside of the nares. The Nasostat nasal balloon is placed into the affected nares and inflated with 15 to 20 cc of air (normal saline is inserted if bleeding stops). Gelfoam is an absorbable hemostatic agent that stimulates coagulation. The Merocel nasal tampon, the Nasostat nasal balloon, and the Gelfoam hemostatic agent are used for anterior epistaxis.
Nursing process step: Intervention

34. A 25-year-old client presents to the emergency department complaining of fever and severe sore throat, which he describes as worse on one side and seeming to cause ear pain as well. He complains he can't swallow, he speaks with a "muffled" voice, and he is noted to have rancid breath. What is the most likely cause of his symptoms?
[ ] **A.** Peritonsillar abscess
[ ] **B.** Oral thrush
[ ] **C.** Dental abscess
[ ] **D.** Paralyzed vocal cords

Correct answer—A. *Rationales:* Peritonsillar abscess is usually found in clients 20 to 30 years of age. It's located on one side, and the pain can radiate to the unilateral ear. Clients often complain of pain or difficulty swallowing secondary to the abscess and inflammation. A muffled, or "hot potato," voice is common. The foul breath is a result of the abscess. Oral thrush will cause pain but not significant pain on one side only. Dental abscess doesn't cause voice changes. Paralyzed vocal cords wouldn't cause fever or rancid breath.
Nursing process step: Assessment

35. Which of the following is an inappropriate treatment for a client with a peritonsillar abscess?
[ ] **A.** Incision and drainage
[ ] **B.** Needle aspiration
[ ] **C.** Peroxide gargles
[ ] **D.** Empiric antibiotics

Correct answer—C. *Rationales:* Gargling will cause further irritation and potential aspiration because the client is already having difficulty managing his secretions. Incision and drainage, needle aspiration, and empiric antibiotics are all appropriate treatments for a client with a peritonsillar abscess.
Nursing process step: Intervention

36. A 4-year-old child is brought to the emergency department by his mother after she noted he seemed to have noisy breathing. The child's history includes a normal development, up-to-date immunizations, and no history of other medical problems. Prior to noting the noisy breathing, the mother said the child was playing with small building blocks with his older brother. The client is alert, with slightly increased respirations and a "crowing" type of sound is noted with each inspiration. What might be a likely cause of the noisy respirations?
[ ] **A.** Lower airway disease
[ ] **B.** Nasal passage obstruction
[ ] **C.** Narrowed upper airway passage
[ ] **D.** Normal for a 4-year-old

Correct answer—C. *Rationales:* The "crowing" type of sound is an indication of narrowed upper airway passages caused by edema or obstruction. Lower airway disease is indicated by breath sounds that are diminished, by wheezing, or by crackles. Nasal passage obstruction wouldn't produce noisy respirations. This noise is never normal in any age-group.
Nursing process step: Analysis

37. Which of the following interventions is the *first* priority for a client experiencing a possible upper airway obstruction?
[ ] **A.** Initiating an I.V. line
[ ] **B.** Checking the client's blood pressure
[ ] **C.** Ensuring a patent airway
[ ] **D.** Checking the client's oral temperature

Correct answer—C. *Rationales:* Maintaining a patent airway is vital in order to ensure adequate oxygenation and ventilation. Initiating an I.V. line and checking the client's blood pressure or oral temperature don't take priority in a suspected airway obstruction.
Nursing process step: Intervention

38. Discharge instructions have been given to a client diagnosed with a ruptured tympanic membrane. Which of the following statements demonstrates the client's understanding of the instructions?
[ ] **A.** "I need to clean my ear canal with a cotton-tipped applicator two times per day."
[ ] **B.** "I should avoid swimming or exposing my ear canal to water until my provider tells me it is OK."
[ ] **C.** "I can take aspirin 325 mg every 4 hours for pain or discomfort."
[ ] **D.** "I can irrigate my ear canal with forced pressure three times per day."

Correct answer—B. *Rationales:* A ruptured tympanic membrane leaves the middle ear exposed and at high risk for infection. Applicators shouldn't be inserted or irrigation forced into the canal because of the risk of infection or further damage to the membrane. Aspirin can cause tinnitus and mask inflammatory symptoms if infection develops.
Nursing process step: Evalution

39. A 72-year-old client arrives in the emergency department accompanied by his wife. The wife states her husband has been weaving all over the house when he walks and has complained of a spinning sensation for the last 24 hours. The client complains of nausea, continuous dizziness, hearing loss in the affected ear, and fever. He attributes the symptoms to the "cold" he has had for the past week. He denies recent changes in medications. The client vomits during triage and is having difficulty sitting upright in a chair. What is the probable cause of this client's symptoms?

[ ] **A.** Benign positional vertigo
[ ] **B.** Intoxication
[ ] **C.** Labyrinthitis
[ ] **D.** Intracerebral hemorrhage

Correct answer—C. *Rationales:* Labyrinthitis presents with the noted symptoms and can be caused by viral or bacterial inner ear infections. It would not be benign positional vertigo because this occurs with certain movements and can be relieved by sitting upright. There's no mention of alcohol use or abuse to indicate the client is intoxicated. Intracerebral hemorrhage would cause severe headache and an altered level of consciousness.
Nursing process step: Analysis

40. The physician prescribes diazepam for a client diagnosed with labyrinthitis. What is the rationale for the use of diazepam?

[ ] **A.** To relieve anxiety
[ ] **B.** To prevent muscle spasms when the client vomits
[ ] **C.** To provide sedation
[ ] **D.** To suppress the vestibular area to prevent further symptoms

Correct answer—D. *Rationales:* Diazepam has been shown to suppress vestibular response and relieve symptoms in clients presenting with labyrinthitis. Diazepam does relieve anxiety and muscle spasm and provides sedation, but those aren't the indications for its use with this client.
Nursing process step: Intervention

41. A client comes to the emergency department with severe facial trauma from a motor vehicle crash. What is the *first* priority in treatment of a client with facial trauma?

[ ] **A.** Provide pain management.
[ ] **B.** Provide airway management.
[ ] **C.** Administer I.V. fluids.
[ ] **D.** Arrange for facial bone X-rays.

Correct answer—B. *Rationales:* A client with facial trauma can develop airway compromise as a possible complication, and airway management must be addressed continuously. Providing pain management, administering I.V. fluids, and arranging for facial bone X-rays are indicated in the treatment of facial injuries but aren't the first priority.
Nursing process step: Intervention

6 Medical emergencies and communicable diseases

1. Signs and symptoms associated with diphtheria include:
[ ] **A.** high fever, cervical adenopathy, and a beefy red pharynx.
[ ] **B.** sore throat, fever, lymphedema, fatigue, and an enlarged spleen.
[ ] **C.** fever and enlarged cervical nodes with a gray membrane attached to the pharynx.
[ ] **D.** sore throat, voice changes, dysphagia, and white lesions in the pharynx.

Correct answer—C. *Rationales:* Option C strongly indicates a diagnosis of diphtheria, especially in the client who has an incomplete or questionable immunization status. Option A is associated with a diagnosis of group A streptococcal infections. Option B is commonly found in the client diagnosed with infectious mononucleosis. Option D is more likely with thrush or streptococcal infection.
Nursing process step: Assessment

2. Hepatitis A is least likely to be transmitted through:
[ ] **A.** sexual contact.
[ ] **B.** oral-fecal route.
[ ] **C.** contaminated food, shellfish, or milk products.
[ ] **D.** blood.

Correct answer—D. *Rationales:* Blood is the primary mode of transmission for hepatitis B and C. The primary mode of transmission for hepatitis A is through fecal contamination of food or water. Hepatitis A is also commonly transmitted through sexual contact with people previously diagnosed with hepatitis A.
Nursing process step: Assessment

3. A client has diffuse urticaria, facial swelling, and mild respiratory distress after eating at a friend's house. What's the nurse's priority in caring for this client?
[ ] **A.** Administer epinephrine solution subcutaneously.
[ ] **B.** Obtain vital signs.
[ ] **C.** Deliver high-flow oxygen.
[ ] **D.** Initiate I.V. access.

Correct answer—C. *Rationales:* The priority in treating a medical emergency is establishing or maintaining an airway and supplementing respiratory effort. The other options are also appropriate interventions for a client having an allergic or anaphylactic reaction. These interventions should follow airway and breathing interventions.
Nursing process step: Intervention

4. To prevent transmission of hepatitis, the health care worker should do all of the following *except:*
[ ] **A.** wash hands after every client contact.
[ ] **B.** obtain a single hepatitis B virus (HBV) vaccine immunization before exposure.
[ ] **C.** place all clients with hepatitis A on enteric precautions.
[ ] **D.** avoid recapping needles.

Correct answer—B. *Rationales:* A single dose of the vaccine HBV alone doesn't give an employee active immunity. The employee should obtain a series of three HBV vaccines, with the second and third doses being given 1 and 6 months after the first dose. Standard precautions and hand washing should be practiced during the treatment of all clients. Because transmission of hepatitis A is primarily through the fecal route, enteric precautions should be initiated. Recapping needles greatly increases the employee's risk of getting unintentional puncture wounds.
Nursing process step: Intervention

5. Clinical manifestations of acquired immunodeficiency syndrome (AIDS) include all of the following *except:*

[ ] **A.** sore throat.
[ ] **B.** trismus.
[ ] **C.** Kaposi's sarcoma.
[ ] **D.** dementia.

Correct answer—B. *Rationales:* Trismus isn't a symptom of AIDS. Trismus, present in a client with tetany, is marked by painful spasms of the masticatory muscles. The other options are common developments of AIDS-related diseases. A sore throat suggests oral candidiasis. Kaposi's sarcoma, the most common neoplasm found in a client with AIDS, appears as blue to violet lesions. Dementia occurs from cortical atrophy.

Nursing process step: Assessment

6. Toxic effects of zidovudine (Retrovir) may be indicated by which laboratory result?

[ ] **A.** Platelet count: 300,000 µL
[ ] **B.** White blood cell (WBC) count: $2.9 \times 10^3/\mu L$
[ ] **C.** Hematocrit: 44%
[ ] **D.** Potassium level: 5 mEq/L

Correct answer—B. *Rationales:* The toxic effects of zidovudine result in reduced WBC count, bone marrow suppression, anemia, and low platelet count. The normal platelet range is 100,000 to 500,000/µL. Hematocrit, an indicator of anemia, is normal in the range of 36% to 50%. Potassium levels, normally 3.5 to 5.5 mEq/L, are unaffected by zidovudine.

Nursing process step: Evaluation

7. Laboratory findings on the cerebrospinal fluid (CSF) of a client diagnosed with meningitis show all of the following *except:*

[ ] **A.** elevated protein level.
[ ] **B.** elevated glucose level.
[ ] **C.** purulent appearance.
[ ] **D.** leukocytes.

Correct answer—B. *Rationales:* The glucose level in a client diagnosed with bacterial meningitis is decreased. It may be normal in viral meningitis. An elevated protein level is seen in most cases of meningitis. Protein levels are higher in bacterial meningitis than in viral meningitis. Generally, cerebrospinal fluid (CSF) is purulent or turbid. Trauma during a lumbar puncture may cause the sample to appear bloody. Polymorphonuclear leukocytes are the predominant cells identified in a positive CSF sample from a client with bacterial meningitis; in viral meningitis, lymphocytes predominate.

Nursing process step: Analysis

8. Signs of meningitis include which of the following?

[ ] **A.** Cullen's sign
[ ] **B.** Koplik's spots
[ ] **C.** Kernig's sign
[ ] **D.** Homans' sign

Correct answer—C. *Rationales:* In Kernig's sign, the client is in the supine position with knees flexed; a leg is flexed then at the hip so that the thigh is brought to a position perpendicular to the trunk. An attempt is then made to extend the knee. If meningeal irritation is present, the knee can't be extended and attempts to extend the knee result in pain. Other common symptoms include stiff neck, headache, and fever. Cullen's sign is the bluish discoloration of the periumbilical skin due to intraperitoneal hemorrhage. Koplik's spots are reddened areas with grayish blue centers that are found on the buccal mucosa of a client with measles. Homans' sign is used to evaluate the presence of deep vein thrombosis.

Nursing process step: Assessment

9. Diuretics are indicated as part of the treatment regimen for edema and hypertension. Which of the following is one of the most potent types of loop diuretic?
[ ] **A.** Mannitol (Osmitrol)
[ ] **B.** Furosemide (Lasix)
[ ] **C.** Hydrochlorothiazide
[ ] **D.** Spironolactone (Aldactone)

Correct answer—B. *Rationales:* Furosemide acts by blocking the reabsorption of sodium chloride, which causes a significant diuresis of isotonic urine. Loop diuretics also cause the renal vasculature to vasodilate, which increases their effect. Mannitol is an osmotic diuretic, which, when present, exerts an osmotic effect, causing water diuresis. Hydrochlorothiazide inhibits the reabsorption of sodium in the loop of Henle. One of the potassium-sparing diuretics, spironolactone, promotes potassium reabsorption and sodium secretion, which produces a mild diuretic effect.
Nursing process step: Intervention

10. A client on diuretic therapy is instructed to eat foods that are high in potassium. The selection of which food indicates the need for further client education?
[ ] **A.** Potatoes
[ ] **B.** Honey
[ ] **C.** Beef
[ ] **D.** Cheese

Correct answer—B. *Rationales:* Excellent sources of potassium are cheese, beans, potatoes, broccoli, milk, and beef. Honey has a moderate amount of iron but has insignificant amounts of potassium.
Nursing process step: Evaluation

11. The use of isoniazid (Laniazid) is contraindicated in which client?
[ ] **A.** A client diagnosed with coronary artery disease
[ ] **B.** A client receiving diuretic therapy
[ ] **C.** A client taking phenytoin (Dilantin)
[ ] **D.** A client with glaucoma

Correct answer—C. *Rationales:* Isoniazid is contraindicated in a client who takes phenytoin. Isoniazid can decrease the excretion of phenytoin or may enhance its effects. To avoid phenytoin intoxication, adjustments to the anticonvulsant should be initiated. Indications or contraindications for a client in the other options haven't been documented.
Nursing process step: Evaluation

12. Which of the following demonstrates proper administration of the tuberculin skin test?
[ ] **A.** Administration of the purified protein derivative (PPD) through a 21G steel needle
[ ] **B.** Administration of 5 tuberculin units in adult clients and 2 tuberculin units in pediatric clients
[ ] **C.** An immediate wheal 6 to 10 mm in diameter at the site of injection
[ ] **D.** Follow-up appointment within 24 hours to record test results

Correct answer—C. *Rationales:* Injection of the tuberculin test should result in a wheal about 6 to 10 mm in diameter. If no wheal appears, the injection was probably too deep. Another injection should be repeated at least 5 mm away from the initial site. PPD administration should be through a short (½″) 26G or 27G needle. The amount of PPD injection doesn't vary from 5 tuberculin units, regardless of the age or weight of the client. Reading the tuberculin skin test at the end of 24 hours results in an inaccurate diagnosis. The tuberculin skin tests are tests of delayed hypersensitivity and should be read in 48 to 72 hours.
Nursing process step: Intervention

13. The education of a client diagnosed with tuberculosis should include which of the following.
[ ] **A.** Informing the client that he'll no longer be infectious after 4 to 6 weeks of chemotherapy.
[ ] **B.** Informing the client that sputum smears will remain positive for 3 to 5 months.
[ ] **C.** Informing the client that he'll no longer be infectious after 1 to 2 weeks of chemotherapy.
[ ] **D.** Informing the client that sputum smears will remain positive for 1 to 2 months.

Correct answer–B. *Rationales:* The client with tuberculosis should be informed that his sputum smears will remain positive for 3 to 5 months. The client should also be informed that he will no longer be infectious after 2 to 4 weeks of chemotherapy.
Nursing process step: Intervention

14. Pheochromocytoma is most commonly found in a client in what age-group?
[ ] **A.** Under age 10
[ ] **B.** Between ages 20 and 30
[ ] **C.** Between ages 30 and 60
[ ] **D.** Over age 65

Correct answer–C. *Rationales:* Pheochromocytoma is a neoplasm associated with hyperfunction of the adrenal medulla. Although all age-groups can be affected, the disease primarily occurs in people between ages 30 and 60. It seldom occurs in clients over age 65. Common symptoms include sustained hypertension, vision disturbances, headaches, hyperglycemia, and excessive perspiration.
Nursing process step: Analysis

15. Excessive weight gain, moon face, muscle wasting, truncal obesity, and the appearance of a "buffalo hump" in the neck and supraclavicular area are manifestations of which diagnosis?
[ ] **A.** Addison's disease
[ ] **B.** Syndrome of inappropriate antidiuretic hormone (SIADH)
[ ] **C.** Graves' disease
[ ] **D.** Cushing's syndrome

Correct answer–D. *Rationales:* The symptoms described are common manifestations of Cushing's syndrome, a disorder of increased levels of glucocorticoids and corticotropin. Addison's disease presents with hyperpigmentation, changes in sexual characteristics, and dehydration from sodium and fluid volume deficit. SIADH results in emotional and behavioral changes, hostility, anorexia, nausea, and weight gain. Graves' disease, a result of hyperthyroidism, is evidenced by exophthalmos (protrusion of both eyeballs), fluid accumulation, tremors, and goiters.
Nursing process step: Assessment

16. Initial management of a client with diabetic ketoacidosis should include:

[ ] **A.** establishing I.V. dextrose 5% in water (D_5W) at a rate of 500 mL/hour.

[ ] **B.** administering sodium bicarbonate ($NaHCO_3$) I.V.

[ ] **C.** administering regular insulin I.V.

[ ] **D.** administering potassium 50 mEq in 250 mL of normal saline.

Correct answer—C. *Rationales:* Regular insulin should be administered I.V. or S.C. and followed by an insulin drip to increase glucose use and decrease lipolysis. Hourly glucose levels should be obtained to monitor client response to interventions. The rate of insulin administration should be slowed as glucose levels near 200 to 300 mg/dl. Infusing additional dextrose products during diabetic ketoacidosis will worsen the client's condition. I.V. replacement should initially be an infusion of isotonic saline to rehydrate the client, who is usually volume depleted. After hypovolemia and hyperglycemia have been addressed, the solution should be changed to D_5W and half-normal saline. Although $NaHCO_3$ is indicated for the correction of acidosis, it shouldn't be initiated until decreased pH is confirmed by arterial blood gas analysis. If the client's pH is less than 7.0, $NaHCO_3$ should be administered according to the physician's orders until $NaHCO_3$ levels are adjusted. Potassium replacement isn't always indicated in the treatment of diabetic ketoacidosis. Initially, potassium measurements can range from low to high. When levels are abnormal, cardiac monitoring should detect hypokalemia or hyperkalemia. Potassium replacement shouldn't be initiated until urine output is established. If the client is suffering from acute renal failure, potassium replacement could produce toxic levels.

Nursing process step: Intervention

17. Based on a diagnosis of ketoacidosis in a client with diabetes mellitus, the nurse should expect which blood gas values at room air (fraction of inspired oxygen [FIO_2] of .21)?

[ ] **A.** pH, 7.14; partial pressure of arterial oxygen (PaO_2), 70 mm Hg; partial pressure of arterial carbon dioxide ($PaCO_2$), 58 mm Hg; and bicarbonate (HCO_3^-), 26 mEq/L

[ ] **B.** pH, 7.50; PaO_2, 100 mm Hg; $PaCO_2$, 36 mm Hg; and HCO_3^-, 30.5 mEq/L

[ ] **C.** pH, 7.56; PaO_2, 90 mm Hg; $PaCO_2$, 16 mm Hg; and HCO_3^-, 24 mEq/L

[ ] **D.** pH, 7.12; PaO_2, 100 mm Hg; $PaCO_2$, 35 mm Hg; and HCO_3^-, 12.5 mEq/L

Correct answer—D. *Rationales:* Metabolic acidosis is a diagnostic finding in a client with diabetic ketoacidosis. Arterial blood gas analysis indicates a pH below 7.35 (normal range is 7.35 to 7.45), a condition that indicates acidosis. The respiratory component ($PaCO_2$) is normal (normal range is 35 to 45 mEq/L), and the metabolic component (HCO_3^-) is low (normal range, 22 to 26 mEq/L). Option A reveals respiratory acidosis because the $PaCO_2$ is greater than 45 mm Hg and the pH is less than 7.35. Option B reveals metabolic alkalosis, as indicated by a pH greater than 7.45, an HCO_3^- level greater than 26 mEq/L, and a normal $PaCO_2$. Option C indicates respiratory alkalosis because the pH is above 7.45 and the $PaCO_2$ is low. The HCO_3^-, which is the metabolic component, is normal.

Nursing process step: Assessment

18. Which respiratory pattern is associated with a diagnosis of diabetic ketoacidosis?
[ ] **A.** Cheyne-Stokes
[ ] **B.** Kussmaul's
[ ] **C.** Apneustic
[ ] **D.** Biot's

Correct answer—B. *Rationales:* Commonly seen in clients with diabetic ketoacidosis, Kussmaul's respiration is a hyperventilation that tries to correct the respiratory component of metabolic acidosis through deep respirations. Cheyne-Stokes respiration, associated with brain injury, is characterized by periods of apnea lasting for 10 to 60 seconds, followed by increasing depth and frequency of respirations. Apneustic breathing indicates lower pontine injury. The respiratory cycle consists of a prolonged inspiratory phase followed by apnea. Biot's respiration is a variation of Cheyne-Stokes in which periods of apnea alternate irregularly with periods of breath of equal depth.
Nursing process step: Assessment

19. Which statement about the administration of dextrose in a client with confirmed hypoglycemia *isn't* true?
[ ] **A.** Administration of 50% dextrose should be delivered with a slow I.V. push.
[ ] **B.** It isn't necessary to ensure I.V. placement before administration.
[ ] **C.** In the alcohol-dependent client, thiamine (vitamin B_1) should be administered before dextrose.
[ ] **D.** Hypoglycemic neonates should receive a 10% concentration of dextrose.

Correct answer—B. *Rationales:* Because dextrose can sclerose subcutaneous tissues, the nurse must make sure that the I.V. catheter is in the vein. Dextrose is administered in a 50-mL dose, initially given in a slow I.V. push and followed by a continuous infusion. Administering dextrose to an alcohol-dependent client who's deficient in thiamine can precipitate Korsakoff's syndrome or Wernicke's encephalopathy; thiamine is necessary for carbohydrate metabolism. When used to treat hypoglycemia, dextrose should be given in these concentrations: adults, 50%; children, 25%; and neonates, 10%.
Nursing process step: Intervention

20. What is the current Centers for Disease Control and Prevention (CDC) recommendation for the vaccination for shingles (herpes zoster)?
[ ] **A.** Adults aged 60 years and older should receive the immunization.
[ ] **B.** Clients should receive the immunization within 72 hours after vesicle eruption.
[ ] **C.** The immunization also prevents herpes simplex.
[ ] **D.** Elderly clients who had chickenpox as a child don't need the immunization.

Correct answer—A. *Rationales:* The CDC recommends the vaccination for shingles (herpes zoster) for clients aged 60 years and older, regardless of whether they had chickenpox earlier in their life, because immunity wanes with aging. The vaccine shouldn't be given when an active infection is present. The immunization doesn't prevent herpes simplex.
Nursing process step: Analysis

21. As a result of thiamine deficiency, a client with alcoholism may develop what condition?
[ ] **A.** Wernicke-Korsakoff syndrome
[ ] **B.** Delirium tremens
[ ] **C.** Vincent's angina
[ ] **D.** Achalasia

Correct answer—A. *Rationales:* Wernicke-Korsakoff syndrome occurs from reduced absorption of thiamine. Wernicke's encephalopathy progresses to the degenerative brain lesions of Korsakoff's psychosis. The syndrome presents with confusion, nystagmus, ataxia, memory loss, and dementia. Delirium tremens may occur 2 to 5 days after the last drink and is characterized by disorientation, hallucinations, and gross tremors. Vincent's infection is a necrotic ulcerative inflammation of the gums that may result from inadequate diet and sleep, alcoholism, and infectious diseases. Achalasia is a condition in which there's an absence of peristalsis in the esophagus and in which the esophageal sphincter fails to relax after swallowing.
Nursing process step: Analysis

22. Which statement about administering insulin *isn't* true?
[ ] **A.** All insulin may be administered through the I.V. route.
[ ] **B.** NPH insulin action peaks 4 to 12 hours after injection.
[ ] **C.** The appearance of regular insulin is clear.
[ ] **D.** Protamine zinc is a long-acting insulin.

Correct answer—A. *Rationales:* Only regular insulin may be administered through the I.V. route. All other insulins (NPH, Lente) can be administered only subcutaneously. NPH, an intermediate-acting insulin, peaks in 4 to 12 hours and lasts for 18 to 26 hours. Regular insulin, crystalline zinc insulin, and globin zinc insulin are clear; the other types are cloudy. Protamine zinc peaks in 14 to 20 hours, and ultralente peaks in 10 to 30 hours.
Nursing process step: Evaluation

23. Which of the following are major adverse effects of thyroid replacement?
[ ] **A.** Nervousness and tremors
[ ] **B.** Muscle and joint discomfort
[ ] **C.** Obesity
[ ] **D.** Adversity to cold

Correct answer—A. *Rationales:* Nervousness and tremors reflect the hypermetabolic effect of thyroid replacement medications. Options B and D are clinical manifestations of hypothyroidism. Thyroid hormones—alone or in combination with other medicines—have been used to treat obesity.
Nursing process step: Evaluation

24. Which of the following are symptoms of psychogenic polydipsia?
[ ] **A.** Increased specific gravity
[ ] **B.** Elevated serum sodium level
[ ] **C.** Behavioral changes, confusion
[ ] **D.** Hypoventilation

Correct answer—C. *Rationales:* Because brain cells are extremely sensitive to increases in cellular water, mental changes are the first observed symptoms. The dilution of body fluids causes the specific gravity of urine to be significantly decreased. Serum sodium levels are critically depressed in water intoxication (116 mEq/L). Vital signs reflect hyperventilation, slow bounding pulses, increased systolic blood pressure, and decreased diastolic pressure.
Nursing process step: Assessment

25. A client presents with complaints of fever (105.4° F [40.8° C]) and rapid pulse (168 beats/minute). Client history reveals that he's taking levothyroxine (Synthroid). Based on this information, the nurse should suspect:
[ ] **A.** Graves' disease.
[ ] **B.** myxedema coma.
[ ] **C.** thyroid storm.
[ ] **D.** subacute thyroiditis.

Correct answer—C. *Rationales:* Thyroid storm is hyperthyroidism that's exaggerated by stress or infection. It's manifested by fever and increased pulse rate. Other symptoms include hypotension, vomiting, hyperreflexia, and extreme irritability. Graves' disease is characterized by hyperthyroidism, diffuse goiter, and exophthalmos. Myxedema coma represents a severe form of hypothyroidism and is manifested by coma, hypothermia, and hyponatremia. Subacute thyroiditis is a self-limiting inflammation of the thyroid gland from a viral infection.
Nursing process step: Assessment

26. What does a positive Chvostek's sign indicate?
[ ] **A.** Hypocalcemia
[ ] **B.** Hyponatremia
[ ] **C.** Hypokalemia
[ ] **D.** Hypermagnesemia

Correct answer—A. *Rationales:* Chvostek's sign is elicited by tapping the client's face lightly over the facial nerve, just below the temple. A calcium deficit is suggested if the facial muscles twitch. Hyponatremia is identified by the symptoms of weight loss, abdominal cramping, muscle weakness, headache, and postural hypotension. Hypokalemia presents with paralytic ileus and muscle weakness. Hypermagnesemia is marked by loss of deep tendon reflexes, coma, and cardiac arrest.
Nursing process step: Analysis

27. Signs and symptoms of dehydration include all of the following *except:*
[ ] **A.** increased hematocrit (HCT).
[ ] **B.** tachycardia.
[ ] **C.** decreased body temperature.
[ ] **D.** oliguria.

Correct answer—C. *Rationales:* Body temperature increases in a client with water deficit because less water is available for thermoregulation. Signs and symptoms of dehydration include flushed and dry skin, dry mucosa, decreased blood pressure, increased pulse rate, elevated blood urea nitrogen level and HCT, abnormal electrolyte levels, thirst, weight loss, and decreased urine output.
Nursing process step: Assessment

28. What's the primary treatment for a client diagnosed with hypernatremia?
[ ] **A.** Administer sodium polystyrene sulfonate (Kayexalate).
[ ] **B.** Replace fluid.
[ ] **C.** Administer diuretics.
[ ] **D.** Administer activated charcoal.

Correct answer—B. *Rationales:* The primary treatment for a client with hypernatremia is fluid replacement. The choice of fluid should be determined by the cause of the imbalance. If the client is hypovolemic, fluid replacement should begin with normal saline and proceed to half-normal saline. If the cause of hypernatremia is pure water loss, the fluid of choice is dextrose 5% in water. Administering Kayexalate, which contains up to 10 g of sodium, will increase the serum sodium level. Hypernatremia is associated with using diuretics. Activated charcoal is ineffective in absorbing sodium and other small electrolytes.
Nursing process step: Intervention

29. A black male child weighing 39.7 lb (18 kg) is brought to the emergency department by his mother for evaluation. The child is inconsolable and has a rectal temperature of 102.8° F (39.3° C). Nursing assessment reveals swollen hands, primarily over the joints. Based on the information above, the child is evaluated for which potential diagnosis?
[ ] **A.** Meningitis
[ ] **B.** Hepatitis
[ ] **C.** Discoid lupus
[ ] **D.** Sickle cell disease

Correct answer—D. *Rationales:* Sickle cell disease is an inherited disorder that primarily affects West African and African-Americans. Children generally don't show sickled cells until late in the first year of life. The pain is caused by localized bone marrow necrosis that commonly affects the long bones, spine, pelvis, and chest. Children primarily complain of pain in their hands or feet; the pain is usually accompanied by swelling. A diagnosis of meningitis isn't consistent with findings of joint swelling and jaundice. Signs of meningitis include fever, petechial rash, nuchal rigidity, and irritability. Hepatitis is manifested by low-grade fever, jaundice, clay-colored stool, concentrated urine, and hepatomegaly. Discoid lupus affects the connective tissue of the skin. It's identified by malar erythema (butterfly rash), arthralgia, fever, and changes in behavior.
Nursing process step: Analysis

30. A child who weighs 39.7 lb (18 kg) continues to be febrile, so an antipyretic is ordered. The nurse should administer which drug?
[ ] **A.** Acetaminophen (Tylenol), 80 mg
[ ] **B.** Ibuprofen (Motrin), 180 mg
[ ] **C.** Aspirin (salicylate), five chewable children's aspirin (1 tablet = 81 mg)
[ ] **D.** Ketorolac, 10 mg

Correct answer—B. *Rationales:* The standard dose for children's ibuprofen is 10 mg/kg (18 kg × 10 mg = 180 mg). Acetaminophen 80 mg is below the recommended dose. For a child weighing 18 kg, the dose should be about 240 mg. Each children's aspirin contains 81 mg of medication, so five tablets would equal 405 mg, which is 75% more than recommended. Aspirin isn't recommended for children or teenagers with chickenpox or flu symptoms because of the risk of their developing Reye's syndrome. Ketorolac isn't for children.
Nursing process step: Intervention

31. The parents of a child with sickle cell crisis involving the joints should be instructed to:
[ ] **A.** apply cold to the affected areas to reduce the child's discomfort.
[ ] **B.** restrict the child's fluid intake during crisis situations.
[ ] **C.** avoid areas of low oxygen concentration (high-altitude areas).
[ ] **D.** encourage exercise to reduce the likelihood of crisis.

Correct answer—C. *Rationales:* Areas of low oxygen (high altitude) should be avoided because they may precipitate sickle cell crisis. Applying warm compresses reduces discomfort in the affected area; cold may add to discomfort by impairing circulation. Fluids to rehydrate cells should be encouraged. Strenuous exercise, emotional stress, cigarette smoking, and alcohol can induce crisis situations.
Nursing process step: Intervention

32. A client with heatstroke may develop:
[ ] **A.** hyperkalemia.
[ ] **B.** respiratory acidosis.
[ ] **C.** metabolic alkalosis.
[ ] **D.** hypokalemia.

Correct answer—A. *Rationales:* Hyperkalemia may indicate damage to muscle cells and may result in renal failure. Hyperventilation may result in respiratory alkalosis. Metabolic acidosis may occur from decreased tissue perfusion.
Nursing process step: Assessment

33. A client with a tar burn is brought to the emergency department. What's the best method for removing tar?
[ ] **A.** Softening it with warm compresses
[ ] **B.** Peeling it off the skin after administering analgesia
[ ] **C.** Flushing the area with cool water and peeling off the tar
[ ] **D.** Removing it with an acetone-based product

Correct answer—C. *Rationales:* The tar should be flushed with cool water and peeled off the skin. If some tar remains, it may be dissolved with mineral oil. The other options aren't appropriate.
Nursing process step: Intervention

34. An adolescent female presents to the emergency department complaining of fever, sneezing, and coughing. Further assessment reveals conjunctivitis, small white spots on the inside of her cheek, and a red blotchy rash. The client states the rash began today, after 3 days of having the upper respiratory symptoms. What's the suspected diagnosis based on this information?
[ ] **A.** Chickenpox
[ ] **B.** Pertussis
[ ] **C.** Rubella
[ ] **D.** Measles

Correct answer—D. *Rationales:* The early signs and symptoms of measles are fever, sneezing and coughing, conjunctivitis, small white spots on the inside of the cheek (Koplik spots), and a blotchy red rash that begins several days after the initial upper respiratory infection symptoms. Chickenpox presents with low-grade fever, general malaise, and anorexia. The lesions begin as a red maculopapular rash, which then turn almost immediately into vesicles. Pertussis, otherwise known as whooping cough, begins as a mild upper respiratory infection and progresses to an irritating "chronic" cough that becomes spasmodic (repeated, continuous coughs without interrupting breaths) followed by inspiration sounding like a "whoop." Rubella (German measles) is characterized by low-grade fevers, enlarged lymph nodes, and a tiny pink rash.
Nursing process step: Assessment

35. Complications of mumps include all of the following *except:*
[ ] **A.** orchitis.
[ ] **B.** meningoencephalitis.
[ ] **C.** pancreatitis.
[ ] **D.** secondary skin infection.

Correct answer—D. *Rationales:* Secondary skin infections are associated with chickenpox because of the vesicles involved. The other options are all associated with mumps.
Nursing process step: Assessment

36. What parasitic infection can be caused by improper cooking of pork or beef?
[ ] **A.** Tapeworm
[ ] **B.** Roundworm
[ ] **C.** Ringworm
[ ] **D.** Hookworm

Correct answer—A. *Rationales:* Tapeworm larvae live in uncooked beef and pork. Transmission occurs from ingesting improperly cooked meat. Roundworm is transmitted through dirt or inadequately cleaned fruits and vegetables. Ringworm is a skin fungal infection transmitted from contaminated humans or animals. Hookworm originates in warm sandy soil, especially in areas of poor sanitation. Infection occurs through the skin or by drinking contaminated water.
Nursing process step: Assessment

37. A mother brings her 8-year-old daughter to the emergency department; the child is diagnosed with head lice. Upon discharge, the mother makes all of the following statements to indicate her understanding of the spread and treatment of head lice *except:*
[ ] **A.** "I'll tell my daughter not to exchange combs, hats, other headgear, or clothing with other children."
[ ] **B.** "I'll bleach my daughter's hair because the lighter the child's hair the better to see the nits."
[ ] **C.** "My daughter may return to school 24 hours after completion of treatment."
[ ] **D.** "I should have all my family members treated at the same time because louse infestation is generally widespread."

Correct answer—B. *Rationales:* The color of the hair isn't generally a factor. The other options are all recommendations to impress upon students and their families to prevent the spread of lice.
Nursing process step: Evaluation

38. A client presents to the emergency department with abdominal cramping and persistent, foul-smelling diarrhea. During the social history, the client states that he has recently been "roughing it" by camping and "living off the land" in Montana. What protozoan infection would the nurse consider to be the cause of the symptoms?
[ ] **A.** Malaria
[ ] **B.** Amebiasis
[ ] **C.** Giardiasis
[ ] **D.** Amebic liver abscess

Correct answer—C. *Rationales:* Giardiasis is a waterborne parasite spread by the ingestion of untreated or inadequately treated water. It occurs in underdeveloped as well as modern countries. Malaria isn't characterized by diarrhea, but by nausea, fever, chills, and sweating. Amebiasis is a disease of the large intestine that's transmitted by ingestion of the protozoa in the cyst stage in food or water contaminated by feces. Its symptoms are usually chronic, not acute; diarrhea alternates with constipation. Amebic liver abscess is an extraintestinal complication of amebiasis. Associated symptoms don't include diarrhea.
Nursing process step: Assessment

39. A 21-year-old male presents to the emergency department with symptoms of general malaise, intermittent fevers ranging from 98.6° F (37° C) to 104° F (40° C), and enlargement of the submandibular and posterior cervical lymph nodes for the past 3 months. Blood work is obtained and he's found to have an elevated eosinophil count and anemia. Which diagnosis do these symptoms indicate?
[ ] **A.** Acute lymphatic leukemia (ALL)
[ ] **B.** Hodgkin's disease
[ ] **C.** Mycosis fungoides
[ ] **D.** Chronic lymphocytic leukemia (CLL)

Correct answer—B. *Rationales:* Hodgkin's disease symptoms are vague and gradual. Lymph nodes, although swollen, are seldom painful. Fevers are intermittent, lasting from 3 to 14 days and then returning to normal. Hodgkin's usually occurs in young men in their early 20s or after age 50. ALL is most common in young children. It's characterized by low erythrocyte and platelet counts. Mycosis fungoides is a rare lymphoma of the skin, which begins as a pruritic, red rash and develops into tumors of lymphoma on the skin. CLL generally affects persons over 35. Most clients are asymptomatic. Erythrocyte and platelet counts may be normal or decreased.
Nursing process step: Assessment

40. A client rapidly develops a rash and hives while receiving an I.V. antibiotic. After stopping the drug, what drug does the nurse anticipate administering first?

[ ] **A.** Corticosteroid
[ ] **B.** Epinephrine (Adrenalin)
[ ] **C.** Mast-cell stabilizers
[ ] **D.** Leukotriene receptor antagonists

Correct answer—B. *Rationales:* Epinephrine, a sympathomimetic, is the first drug of choice to treat an anaphylactic reaction. It stimulates alpha- and beta-adrenergic receptors. This results in vasoconstriction of peripheral blood vessels and relaxation of bronchial smooth muscles. Corticosteroids wouldn't be used because they have a longer onset. Mast-cell stabilizers and leukotriene receptor antagonists are used to treat asthma, not anaphylaxis.
Nursing process step: Intervention

41. What information obtained from the client's history would make the nurse suspect the client had an allergy to latex?

[ ] **A.** History of seasonal watery eyes and rhinorrhea
[ ] **B.** Allergy to penicillin
[ ] **C.** Allergy to bananas and avocados
[ ] **D.** History of blood transfusion reaction

Correct answer—C. *Rationales:* Some proteins in rubber are similar to proteins found in food; therefore, some foods may cause an allergic reaction in people who are allergic to latex. The most common of these foods are bananas, avocados, chestnuts, kiwis, tomatos, water chestnuts, guava, hazelnuts, potatoes, peaches, grapes, and apricots. A history of seasonal watery eyes and rhinorrhea, an allergy to penicillin, or a history of a blood transfusion reaction wouldn't indicate the client may also have a latex allergy.
Nursing process step: Assessment

42. The trauma victim is bleeding from multiple orifices, and disseminated intravascular coagulation (DIC) is suspected. What would the nurse anticipate administering?

[ ] **A.** Depleted clotting factors through packed red blood cells and platelets
[ ] **B.** Iron supplements
[ ] **C.** Factor VIII through fresh frozen plasma
[ ] **D.** Folic acid

Correct answer—A. *Rationales:* DIC is a dysfunction of the clotting system with excessive thromboses and a depletion of the fibrinolysis system. Treatment includes oxygen, fluids, and replacement of the depleted clotting factors. Use of heparin is currently considered controversial. Factor VIII is related to hemophilia A. Iron supplements are used for iron deficiency anemia. Folic acid is used for the anemia with sickle cell crisis.
Nursing process step: Intervention

43. Which diagnostic test would the nurse anticipate for a client with disseminated intravascular coagulation (DIC)?

[ ] **A.** Hemoglobin
[ ] **B.** Hematocrit
[ ] **C.** D-dimer assay
[ ] **D.** Factor VIII

Correct answer—C. *Rationales:* D-dimer is a specific polymer resulting from the breakdown of fibrin (and not fibrinogen). It's a specific marker for the degree of fibrinolysis. Hemoglobin measures the oxygen-carrying capacity of blood. Hematocrit measures the percentage of whole blood that is made up of red blood cells. Factor VIII is used to diagnose hemophilia A.
Nursing process step: Analysis

44. A client with hemophilia A fell and has active bleeding into the knee joint. What action should the nurse anticipate?

[ ] **A.** Rest the affected joint.
[ ] **B.** Apply a continuous passive motion apparatus.
[ ] **C.** Apply heat.
[ ] **D.** Apply direct pressure.

Correct answer—A. *Rationales:* During an acute attack, the joint should be totally rested to prevent crippling deformities from hemarthrosis. After the bleeding ceases, mobilization is then encouraged through range-of-motion exercises and physical therapy—not a continuous passive-motion apparatus. The joint should be packed in ice—not heat—and aspirin should be avoided. Weight bearing is avoided until all swelling has resolved and muscle strength has returned. Direct pressure is used for active external bleeding.
Nursing process step: Intervention

45. The client with hemophilia A presents with active joint bleeding. What treatment would the nurse anticipate?

[ ] **A.** Heparin
[ ] **B.** Vitamin K
[ ] **C.** Protamine sulfate
[ ] **D.** Fresh frozen plasma

Correct answer—D. *Rationales:* Fresh frozen plasma is used to treat the deficiency of factor VIII present in hemophilia A. Heparin inhibits clotting processes, so it wouldn't be given to a client with hemophilia. Hemophilia A is a deficiency of factor VIII. Vitamin K is not indicated for hemophilia. Protamine sulfate is an antidote for heparin and would not be used to treat hemophilia.
Nursing process step: Intervention

46. The client reports frequent, foul-smelling, watery diarrhea with fever and abdominal cramping. What question should the nurse ask this client to determine whether *Clostridium difficile* is involved?

[ ] **A.** "Have you recently taken an antiviral medication?"
[ ] **B.** "Have you recently been hospitalized for surgery?"
[ ] **C.** "Have you recently received any immunizations?"
[ ] **D.** "Have you ever been diagnosed with hepatitis A?"

Correct answer—B. *Rationales:* The classic clients with *C. difficile* have had a recent hospitalization and surgery, are elderly, and have had antibiotics in the past 2 months. Recent antiviral medication, recent immunizations, and a history of hepatitis A aren't known risk factors for developing a *C. difficile* infection.
Nursing process step: Assessment

47. What will help determine whether the client is colonized with methicillin-resistant *Staphylococcus aureus* (MRSA) after being transferred from a long-term-care facility where MRSA is present?

[ ] **A.** Nasal secretion specimen
[ ] **B.** Blood specimen
[ ] **C.** Urine sample
[ ] **D.** Patch testing

Correct answer—A. *Rationales:* Doctors diagnose MRSA by checking a tissue sample or nasal secretions for signs that a client is colonized if the client has signs of infection or has transferred into a hospital from another health care setting where MRSA is known to be present. A blood sample, a urine sample, and a skin patch testing aren't used to diagnose MRSA infection or colonization.
Nursing process step: Analysis

48. A client is complaining of intense itching and pain in his lumbosacral area. Inspection of the area reveals vesicles and pustules in a linear pattern along a dermatome on his trunk. What treatment does the nurse anticipate will be ordered for this client?

[ ] **A.** Acyclovir
[ ] **B.** Topical immunotherapy
[ ] **C.** Topical antifungal
[ ] **D.** Amoxicillin

Correct answer—A. *Rationales:* This client more than likely has herpes zoster (shingles), which appears as grouped vesicles and pustules on an erythematous base in a linear pattern along a dermatome and resembles chickenpox. It is usually unilateral on the trunk, face, and lumbosacral area. Treatment with an antiviral agent such as acyclovir within 72 hours is the usual protocol. Topical immunotherapy is a therapy used to treat cancer, not herpes zoster. Herpes zoster is a viral infection, so an antifungal agent or an antibiotic such as amoxicillin would not be effective.
Nursing process step: Intervention

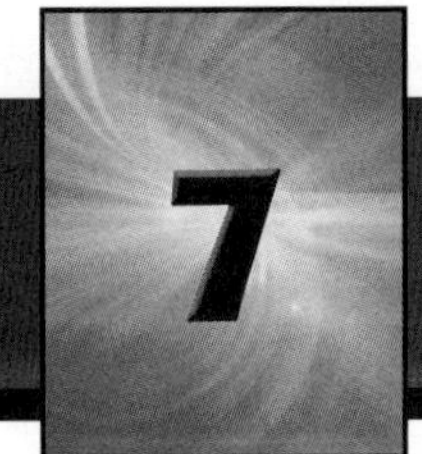

7 Genitourinary and gynecologic emergencies

1. A client enters the emergency department complaining of nausea, vomiting, restlessness, and severe right-sided lower back pain with sudden onset 1 hour ago. The client appears slightly pale and is diaphoretic. Vital signs are blood pressure, 140/92 mm Hg; pulse, 120 beats/minute; respirations, 32 breaths/minute; and temperature, 98° F (36.7° C). Subjective data supporting a diagnosis of renal calculi would include:

[ ] **A.** a history of mild flu symptoms last week.
[ ] **B.** coffee-ground vomitus.
[ ] **C.** dark, scant urine output.
[ ] **D.** pain radiating to the right upper quadrant.

Correct answer–C. *Rationales:* Most clients with renal calculi have blood in their urine from the stone's passing. The urine is dark, tests Hemoccult positive, and is usually scant. Option B refers to an upper GI bleed, and option D refers to cholecystitis. Option A isn't a precipitating factor relating to renal calculi.
Nursing process step: Assessment

2. Which laboratory value supports a diagnosis of pyelonephritis?

[ ] **A.** Myoglobinuria
[ ] **B.** Ketonuria
[ ] **C.** Pyuria
[ ] **D.** Low white blood cell (WBC) count

Correct answer–C. *Rationales:* Pyelonephritis is diagnosed by the presence of leukocytosis, hematuria, pyuria, and bacteriuria. The client presents with fever, chills, and flank pain. Because the client is usually septic, the WBC count is more likely to be elevated, not low as indicated in option D. Ketonuria indicates a diabetic state as indicated in option B. Myoglobinuria, option A, indicates muscle wasting in rhabdomyolysis.
Nursing process step: Assessment

3. A 27-year-old paraplegic with a pounding, severe headache is admitted to the emergency department. Vital signs are blood pressure, 240/110 mm Hg; pulse, 60 beats/minute; respirations, 28 breaths/minute; and temperature, 99° F (37.2° C). The client seems anxious. An indwelling urinary catheter was inserted 30 minutes ago, and 100 mL of urine is in the bag. The client also has pressure ulcers in varying stages. What's a priority medication for this client?

[ ] **A.** Nifedipine (Procardia)
[ ] **B.** Meperidine (Demerol)
[ ] **C.** Verapamil (Calan)
[ ] **D.** Heparin

Correct answer–A. *Rationales:* Autonomic dysreflexia is a potentially life-threatening emergent situation that occurs in quadriplegics and high-cord-lesion (above T6) paraplegics. The priority is to lower the blood pressure by using nifedipine. Lowering the blood pressure should eliminate the headache. Meperidine doesn't lower blood pressure. Verapamil is contraindicated because it's used to treat supraventricular tachycardia. Heparin shouldn't be used because of the potential for a cerebral or subarachnoid bleed from hypertension.
Nursing process step: Analysis

4. A paraplegic who's experiencing autonomic dysreflexia comes to the emergency department with a pounding, severe headache. What's another symptom that might occur in this client?
[ ] **A.** Flushing of skin below the lesion
[ ] **B.** Pale, cool skin above the cord lesion
[ ] **C.** Diaphoresis above the cord lesion
[ ] **D.** Increased temperature below the cord lesion

Correct answer—C. *Rationales:* Autonomic dysreflexia occurs as a result of autonomic responses to stimuli, after which sympathetic responses above the splanchnic outflow level are increased. The increase in turn causes cutaneous vasodilation above the cord lesion (flushing and excessive sweating) and cutaneous vasoconstriction below the lesion (pallor, coolness). Thus, the other options are incorrect.
Nursing process step: Assessment

5. A paraplegic client admitted to the emergency department had an indwelling catheter inserted 30 minutes ago. It's patent and draining urine. The client experiences autonomic dysreflexia. Potential precipitating factors for this client with autonomic dysreflexia include all of the following *except:*
[ ] **A.** rectal impaction.
[ ] **B.** skin lesions.
[ ] **C.** catheter manipulation.
[ ] **D.** bladder distention.

Correct answer—D. *Rationales:* The most common cause of autonomic dysreflexia is bladder distention, but this client had an indwelling urinary catheter inserted 30 minutes before admission. Urine return was 100 mL, indicating that the bladder has been drained. The second most common cause of this condition is rectal distention from an impaction. Other causes include catheterization and catheter manipulation, cleansing enemas, acute abdominal or genitourinary pathology, temperature extremes, and skin lesions, such as pressure ulcers and ingrown toenails.
Nursing process step: Evaluation

6. A client with a history of heart failure and sepsis is at risk for what genitourinary complication?
[ ] **A.** Renal calculi
[ ] **B.** Urinary retention
[ ] **C.** Acute renal failure
[ ] **D.** Urethral stricture

Correct answer—C. *Rationales:* Heart failure and sepsis can decrease cardiac output. This decreased perfusion to the kidney can lead to acute renal failure. Renal calculi, urinary retention, and urethral strictures can be caused by obstruction in the renal urine collection system.
Nursing process step: Assessment

7. Which of the following is an appropriate intervention for a client with renal calculi?
[ ] **A.** I.V. fluids at a keep-vein-open (KVO) rate
[ ] **B.** Opioid analgesics, preferably I.V.
[ ] **C.** Indwelling urinary catheter, gravity drainage
[ ] **D.** Nasogastric (NG) tube, low suction

Correct answer—B. *Rationales:* The rule of therapy for a client with renal calculi is hydration and analgesia. Opioids are usually required to control the pain. The I.M. route may be used, but I.V. is preferred. I.V. fluids are provided to hydrate the client and help flush out the calculus. Option A provides only for a KVO rate; a faster rate is necessary to accomplish the goals. An indwelling urinary catheter and an NG tube are usually unnecessary.
Nursing process step: Analysis

8. Possible causes of priapism include all of the following *except:*
[ ] **A.** spinal cord injury.
[ ] **B.** leukemia.
[ ] **C.** bacterial infection.
[ ] **D.** sickle cell disease.

Correct answer—C. *Rationales:* Bacterial infections aren't a cause of priapism. Causes of priapism (a prolonged and painful penile erection that isn't usually associated with sexual desire) include spinal cord injury, leukemia, and sickle cell disease. Other causes are psychotropic drugs, multiple sclerosis, prolonged sexual stimulation, penile or urethral tumor, anticoagulant therapy, and treatments for impotence.
Nursing process step: Assessment

9. A client with scrotal pain that has been present for 2 days is admitted to the emergency department. Which result would indicate a diagnosis of epididymitis rather than testicular torsion?
[ ] **A.** Hypoperfusion on testicular scan
[ ] **B.** Leukopenia on complete blood count
[ ] **C.** Bacteriuria on urinalysis
[ ] **D.** Elevated creatinine level on electrolyte study

Correct answer—C. *Rationales:* Epididymitis is suggested by hyperperfusion on testicular scan, an elevated white blood cell count, and the presence of bacteria in the urine. An elevated creatinine level is an indicator of renal, not scrotal, disease.
Nursing process step: Assessment

10. Which orthostatic reading would be of concern for a client suspected of hemorrhage?
[ ] **A.** Lying: blood pressure, 120/64 mm Hg; heart rate, 82 beats/minute. Sitting: blood pressure, 114/60 mm Hg; heart rate, 86 beats/minute. Standing: blood pressure, 132/84 mm Hg; heart rate, 92 beats/minute
[ ] **B.** Lying: blood pressure, 92/40 mm Hg; heart rate, 64 beats/minute. Sitting: blood pressure, 94/60 mm Hg; heart rate, 72 beats/minute. Standing: blood pressure, 86/54 mm Hg; heart rate, 78 beats/minute
[ ] **C.** Lying: blood pressure, 128/52 mm Hg; heart rate, 74 beats/minute. Sitting: blood pressure, 96/48 mm Hg; heart rate, 94 beats/minute. Standing: blood pressure, 72/40 mm Hg; heart rate, 120 beats/minute
[ ] **D.** Lying: blood pressure, 116/80 mm Hg; heart rate, 76 beats/minute. Sitting: blood pressure, 120/76 mm Hg; heart rate, 82 beats/minute. Standing: blood pressure, 130/64 mm Hg; heart rate, 88 beats/minute

Correct answer—C. *Rationales:* Orthostatic hypotension can be a sign of hemorrhage and a precursor to hypovolemic shock. It's a good test to use in the early phases of hemorrhage, when other symptomatology may be absent (a negative orthostatic test doesn't rule out the possibility of bleeding). An increase in the pulse of 20 beats/minute or a systolic drop of 10 to 20 mm Hg is a positive indicator of occult blood loss. Some experts say a drop in systolic blood pressure of 25 mm Hg or a drop in diastolic of 10 mm Hg is positive. Option C has both of these present. The other options don't represent positive orthostatics.
Nursing process step: Evaluation

11. A client's urine pH is 4.8. What type of renal calculi might this client have?
[ ] **A.** Magnesium, ammonia, phosphate
[ ] **B.** Calcium oxalate
[ ] **C.** Uric acid
[ ] **D.** Calcium phosphate

Correct answer—C. *Rationales:* In acid urine (pH less than 5.5), uric acid crystals precipitate, leading to stone formation. Magnesium, ammonia, and phosphate stones (also called triple phosphate, struvite, or infection stones) develop when the urine pH is higher than 7.2 and ammonia is present in the urine. Calcium oxalate stones develop in acid urine (pH less than 6.0). Calcium phosphate stones develop in alkaline urine (pH greater than 7.2).
Nursing process step: Analysis

12. All of the following are possible complications from an ovarian cyst *except:*
[ ] **A.** adhesions.
[ ] **B.** peritonitis.
[ ] **C.** ischemic ovary.
[ ] **D.** mittelschmerz.

Correct answer—D. *Rationales:* An ovarian cyst can cause adhesions and peritonitis from leakage of cystic contents. An ovary can become ischemic from torsion that occurs when a cyst is twisted on its pedicle. Mittelschmerz occurs in the form of abdominal pain at ovulation; it needs to be considered in the differential diagnosis of an ovarian cyst.
Nursing process step: Evaluation

13. Which of the following medication use in the client's medical history can increase the risk of dysfunctional uterine bleeding (DUB)?
[ ] **A.** Oral contraceptives and antibiotics
[ ] **B.** Nonsteroidal anti-inflammatory drugs (NSAIDS) and muscle relaxers
[ ] **C.** Digoxin and steroids
[ ] **D.** Injectable anticoagulants and angiotensin-converting enzyme (ACE) inhibitors

Correct answer—C. *Rationales:* DUB can be caused by hormone replacement therapy, steroids, androgens, digitalis, and anticoagulants. NSAIDs may increase bleeding after it has started. Antibiotics, muscle relaxers, and ACE inhibitors aren't known to cause DUB.
Nursing process step: Assessment

14. What position should the client assume to achieve the most accurate diagnostic bladder ultrasound result?
[ ] **A.** Prone
[ ] **B.** Supine
[ ] **C.** High Fowler's
[ ] **D.** Lithotomy

Correct answer—B. *Rationales:* Diagnostic bladder ultrasound is performed to determine bladder volume. With the client in a supine or reclining position, the bladder is most easily accessed. Accurate determination of bladder volumes can guide the need for bladder aspiration or catheterization. The prone, High-Fowler's, and lithotomy positions won't achieve the most accurate results.
Nursing process step: Intervention

15. In the treatment of genital herpes lesions, oral acyclovir (Zovirax) is the drug of choice. It works by accomplishing all of the following *except:*
[ ] **A.** providing bactericidal functions.
[ ] **B.** relieving local and systemic pain.
[ ] **C.** diminishing the interval of viral shedding.
[ ] **D.** decreasing the formation of new lesions.

Correct answer—A. *Rationales:* Herpes is a viral, not a bacterial, infection (although a secondary bacterial infection can occur), and acyclovir isn't a bactericide. Acyclovir relieves systemic pain, diminishes the interval of viral shedding, and decreases the formation of new lesions.
Nursing process step: Analysis

16. Which of the following is an ovarian cyst that usually contains hair and teeth?
[ ] **A.** Corpus luteum
[ ] **B.** Teratoma
[ ] **C.** Endometrioma
[ ] **D.** Chocolate cyst

Correct answer—B. *Rationales:* A teratoma, or dermoid cyst, is produced from all three germ layers and usually contains hair and teeth, although it can contain tissue from any body structure. Teratoma cysts usually occur during active reproductive years. A corpus luteum cyst is caused by cystic changes in an ovary from hemorrhage in a mature corpus luteum. It can cause bleeding and hemorrhage. An ovarian endometrioma is a chocolate cyst and occurs when endometrial tissue in an ovary cyclically bleeds with monthly periods and collects blood and blood clots.
Nursing process step: Assessment

17. Which statement regarding treatment regimens for herpetic lesions is true?
[ ] **A.** Systemic antibiotics aren't necessary.
[ ] **B.** Topical acyclovir (Zovirax) assists with pain relief.
[ ] **C.** Oral acyclovir (Zovirax) should be taken continuously.
[ ] **D.** The use of condoms allows immediate return of sexual relations.

Correct answer—B. *Rationales:* Topical acyclovir only relieves pain and itching. Unlike oral acyclovir, it doesn't help prevent new lesions and reduce the duration of viral shedding. Systemic antibiotics may be necessary to treat secondary infections caused by scratching the lesions. Oral acyclovir should be taken from the onset of prodromal symptoms for 5 days. Lesions may occur in areas left uncovered by condoms, such as the base of the penis and around the labia. Sexual activity should cease from the onset of prodromal symptoms until lesions are healed.
Nursing process step: Evaluation

18. A hydatidiform mole shows what human chorionic gonadotropin level?

[ ] **A.** Zero

[ ] **B.** Very low

[ ] **C.** Very high

[ ] **D.** Normal for gestational age

Correct answer—C. *Rationales:* A hydatidiform mole or gestational trophoblastic tumor demonstrates an extremely elevated human chorionic gonadotropin level. Other signs include snowstorm pattern on ultrasound, early preeclampsia, absence of fetal heart tones, bleeding or spotting, and enlarged uterus.

Nursing process step: Assessment

19. Which test result provides information that's important immediately after sexual assault for treatment purposes?

[ ] **A.** Negative serologic test for syphilis

[ ] **B.** Complete blood count (CBC) within normal limits

[ ] **C.** Positive Rh factor

[ ] **D.** Negative pregnancy test

Correct answer—D. *Rationales:* Treatment for a client who has been sexually assaulted includes prophylactic antibiotic therapy. Cultures and tests for syphilis won't be finished for several days, so antibiotics may be routinely started. A CBC doesn't provide vital information for this client. It might be useful if trauma were relevant to the situation and hypovolemia was suspected. The positive Rh factor doesn't require treatment. It's important to know whether the client was pregnant before the attack so that pregnancy prevention medication can be started, if appropriate. Ovral (ethinyl estradiol and norgestrel) may be used but must be given within 72 hours to prevent pregnancy.

Nursing process step: Analysis

20. After evidence is collected after a sexual assault, what should be done with the client's clothing?

[ ] **A.** Shake it out carefully to look for hidden evidence.

[ ] **B.** Return it to the client after determining no evidence is present.

[ ] **C.** Place it in a plastic bag and label it with the client's name.

[ ] **D.** Place it in a paper bag and seal it with evidence tape.

Correct answer—D. *Rationales:* Evidence obtained in a rape examination, including the clothing, should be placed in a paper bag and secured with evidence tape to ensure that no tampering occurs. The client's clothing should be carefully removed but not shaken out; microscopic evidence may be lost. All clothing should be given to the police; it's their responsibility to determine if evidence is present. Clothing shouldn't be placed in plastic bags, which cause mildewing and moisture retention, both of which can cause loss of evidence. All evidence collected should be labeled with the client's name, site of collection, date and time of collection, and the name of the person collecting the evidence.

Nursing process step: Intervention

21. Which of the following shouldn't be collected during a rape examination?

[ ] **A.** Fingernail scraping and clippings

[ ] **B.** Pubic hair

[ ] **C.** Saliva specimen

[ ] **D.** Upper thigh scrapings

Correct answer—D. *Rationales:* As a rule, any potential foreign material, such as suspected semen, blood, or saliva, should be collected with a cotton swab moistened with saline, not by scraping. However, evidence under fingernails must be obtained by scraping or clipping. The other options are all part of the routine evidence collection.

Nursing process step: Intervention

22. A male client has been involved in a motorcycle accident. He presents with abdominal pain and an inability to void. Guarding is present with slight abdominal rigidity. He has a laceration across the upper thigh and blood at the urinary meatus. Gentle compression of the iliac crests medially and posteriorly invokes pain. Vital signs are blood pressure, 108/62 mm Hg; pulse, 116 beats/minute; respirations, 32 breaths/minute; temperature, 99° F (37.2° C); and pulse oximetry, 96% (on room air). Which intervention is appropriate at this time?

[ ] **A.** Insert an indwelling urinary catheter.
[ ] **B.** Perform a peritoneal lavage.
[ ] **C.** Schedule an immediate retrograde urethrogram.
[ ] **D.** Schedule an immediate cystogram.

Correct answer—C. *Rationales:* The absence of urine production and the presence of blood at the meatus indicate a ruptured urethra. A retrograde urethrogram can be used to determine injury. An indwelling urinary catheter shouldn't be inserted prior to a urologic consultant's examination. Peritoneal lavage requires the use of an indwelling urinary catheter, so it can't be done until urethral injury has been ruled out. A cystogram may be necessary, but again, an indwelling urinary catheter is needed for this diagnostic tool.
Nursing process step: Assessment

23. A direct blow to the male groin will most likely result in:

[ ] **A.** right testicular injury.
[ ] **B.** left testicular injury.
[ ] **C.** penile fracture.
[ ] **D.** urethral tear.

Correct answer—A. *Rationales:* Possibly due to its higher position, the right testicle is more prone to injury following a blow to the male groin. Penile fracture occurs following trauma while engorged. Urethral tear is more likely with a sheering injury as opposed to a direct blow.
Nursing process step: Assessment

24. A trauma client with a diagnosis of a ruptured bladder has two large-bore I.V. lines, oxygen, a nasogastric tube, and an indwelling urinary catheter in place. Initial vital signs are blood pressure, 120/54 mm Hg; pulse, 120 beats/minute; respirations, 32 breaths/minute; pulse oximetry, 95% (on room air); and temperature, 98.2° F (36.8° C). Which of the following might indicate impending hypovolemic shock?

[ ] **A.** Pulse of 100 beats/minute
[ ] **B.** Restlessness
[ ] **C.** Blood pressure, 106/64 mm Hg
[ ] **D.** Request for pain relief

Correct answer—B. *Rationales:* Restlessness is typically the first sign of impending hypovolemic shock or hypoxia. A pulse rate of 100 beats/minute is actually a decrease compared with the original 120 beats/minute, and the blood pressure is close to the initial reading. Requests for pain relief are normal for a trauma client.
Nursing process step: Evaluation

25. Which of the following would be further evidence of a urethral injury in a client during a rectal examination?

[ ] **A.** A low-riding prostate
[ ] **B.** The presence of a high-riding, boggy mass
[ ] **C.** Absent sphincter tone
[ ] **D.** A positive Hemoccult

Correct answer—B. *Rationales:* When the urethra is ruptured, a hematoma or collection of blood separates the two sections of urethra. This may feel like a boggy mass on rectal examination. Because of the rupture and hematoma, the prostate becomes high-riding. A palpable prostate gland usually indicates a nonurethral injury. Absent sphincter tone would refer to a spinal cord injury. The presence of blood would probably correlate with a GI bleed or colon injury.
Nursing process step: Assessment

26. After falling 8′ (2.4 m) and landing on his buttocks, a client is brought to the emergency department. Along with possible spinal compression fractures, what signs may be present indicating possible genitourinary vasculature trauma?

[ ] **A.** Bruit at the second lumbar vertebra
[ ] **B.** Suprapubic pain on palpation
[ ] **C.** Slowly escalating hypertension
[ ] **D.** Decreased or absent bowel sounds

Correct answer—A. *Rationales:* A contrecoup injury can occur to the kidney after a fall that exerts force from above the kidney. The force tears the renal pedicle and causes a bruit that can be auscultated at the first or second lumbar vertebra. Suprapubic pain accompanies a bladder injury, not a vascular disruption. Hypertension may occur after an injury has been repaired. Decreased or absent bowel sounds would occur with an abdominal insult that created an ileus.
Nursing process step: Assessment

27. Which vaginal infection doesn't require treatment of sexual partners?

[ ] **A.** *Neisseria gonorrhoeae*
[ ] **B.** *Candida albicans*
[ ] **C.** *Trichomonas vaginalis*
[ ] **D.** *Chlamydia trachomatis*

Correct answer—B. *Rationales: Candida* is treated with Mycostatin (nystatin) and doesn't require sexual partner treatment. The other options are sexually transmitted diseases that necessitate partner treatment.
Nursing process step: Analysis

28. Which diluent is best to use when giving an I.M. injection of ceftriaxone (Rocephin)?

[ ] **A.** Sterile water
[ ] **B.** Dextrose 5% in water (D_5W)
[ ] **C.** Sterile saline
[ ] **D.** 1% lidocaine

Correct answer—D. *Rationales:* Because injections of ceftriaxone cause discomfort, 1% lidocaine is recommended as the diluent of choice. Sterile water, D_5W, and sterile saline will increase discomfort.
Nursing process step: Analysis

29. For mothers with chlamydial infections, cesarean birth is usually the delivery method of choice because it decreases the infant's risks of developing:

[ ] **A.** blindness.
[ ] **B.** hepatitis.
[ ] **C.** pneumonia.
[ ] **D.** encephalitis.

Correct answer—C. *Rationales:* A mother infected with *Chlamydia* can pass the organisms to her infant during its passage through the cervix. Potential complications for the infant include conjunctivitis and *Chlamydia* pneumonia. Blindness, hepatitis, and encephalitis aren't passed by *Chlamydia.*
Nursing process step: Analysis

30. A client complains of foul-smelling vaginal discharge and intermittent vaginal bleeding. She normally has irregular menses and doesn't remember the date of her last normal menstrual cycle. Her triage vital signs are as follows: oral temperature, 102.4° F (39.1° C); pulse, 118 beats/minute; respirations, 22 breaths/minute; blood pressure, 104/62 mmHg; and pulse oximetry, 99% on room air. What would the nurse suspect?

[ ] **A.** Septic abortion
[ ] **B.** Pyelonephritis
[ ] **C.** Vaginitis
[ ] **D.** Ovarian cyst

Correct answer—A. *Rationales:* A client with septic abortion will present with prolonged retained products of conception, resulting in foul-smelling vaginal bleeding or discharge, fever, and a closed cervical os. She won't experience uterine contractions. Pyelonephritis wouldn't have foul-smelling discharge. Vaginitis isn't generally associated with bleeding, and the discharge is typically either frothy or curd-like. Ovarian cysts aren't generally associated with discharge.
Nursing process step: Assessment

31. A 14-year-old boy comes to the emergency department with severe pain to his left testicle, which woke him out of sleep. On physical examination, his heart rate is 120 beats/minute, respiratory rate is 30 breaths/minute, blood pressure is 110/72 mm Hg, and temperature is 98.5° F (36.9° C). His left testicle is slightly elevated and firm. He has been diagnosed with testicular torsion. The most appropriate intervention is to:

[ ] **A.** establish an I.V. for crystalloid fluid administration and analgesia.
[ ] **B.** apply ice packs to scrotum.
[ ] **C.** prepare to transfuse blood products.
[ ] **D.** elevate scrotum at 45-degree angle.

Correct answer—A. *Rationales:* Testicular torsion results from congenital maldevelopment between the testis and the posterior scrotal wall. The pain level associated with this diagnosis is severe and isn't relieved by ice or elevation. Twisting of the spermatic cord compromises testicular circulation. There's no blood volume lost with testicular torsion, so blood products aren't indicated.
Nursing process step: Intervention

32. A 68-year-old man with a history of benign prostatic hyperplasia reports an inability to void for 12 hours. Which medication could contribute to acute urinary retention?

[ ] **A.** Ibuprofen
[ ] **B.** Terazosin
[ ] **C.** Vitamin C
[ ] **D.** Pseudoephedrine

Correct answer—D. *Rationales:* Pseudoephedrine is an alpha-adrenergic agonist that increases urinary resistance. The effect is minimal but can contribute to urinary retention in combination with bladder outlet obstruction (enlarged prostate gland). Nonsteroidal anti-inflammatory drugs are associated with cystitis, hematuria, and acute renal failure but not urinary retention. Terazosin is an alpha-adrenergic blocker used to improve bladder neck dyssynergia (improve bladder outlet). Vitamin C adverse effects include acidic urine, oxaluria, and renal stones.
Nursing process step: Assessment

33. The nurse would expect which client to require admission to an inpatient unit?

[ ] **A.** A 3-year-old child diagnosed with a grade I kidney contusion and microscopic hematuria
[ ] **B.** A 19-year-old woman diagnosed with a urinary tract infection (UTI) (second occurrence within 12 months)
[ ] **C.** A 45-year-old man who's hypertensive (150/100 mm Hg) diagnosed with urethritis
[ ] **D.** A 32-year-old woman who's 30 weeks' pregnant, diagnosed with pyelonephritis

Correct answer—D. *Rationales:* A pregnant client with pyelonephritis requires aggressive treatment. Pregnancy is an immunocompromised state, and pyelonephritis could quickly develop to acute renal failure. Children with renal injury can be managed similarly to adults under nonsurgical management. A client with uncomplicated UTI infection would be discharged with instructions for prevention of UTI (hydration, review hygiene practices, conditions to return to the emergency department). Urethritis in a male client is likely caused by a sexually transmitted disease (gonococcal, nongonococcal, or chlamydial). Treatment includes testing for syphilis, oral or intramuscular anti-infective therapy, and instruction to treat sexual partners.
Nursing process step: Analysis

34. A 39-year-old white female comes to the emergency department stating that she was raped multiple times over the past 12 hours. She's awake and alert, and she's with a friend. She's tearful upon presentation. The nurse knows that important assessment information for this client includes which of the following?

[ ] **A.** Whether the police were notified
[ ] **B.** Whether the client used a method of birth control
[ ] **C.** Whether the client has brushed her teeth or changed clothing since the attack
[ ] **D.** Whether the client has been raped before

Correct answer–C. *Rationales:* Whether the client has brushed her teeth or changed her clothes since the attack is critical to evidence collection and preservation for this client. It's important that the client hasn't showered, urinated, or defecated since the attack. It's also important for the client to notify the police, but this doesn't affect your assessment. It isn't relevant whether the client has been previously raped or if she used a method of birth control.
Nursing process step: Assessment

35. What's the highest priority in the nursing care of a client who has been raped?

[ ] **A.** Evidence preservation
[ ] **B.** Report of crime to the appropriate law enforcement agency
[ ] **C.** Caring for injuries sustained in the assault
[ ] **D.** Ensuring that her family understands the situation

Correct answer–C. *Rationales:* The client's well-being always takes precedence over evidence preservation. Each of the other choices is important but doesn't affect the client's well-being.
Nursing process step: Analysis

36. For a client who has been raped, which response demonstrates the client's understanding of the discharge instructions?

[ ] **A.** "I'll follow up with the local health department unit in 10 days for testing for sexually transmitted diseases."
[ ] **B.** "I'll stay home with my family and friends for the next 10 days."
[ ] **C.** "I'll follow up with my regular physician if I feel the need to."
[ ] **D.** "This is all my fault. I am ashamed of myself."

Correct answer–A. *Rationales:* Clients typically receive prophylaxis for sexually transmitted disease and pregnancy when undergoing treatment for a sexual assault. To ensure treatment was adequate, follow-up with either the local health department unit or the client's primary care physician for repeat sexually transmitted diseases testing is essential. While some sexual assault victims blame themselves for the attack, this certainly isn't a healthy coping mechanism.
Nursing process step: Evaluation

8 Neurologic emergencies

1. Receptive aphasia results from damage to which area of the brain?
[ ] **A.** Parietal lobe
[ ] **B.** Occipital lobe
[ ] **C.** Temporal lobe
[ ] **D.** Frontal lobe

Correct answer—C. *Rationales:* The temporal lobe contains the auditory association area. If the area is damaged in the dominant hemisphere, the client hears words but doesn't know their meaning. Damage to the parietal lobe affects the client's ability to identify special relationships with the environment. When damaged, the occipital lobe affects visual associations—the client can visualize objects but can't identify them. The frontal lobe acts as a storage area for memory.
Nursing process step: Analysis

2. During neurosurgical evaluation of an unresponsive client, the physician evaluates the oculo-cephalic reflex (*doll's eye phenomenon*). When the head is rotated to the left, the client's eyes also move to the left. What does this finding indicate?
[ ] **A.** No abnormality
[ ] **B.** Damage to cranial nerve (CN) I
[ ] **C.** Damage to the fovea
[ ] **D.** A lesion at the pontine (midbrain level of the brain stem)

Correct answer—D. *Rationales:* Evaluation of brain stem function can be done in an unconscious client by testing the oculo-cephalic reflex. When the client's head is rotated, the eyes should move in a direction opposite to the head movement. Brain-stem damage is indicated if the eyes move in the same direction as head movement. Evaluation of this reflex is contraindicated in a client with suspected cervical spine injury. CN I is the olfactory nerve; damage to this nerve results in the inability to identify odors. The fovea is the center of the retina's macula, the area of greatest visual acuity.
Nursing process step: Assessment

3. During a neurologic examination, the client can't raise his eyebrows or close his eyes tightly against resistance. Which cranial nerve might be damaged?
[ ] **A.** Cranial nerve (CN) II
[ ] **B.** CN V
[ ] **C.** CN VII
[ ] **D.** CN XII

Correct answer—C. *Rationales:* The facial nerve, CN VII, controls facial expression and taste in the anterior two-thirds of the tongue. CN II, the optic nerve, allows the client to blink and perceive light. CN V, the trigeminal nerve, controls jaw movement and facial sensation. CN XII, the hypoglossal nerve, controls tongue movement.
Nursing process step: Assessment

4. What's the primary intervention for a client who complains of head and neck pain and doesn't recall events leading up to his arrival in the emergency department? On arrival, the client is tested and has a Glasgow Coma Scale of 14. A hematoma is palpated from the occipital to the frontal skull areas.
[ ] **A.** Perform a complete head-to-toe assessment.
[ ] **B.** Apply cervical immobilization.
[ ] **C.** Administer opioid analgesics for complaints of discomfort.
[ ] **D.** Obtain a specimen to determine the blood alcohol level.

Correct answer—B. *Rationales:* Immobilization of the head and neck reduces the risk of further damage to the cervical spine. All clients with suspected head and neck trauma should be immobilized until all seven cervical vertebrae are cleared by X-ray visualization. A complete head-to-toe assessment (secondary survey) should be performed after airway, breathing, and circulation are assessed, the cervical spine is immobilized, and the client is evaluated for potential life-threatening injuries (primary survey). Administering opioid analgesics to a client with altered mental status or head injuries isn't a primary intervention because opioids can increase respiratory depression and hypotension in clients with head injury. Obtaining a specimen for blood alcohol level helps to determine whether the amount of alcohol the client has consumed corresponds with the level of consciousness. Although this is useful information, it isn't a primary intervention.
Nursing process step: Intervention

5. Thirty minutes after admission to the emergency department, the nurse performs a repeat neurologic examination. The client doesn't follow commands, but after several attempts by the nurse to apply noxious stimuli, he opens his eyes and moves the nurse's hand. The client utters a one-word response to the nurse. The nurse determines that the Glasgow Coma Scale score should be:
[ ] **A.** 5.
[ ] **B.** 7.
[ ] **C.** 10.
[ ] **D.** 12.

Correct answer—C. *Rationales:* The client is given 5 points for purposeful movement to pain (motor), 3 points for inappropriate words (verbal), and 2 points for eye opening in response to painful stimuli. The total score is 10.
Nursing process step: Evaluation

6. What signs and symptoms might indicate the presence of a spinal cord injury?
[ ] **A.** Hypertension with tachycardia
[ ] **B.** Numbness and tingling in the extremities
[ ] **C.** Cloudy cerebrospinal fluid (CSF)
[ ] **D.** Exophthalmos

Correct answer—B. *Rationales:* A client with possible spinal cord injury typically complains of numbness and tingling in the extremities or an inability to detect sensation. A client with injury to the spinal cord commonly becomes bradycardic and hypotensive. Cloudy CSF is associated with bacterial infections such as meningitis. Exophthalmos is an abnormal protrusion of the eyeball. It's associated with orbital tumors, thyroid disorders, and orbital cellulitis.
Nursing process step: Assessment

7. An ovoid-shaped pupil indicates which condition?
[ ] **A.** Traumatic orbital injury
[ ] **B.** Intracranial hypertension
[ ] **C.** History of cataract surgery
[ ] **D.** Pontine hemorrhage

Correct answer—B. *Rationales:* An ovoid pupil is the midpoint between a normally round pupil and a fully dilated and fixed pupil and is a sign of increased intracranial pressure. Traumatic orbital injury results in a jagged-appearing pupil. A keyhole-shaped pupil is common in clients who have had an iridectomy as part of cataract surgery. Pontine hemorrhage causes the pupil to be pinpoint.
Nursing process step: Assessment

8. Pharmacologic medications are ordered for a combative client with head injuries. The client, who's awaiting a diagnostic computed tomography scan, responds to noxious stimuli only when his Ramsey score reaches what level?

[ ] **A.** 1
[ ] **B.** 3
[ ] **C.** 5
[ ] **D.** 15

Correct answer—C. *Rationales:* The Modified Ramsey Score for Sedation measures the level of sedation achieved with pharmacologic agents. A Ramsey score of 5 suggests that the client responds only to noxious stimuli. A client who's anxious, agitated, or restless has a Ramsey score of 1. A client who's cooperative, tranquil, and oriented has a score of 2. A client who responds to voice and verbal commands has a Ramsey score of 3. A client who responds to gentle shaking scores a 4. A client who shows no response to noxious stimuli is considered a 6 on the scale.
Nursing process step: Evaluation

9. In an adult client with head injuries, which medication should be administered before sedating the client with succinylcholine (Anectine)?

[ ] **A.** Atropine
[ ] **B.** Ketamine (Ketalar)
[ ] **C.** Lidocaine (Xylocaine)
[ ] **D.** Meperidine (Demerol)

Correct answer—C. *Rationales:* Succinylcholine is a neuromuscular blocking agent that can increase intracranial pressure (ICP) in a client with head injuries. Administering 1 mg/kg of lidocaine provides ICP control. Atropine is the premedication of choice for children receiving succinylcholine because it decreases the bradycardia that occurs with succinylcholine administration. Ketamine and meperidine are contraindicated in a client with head injuries because they increase ICP.
Nursing process step: Intervention

10. Which assessment findings would be associated with a client with an intracranial pressure (ICP) reading of 35 mm Hg?

[ ] **A.** Narrowed pulse pressure
[ ] **B.** Hypothermia
[ ] **C.** Cheyne-Stokes respirations
[ ] **D.** Kussmaul's respirations

Correct answer—C. *Rationales:* Normal ICP should be less than 10 mm Hg when measured at the foramen of Monro. Widening pulse pressure, hyperthermia, and Cheyne-Stokes respirations are signs of increased ICP. Kussmaul's respirations are associated with diabetic ketoacidosis.
Nursing process step: Assessment

11. Which intervention will decrease an elevated intracranial pressure (ICP)?

[ ] **A.** Frequent suctioning of the airway
[ ] **B.** Administering meperidine (Demerol) for pain
[ ] **C.** Maintaining the client in Trendelenburg's position
[ ] **D.** Administering mannitol (Osmitrol)

Correct answer—D. *Rationales:* Mannitol is an osmotic diuretic that decreases ICP. Suctioning the client's airway should be minimized to prevent increased ICP. Meperidine should be used cautiously in a client with head injury or increased ICP; the drug's respiratory depressant effects are considerably enhanced in these situations. A client with a head injury should have his head elevated 30 degrees to promote venous drainage. Placing a client in Trendelenburg's position obstructs venous return from the brain and increases ICP.
Nursing process step: Intervention

12. Early symptoms of multiple sclerosis (MS) include all of the following *except:*

[ ] **A.** diplopia.
[ ] **B.** scotomas.
[ ] **C.** weakness.
[ ] **D.** paralysis.

Correct answer—D. *Rationales:* Paralysis is a late symptom of MS. The earliest clinical sign of MS may be vague, such as weakness, numbness, or tingling in limbs; visual blurring; or urinary changes. Motor symptoms initially present as weakness and then progress to paralysis. Diplopia (double vision) or scotoma (area of depressed vision in the visual field) may also present early in the disease.
Nursing process step: Assessment

13. A client is brought to the emergency department by ambulance; her chief complaint is lethargy. Two days ago, the client was in a high-speed motor vehicle accident and refused care. Since that time, she has complained of headaches and drowsiness. Her friend states that she's now difficult to wake up. Assessment reveals a right pupil that's fixed and dilated with papilledema present. The Glasgow Coma Scale score is 8. What signs does the client exhibit?

[ ] **A.** Subdural hematoma
[ ] **B.** Epidural hematoma
[ ] **C.** Diffuse axonal injury
[ ] **D.** Postconcussion syndrome

Correct answer—A. *Rationales:* A subdural hematoma, occurring between the dura mater and the arachnoid layer of the meninges, is bleeding that causes direct pressure to the surface of the brain. Signs and symptoms appear within 48 hours (acute) and can be delayed as long as several months (chronic). Symptoms of an epidural hematoma include a history of momentary loss of consciousness followed by a lucid period after which the client's mental status deteriorates rapidly due to the presence of bleeding from the middle meningeal artery. The clinical manifestations of a diffuse axonal injury are immediate and prolonged coma with decorticate or decerebrate posturing. Manifestations of postconcussion syndrome include headache, dizziness, irritability, poor judgment, and insomnia.
Nursing process step: Analysis

14. Which area of the brain controls the respiratory and cardiac systems?

[ ] **A.** Medulla
[ ] **B.** Frontal lobe
[ ] **C.** Diencephalon
[ ] **D.** Hypothalamus

Correct answer—A. *Rationales:* The medulla controls the arterioles, the blood pressure, and the rate and depth of respirations. Severe injury to this area generally results in death. The medulla also controls yawning, coughing, vomiting, and hiccoughing. The frontal lobe of the cerebrum controls personality, judgment, thought, and logic. The diencephalon contains the thalamus, which is the sensory pathway between the spinal cord and the cortex of the brain. The hypothalamus regulates body temperature, heart rate, appetite, and sleep.
Nursing process step: Evaluation

15. Which of the following is a delayed sign of a basilar skull fracture?

[ ] **A.** Battle's sign
[ ] **B.** Headache
[ ] **C.** Decreased level of consciousness
[ ] **D.** Respiratory irregularities

Correct answer—A. *Rationales:* All the options listed are symptoms of a basilar skull fracture; however, Battle's sign, a later manifestation, may not become evident until 12 to 24 hours after injury.
Nursing process step: Assessment

16. Which head injury results in a collection of blood between the skull and the dura mater?

[ ] **A.** Subdural hematoma
[ ] **B.** Subarachnoid hemorrhage
[ ] **C.** Epidural hematoma
[ ] **D.** Contusion

Correct answer—C. *Rationales:* An epidural hematoma results from blood collecting between the skull and the dura mater. A subdural hematoma is commonly caused by trauma or violent shaking and results in a collection of venous blood between the dura mater and the arachnoid mater. A subarachnoid hemorrhage is a collection of blood between the pia mater and the arachnoid membrane. A contusion is a bruise on the surface of the brain.
Nursing process step: Evaluation

17. A mother brings her 1-year-old child, who fell down the stairs 2 hours ago, to the emergency department. The child is dirty and wearing clothing that's inappropriate for the cold weather. The child cries when the head and neck are palpated. Bruises at various stages of healing are noted on the buttocks and back. As the physician enters the room, the child begins seizing. The child is evaluated for which condition?

[ ] **A.** Coagulation disorder
[ ] **B.** Meningitis
[ ] **C.** Subarachnoid hemorrhage
[ ] **D.** Leukemia

Correct answer—C. *Rationales:* The child has classic signs of a traumatic head injury such as subarachnoid hemorrhage, which is caused by arterial disruption that leads to the collection of blood between the pia mater and the arachnoid membrane. This injury is frequently associated with child abuse. A client with a history of coagulation or hematologic disorders may present with ecchymoses, petechiae (in platelet disorders), or purpura. Meningitis is associated with lethargy, irritability, fever, seizures, and headache. Petechiae and purpura present in meningococcemia. When assessing any client, the history, psychological findings, and client's appearance must also be considered to determine whether the signs and symptoms are consistent with the client history.

Nursing process step: Assessment

18. What's the primary intervention for a client who is brought to the emergency department after falling down the stairs and who may have had a seizure but is now speaking?

[ ] **A.** Administer lorazepam (Ativan) I.V.
[ ] **B.** Administer oxygen by way of a nonrebreather mask at 15 L/minute.
[ ] **C.** Establish I.V. access.
[ ] **D.** Immobilize the cervical spine.

Correct answer—B. *Rationales:* Because the patient has circulation and airway intact as evidenced by speaking, the next priority is breathing. Administrating oxygen via a nonrebreather mask is a breathing intervention. After circulation, airway, and breathing have been addressed, the next focus would be stabilization and immobilization of the cervical spine. Based on the history of falling down stairs, the cervical spine immobilization must be maintained until fractures are ruled out by X-ray or computed tomography scan. Lorazepam is effective in controlling seizure activity and may be administered either I.M. or I.V. After completing the rapid primary assessment, an I.V. should be established to facilitate resuscitative and pharmacologic interventions.

Nursing process step: Intervention

19. Which of the following would be an ominous sign in a 1-year-old child with a possible neck injury?

[ ] **A.** Heart rate of 60 beats/minute
[ ] **B.** Respiratory rate of 30 breaths/minute
[ ] **C.** Capillary refill time of 3 seconds
[ ] **D.** Positive Babinski's reflex

Correct answer—A. *Rationales:* The normal heart rate for a 1-year-old child ranges from 90 to 120 beats/minute. Bradycardia is a sign of increasing intracranial pressure. Normally, respirations for a child in this age range from 20 to 30 breaths/minute. Capillary refill time less than or equal to 3 seconds is a normal finding. After age 2 or after the child is walking, a positive Babinski's reflex is an abnormal finding.

Nursing process step: Assessment

20. While caring for a client with a ventriculostomy, the nurse notices that the intracranial pressure (ICP) is 30 mm Hg. The nurse assesses the client and the ICP monitor and determines that the drain is open. Immediate interventions should include which of the following?

[ ] **A.** Move the head from a rotated position to the midline.

[ ] **B.** Lower the head of the bed to the Trendelenburg position.

[ ] **C.** Close the stopcock on the ventriculostomy to prevent drainage of cerebrospinal fluid (CSF).

[ ] **D.** Elevate the head of the bed to high Fowler's position.

Correct answer—A. *Rationales:* The head of the bed should be maintained at 30 degrees, and hyperextension, flexion, and rotation of the head should be avoided. A rotated position will prevent venous outflow via the jugular veins and contribute to increased ICP. Lowering the head of the bed would increase the pressure on the brain. Closing the stopcock on the ventriculostomy causes the ICP to rise because there's no longer an outlet for CSF.
Nursing process step: Intervention

21. A client involved in a 20-foot fall sustains a fracture with spinal cord transection at the level of C6. This injury results in which finding?

[ ] **A.** Quadriplegia with diaphragmatic breathing and gross arm movements

[ ] **B.** Quadriplegia with total loss of respiratory function

[ ] **C.** Paraplegia with variable loss of intercostal and abdominal muscle use

[ ] **D.** Bowel and bladder dysfunction

Correct answer—A. *Rationales:* A client with an injury at level C6 has quadriplegia with diaphragmatic breathing and gross arm movements. The client may also suffer from hypotension and an atonic bladder. An injury at level C2 results in total loss of respiratory function and movement from the shoulders down. Paraplegia with loss of portions of intercostal and abdominal muscles is indicative of injury at T1-L2. An injury below L2 results in mixed motor sensory loss and bowel and bladder dysfunction.
Nursing process step: Assessment

22. When administering a loading dose of phenytoin (Dilantin), which of the following is important to remember?

[ ] **A.** Therapeutic blood levels should be between 20 and 30 mg/ml.

[ ] **B.** Rapid administration of phenytoin can lead to cardiac arrhythmias.

[ ] **C.** Phenytoin is normally mixed in dextrose in water solution.

[ ] **D.** Phenytoin potentiates the action of cardiac glycosides.

Correct answer—B. *Rationales:* When phenytoin is administered I.V., it shouldn't be given faster than 50 mg/minute because doing so can depress the myocardium and lead to arrhythmias and cardiac arrest. Therapeutic blood levels should range from 10 to 20 mg/ml. Mixing phenytoin in any solution other than normal saline can cause the drug to precipitate into crystals. Phenytoin inhibits the action of cardiac glycosides and corticosteroids. It does, however, potentiate the actions of propranolol (Inderal), methotrexate (Mexate), and antihypertensives.
Nursing process step: Intervention

23. Discharge instructions for a client taking phenytoin (Dilantin) should include which of the following?

[ ] **A.** Missed doses of phenytoin can't easily be made up without adverse effects.

[ ] **B.** Routine blood studies aren't necessary.

[ ] **C.** Status epilepticus can be precipitated by abrupt anticonvulsant withdrawal.

[ ] **D.** There are so few adverse effects of the medication that none are worth mentioning.

Correct answer—C. *Rationales:* Because of the slow absorption of phenytoin from the GI tract, daily drug routines can be easily adjusted when a dose is missed. One of the most common causes of seizures in a client taking phenytoin is discontinuation of the medication. The client also needs to be made aware of possible adverse effects of his medications. Phenytoin is metabolized in the liver, and both the inactive metabolites and unchanged drug are excreted in the urine. Because phenytoin has many hematopoietic adverse effects, blood work (including complete blood count, liver, and renal function studies) should be obtained on a regular basis. Serum levels should also be monitored because serum concentrations increase disproportionately to dosing regimens.
Nursing process step: Intervention

24. Guillain-Barré syndrome is characterized by which statement?
[ ] **A.** It's most common in children and in young adults under age 18.
[ ] **B.** It causes demyelination of the cranial and spinal nerves.
[ ] **C.** The onset of symptoms is slow and insidious.
[ ] **D.** Paralysis affects the lower extremities exclusively.

Correct answer—B. *Rationales:* Guillain-Barré syndrome is distinguished from other forms of polyneuritis by its acute onset and rapid progression. It's classified as a neuritis because it causes demyelination of the spinal cord, peripheral nerves, root ganglia, and nerve roots. The disease manifests itself by sudden onset of lower-extremity weakness that rapidly progresses to the arms, trunk, and face. It primarily affects people between ages 30 and 50.
Nursing process step: Analysis

25. Clinical manifestations of Parkinson's disease include all of the following *except*:
[ ] **A.** pill-rolling movement when at rest.
[ ] **B.** bradykinesia.
[ ] **C.** rigidity.
[ ] **D.** alopecia.

Correct answer—D. *Rationales:* Alopecia isn't a manifestation of Parkinson's disease. The symptom that typically characterizes this disease is a faint tremor that slowly progresses in intensity. As the client's muscle tone becomes more rigid, the gait takes on a shuffling appearance. The client's face is masklike, and his speech is slow and monotone. It's common for the client to develop dysphagia and drooling. The client's judgment becomes impaired even though actual intelligence remains unaffected.
Nursing process step: Assessment

26. Which medication is commonly used to treat the symptoms of Parkinson's disease?
[ ] **A.** Pramipexole (Mirapex)
[ ] **B.** Reserpine (Serpalan)
[ ] **C.** Haloperidol (Haldol)
[ ] **D.** Benztropine (Cogentin)

Correct answer—A. *Rationales:* Pramipexole (Mirapex) is a dopamine agonist. It activates dopamine receptors, which mimic or copy the function of dopamine in the brain. The use of dopamine-blocking drugs has been linked to pharmacologically increased parkinsonism. Dopamine and acetylcholine are neurotransmitters that act on the input nuclei to the basal ganglia. When dopamine (an inhibitor) is reduced, acetylcholine (an excitatory neurotransmitter) becomes predominant and precipitates tremor.
Nursing process step: Intervention

27. Many clients with myasthenia gravis are treated with anticholinesterase drugs. What's the antidote for anticholinesterase toxicity?
[ ] **A.** Vitamin K analogue (AquaMEPHYTON)
[ ] **B.** Atropine
[ ] **C.** Physostigmine (Antilirium)
[ ] **D.** Pyridostigmine (Mestinon)

Correct answer—B. *Rationales:* Atropine is the antidote for anticholinesterase toxicity and should be available to clients on this pharmacologic routine. It corrects the extreme bradycardia that can be associated with the use of anticholinesterase-type drugs. Vitamin K analogue is the antidote for warfarin (Coumadin) ingestion. Physostigmine and pyridostigmine are anticholinesterase drugs that are used to treat myasthenia gravis.
Nursing process step: Intervention

28. A 28-year-old woman comes to the emergency department with blurred vision and drooping of the right eyelid. She also complains of intermittent episodes of muscle weakness and states that at times her neck doesn't feel strong enough to support her head. She tires when eating and must take frequent breaks during a meal. Several times, she has had to close her mouth using her hand because "the muscles in my face feel so weak." What's the probable diagnosis for this client?

[ ] **A.** Myasthenia gravis
[ ] **B.** Bell's palsy
[ ] **C.** Trigeminal neuralgia
[ ] **D.** Glioblastoma

Correct answer—A. *Rationales:* Myasthenia gravis affects two to three times more women than men until age 40. This disease may result from a defect at the myoneural junction. The primary symptom is weakness of voluntary muscles, especially those of the face. This weakness may temporarily improve with short periods of rest. Bell's palsy is an inflammatory reaction involving the facial nerves. It presents as ipsilateral facial paresis. Trigeminal neuralgia is characterized by sudden episodes of ipsilateral facial pain. Glioblastomas are intracranial tumors that present with symptoms of increased intracranial pressure and focal deficits.
Nursing process step: Analysis

29. Which test is frequently used to diagnose myasthenia gravis?

[ ] **A.** Lumbar puncture
[ ] **B.** Tensilon test
[ ] **C.** Allen's test
[ ] **D.** Magnetic resonance imaging (MRI)

Correct answer—B. *Rationales:* In the Tensilon test, edrophonium is administered by I.V. infusion to a client exhibiting signs of muscle weakness. Significant improvement in the client's muscle tone indicates a positive diagnosis for myasthenia gravis. This effect lasts for about 4 to 5 minutes. A lumbar puncture is frequently performed to assist in diagnosing meningitis. Allen's test is performed to evaluate the circulatory function of the ulnar artery. MRI is effective in detecting degenerative central nervous system diseases, malignant tumors, and oxygen-deprived tissue, but none of these findings are associated with myasthenia gravis.
Nursing process step: Evaluation

30. Medications that reduce the spasticity or pain associated with multiple sclerosis (MS) include all of the following *except*:

[ ] **A.** diazepam (Valium).
[ ] **B.** baclofen (Lioresal).
[ ] **C.** gabapentin (Neurontin).
[ ] **D.** cyclophosphamide (Cytoxan).

Correct answer—D. *Rationales:* Cytoxan is a chemotherapeutic agent used to slow growth of cancer cells and interfere with their spread throughout the body. Diazepam, baclofen, and gabapentin are associated with medical management of the client with MS. Diazepam and baclofen are primarily effective in decreasing the spasms and stiffness associated with the disease, whereas gabapentin relieves pain as well as spasticity.
Nursing process step: Intervention

31. Alzheimer's disease is characterized by profound impairment of cognitive functions. Which of the following is the cause of this disorder?

[ ] **A.** Destruction of motor cells in the anterior gray horns and pyramidal tracts
[ ] **B.** Metabolic disorders
[ ] **C.** Cerebral atrophy and cellular degeneration
[ ] **D.** Degeneration of the basal ganglia

Correct answer—C. *Rationales:* Alzheimer's disease is a neurologic and degenerative disorder resulting from cerebral atrophy and cellular degeneration. Predominating symptoms are mental status changes, increased anxiety, forgetfulness, and eventually, the inability to recognize significant others and to perform activities of daily living. Destruction of motor cells in the anterior gray horns and pyramidal tracts can result in the symptoms associated with amyotrophic lateral sclerosis. Metabolic disorders may cause altered cognitive function but can be reversed by correction of the underlying problem. Degeneration of the basal ganglia is usually associated with Parkinson's disease.
Nursing process step: Evaluation

32. A nurse is caring for a client who has suffered a closed head injury and has elevated intracranial pressure (ICP). Which guideline should the nurse follow when maintaining the patency of the endotracheal tube?

[ ] **A.** Suction every two hours.
[ ] **B.** Instill normal saline prior to suctioning.
[ ] **C.** Lower the head of the bed prior to suctioning.
[ ] **D.** Suction only when needed.

Correct answer–D. *Rationales:* Suctioning will cause coughing, which increases intrathoracic pressure and intracranial pressure. Suctioning shouldn't occur every 2 hours but should be performed in the case of elevated peak pressures or visible secretions accompanied by respiratory assessments that support the need. The instillation of normal saline prior to suctioning increases ventilator-associated pneumonia. Lowering the head of the bed will elevate the ICP. The head of bed should be maintained at 30 degrees.
Nursing process step: Intervention

33. A woman with complaints of seeing "zigzagging lines" in her visual field after waking this morning presents to the emergency department. She now complains of a right temporal headache accompanied by nausea and photosensitivity. Based on the symptoms, the client is evaluated for which condition?

[ ] **A.** Sinusitis
[ ] **B.** Meningitis
[ ] **C.** Migraine
[ ] **D.** Trigeminal neuralgia

Correct answer–C. *Rationales:* The client is experiencing a migraine headache. Migraines are more prevalent in women than in men, and there's usually a familial tendency. Migraines are divided into three phases:

◆ aura (vision disturbances, confusion, paresthesia), which precedes the headache and lasts from 15 to 30 minutes
◆ headache, characterized by a throbbing pain that usually begins as unilateral and progresses to bilateral and is accompanied by nausea or vomiting
◆ postheadache, accompanied by scalp tenderness and muscular aching of the neck.

Sinusitis is described as pain or pressure over the maxillary or frontal sinus areas. The pain can be reproduced by palpation. Meningitis presents with symptoms of fever, headache, severe neck discomfort, and irritability. Typically, there's an altered level of consciousness. Trigeminal neuralgia is characterized by ipsilateral facial pain from the side of the mouth to the ear, eye, or nostril on the same side.
Nursing process step: Assessment

34. Which medication would the client receive as preventative treatment for migraine headache?

[ ] **A.** Propranolol (Inderal)
[ ] **B.** Ondansetron (Zofran)
[ ] **C.** Codeine
[ ] **D.** Diphenhydramine (Benadryl)

Correct answer–A. *Rationales:* Propranolol, a beta blocker, is one of the most commonly prescribed drugs for the prevention of migraines. Ondansetron is an antiemetic used to control the nausea and vomiting associated with a migraine headache. Codeine can be given for the pain of a full-blown migraine. Diphenhydramine is useful in treating cluster headaches.
Nursing process step: Intervention

35. The client is prescribed ergotamine (Cafergot) for treatment of her headache. The drug has a cumulative effect that increases the risk of drug overdose. Clinical manifestations of ergotamine overdose (ergotism) include which symptoms?

[ ] **A.** Altered mental status
[ ] **B.** Hypertension and tachycardia
[ ] **C.** Numbness and tingling in the toes and fingers
[ ] **D.** Ataxia

Correct answer–C. *Rationales:* Symptoms of ergotamine overdose occur in response to intense arterial vasoconstriction, which produces signs and symptoms of peripheral vascular ischemia. In addition to numbness of fingers and toes, the client may experience muscle pain and weakness, gangrene, and blindness. Altered mental status, hypertension and tachycardia, and ataxia aren't associated with ergotamine tartrate overdose.
Nursing process step: Assessment

36. What's the immediate action in establishing an airway in a client with suspected neck injury?
[ ] **A.** Insert a nasopharyngeal airway.
[ ] **B.** Prepare for blind orotracheal intubation.
[ ] **C.** Perform the jaw thrust–chin lift maneuver.
[ ] **D.** Conduct head tilt maneuvers.

Correct answer—C. *Rationales:* The preferred method of opening the airway in a client with a suspected neck injury is the jaw thrust–chin lift maneuver. Options A and B are appropriate methods to maintain or establish an open airway. The head tilt causes the neck to hyperextend, which causes further damage in a client with a cervical spine injury.
Nursing process step: Intervention

37. Appropriate interventions for a client having a seizure include all of the following *except*:
[ ] **A.** administering oxygen.
[ ] **B.** administering I.V. diazepam (Valium).
[ ] **C.** inserting a tongue blade into the mouth.
[ ] **D.** turning the head or body to one side.

Correct answer—C. *Rationales:* Inserting a wooden tongue blade into the mouth of a client having a seizure puts him at risk for oral injury from splinters and for aspiration of the foreign body. Administering oxygen and diazepam and turning the client's head or body to one side are appropriate interventions. Additionally, suction should be available and side rails should be padded and raised to protect the client from self-injury.
Nursing process step: Intervention

38. A client arrives by ambulance for evaluation of seizure activity after falling to the ground while engaged in an argument with his employer. He's screaming and violently flinging his extremities, but there's no evidence of incontinence or tongue biting. Prehospital providers state that this episode has lasted for 40 minutes. Based on this information, the client is diagnosed with what condition?
[ ] **A.** Pseudoseizures
[ ] **B.** Absence (petit mal) seizures
[ ] **C.** Tonic-clonic (grand mal) seizures
[ ] **D.** Focal seizures

Correct answer—A. *Rationales:* Emotional upset usually precedes a pseudoseizure, which generally lasts longer than a true seizure. In a true seizure, the client screams at the onset of the event but repetitive, consistent movement of the extremities is ongoing. Absence, or petit mal, seizures are manifested by an absence of consciousness for 5 to 10 seconds. Tonic-clonic (grand mal) seizures present with the following pattern: aura, cry, loss of consciousness, fall, tonic-clonic movement, and incontinence. Focal seizures involve one area of the body (which varies from client to client) and aren't associated with an altered mental state.
Nursing process step: Assessment

39. Phenytoin (Dilantin) is ineffective in the treatment of which seizure classification?
[ ] **A.** Status epilepticus
[ ] **B.** Absence (petit mal)
[ ] **C.** Psychomotor
[ ] **D.** Tonic-clonic (grand mal)

Correct answer—B. *Rationales:* Phenytoin isn't effective in the treatment of absence (petit mal) seizures. Absence seizures are treated with trimethadione (Tridione), clonazepam (Klonopin), ethosuximide (Zarontin), and valproic acid (Depakene). Phenytoin is effective in the treatment of tonic-clonic (grand mal), psychomotor, and focal seizures.
Nursing process step: Intervention

40. Temporary periods of cerebral ischemia may result in symptoms associated with which condition?
[ ] **A.** Transient ischemic attacks (TIAs)
[ ] **B.** Hypercapneic encephalopathy
[ ] **C.** Disequilibrium syndrome
[ ] **D.** Transtentorial herniation

Correct answer—A. *Rationales:* TIAs are temporary episodes of neurologic dysfunction in response to brief episodes of cerebral ischemia. Most commonly, a TIA presents as weakness of the lower face and upper and lower extremities as well as dysphagia, which may occur multiple times during the day. Between each attack, neurologic findings are normal. Hypercapneic encephalopathy is seen in clients with problems associated with chronic respiratory acidosis. Disequilibrium syndrome is an acute complication of peritoneal dialysis or hemodialysis. Transtentorial herniation occurs as a result of downward pressure from edema in the parietal or frontal lobes.
Nursing process step: Analysis

41. Which drug class is most commonly used in the treatment of a stroke?

[ ] **A.** Thrombolytics
[ ] **B.** Neuroleptics
[ ] **C.** Anticoagulants
[ ] **D.** Vasopressors

Correct answer—A. *Rationales:* Thrombolytics are part of a drug therapy that dissolves clots by fibrinolysis. Tissue plasminogen activator (Activase) is the only approved thrombolytic for use in acute ischemic stroke. Anticoagulants, such as aspirin, heparin, and warfarin (Coumadin), are primarily used in anticoagulation at the tissue level. Neuroleptics, which are antipsychotics, aren't indicated in a stroke. Vasopressors elevate blood pressure and increase oxygen demands, which are contraindicated in the client with a stroke.

Nursing process step: Intervention

42. What's the treatment for a warfarin (Coumadin) overdose?

[ ] **A.** Vitamin K (AquaMEPHYTON)
[ ] **B.** Protamine
[ ] **C.** Acetylcysteine (Mucomyst)
[ ] **D.** Atropine

Correct answer—A. *Rationales:* Vitamin K is used to treat warfarin overdose. Protamine is the reversing agent for heparin overdose. Acetylcysteine is used in the treatment of acetaminophen (Tylenol) overdose. Atropine is used in the treatment of bradycardia.

Nursing process step: Intervention

43. What's the term for difficulty in transforming sound into patterns of understandable speech?

[ ] **A.** Receptive aphasia
[ ] **B.** Dysphagia
[ ] **C.** Expressive aphasia
[ ] **D.** Apraxia

Correct answer—C. *Rationales:* Expressive aphasia is indicative of stroke syndrome on the left side (right-sided hemiplegia). Receptive aphasia is an impaired ability to understand spoken words. Dysphagia refers to difficulty in swallowing, which occurs when injury affects the vertebrobasilar region. Apraxia is the inability to perform a learned movement, such as using a comb, brushing one's teeth, or waving good-bye.

Nursing process step: Analysis

44. Brain tumors of the frontal lobe result in which symptoms?

[ ] **A.** Focal seizures
[ ] **B.** Personality changes
[ ] **C.** Visual hallucinations
[ ] **D.** Loss of right-left discrimination

Correct answer—B. *Rationales:* The frontal lobe provides memory storage, thought expression, and word formation. In addition to personality changes, a person with a brain tumor of the frontal lobe exhibits indifference to bodily functions and inappropriate affects. Focal seizures are indicative of tumors in the precentral gyrus area. Visual hallucinations are manifested in temporal lobe abnormalities. The loss of right-left discrimination is caused by disturbances in the parietal lobe.

Nursing process step: Assessment

45. Which of the following is one of the most malignant and rapidly growing forms of brain tumor?

[ ] **A.** Astrocytoma
[ ] **B.** Meningioma
[ ] **C.** Neuroma
[ ] **D.** Glioblastoma

Correct answer—D. *Rationales:* The glioblastoma and medulloblastoma are two of the most malignant and rapidly growing brain tumors. They are difficult to excise and can cause death within months. An astrocytoma is a slower growing form of glioma. A meningioma is benign and frequently encapsulated. A neuroma is an extremely slow growing tumor that arises from any of the cranial nerves.

Nursing process step: Evaluation

46. Children under age 8 are most likely to injure which portion of the vertebral column?
[ ] **A.** C6 to C7
[ ] **B.** C1 to C3
[ ] **C.** C5 to C6
[ ] **D.** C7 exclusively

Correct answer—B. *Rationales:* When a young child is placed in a safety restraint seat facing the front of the car, the risk of cervical fracture at the C1 to C3 level increases because of the fulcrum effect as the child's head whips forward in an accident. For several reasons, a child's cervical spine is more susceptible to injury than an adult's.
◆ The vertebral bodies of children are wedged anteriorly and tend to slide forward with flexion.
◆ The neck ligaments of children are more lax.
◆ The neck muscles of children are weaker.
◆ The upper cervical spine facets of children are flatter.

The other options are more common injuries in older children and adults.
Nursing process step: Analysis

47. What are the symptoms of a subdural hematoma in a child younger than age 2?
[ ] **A.** Bulging fontanels
[ ] **B.** Hypervolemia
[ ] **C.** Conjunctival hemorrhages
[ ] **D.** Normal ICP readings

Correct answer—A. *Rationales:* A child with a subdural hematoma exhibits bulging fontanels because the sutures separate as intracranial pressure (ICP) increases. An increase in ICP also causes retinal hemorrhages. Hypovolemia may occur if a large amount of blood has been lost due to bleeding from a subdural hematoma.
Nursing process step: Assessment

48. Before applying Crutchfield tongs, the nurse should tell the client which of the following?
[ ] **A.** "You'll experience numbness in the extremities after application of the tongs."
[ ] **B.** "X-rays will be taken after each addition of weight to the traction setup."
[ ] **C.** "The traction and weights should rest against the foot of the bed to prevent unnecessary movement."
[ ] **D.** "The Crutchfield tong application will be done under general anesthesia."

Correct answer—B. *Rationales:* X-rays are taken after the addition of each weight to evaluate progress in reducing cervical spine injury. Neurologic status should be reevaluated at that time and should indicate no worsening of neurologic deficit as a result of traction. The traction and weight should suspend freely to prevent interference with traction. Crutchfield tongs can be applied while the client is under local anesthetic.
Nursing process step: Intervention

49. Clinical symptoms of autonomic dysreflexia include headache, profuse sweating, piloerection (gooseflesh), hypertension, and bradycardia. This syndrome occurs in clients with injuries at or above which of the following levels?
[ ] **A.** S5
[ ] **B.** L1
[ ] **C.** T6
[ ] **D.** T12

Correct answer—C. *Rationales:* Autonomic dysreflexia is most commonly associated with spinal cord injuries at or above the T6 level. This serious hypertensive condition occurs during the rehabilitative phase of spinal cord injury. It's caused by noxious stimuli that create an exaggerated sympathetic response.
Nursing process step: Assessment

50. What's the outermost covering of the brain?
[ ] **A.** Pia mater
[ ] **B.** Galea aponeurotica
[ ] **C.** Dura mater
[ ] **D.** Arachnoid mater

Correct answer—C. *Rationales:* The dura mater is a tough fibrous tissue that makes up the outermost covering of the brain. The pia mater is a delicate layer that adheres to the surface of the spinal cord and the brain. The galea aponeurotica is a dense, fibrous tissue that covers the skull and absorbs the forces of external trauma. The arachnoid mater is a fine fibrous layer that lies between the dura mater and the pia mater.
Nursing process step: Analysis

51. What's the function of cerebrospinal fluid (CSF)?
[ ] **A.** Cushions the brain and spinal cord
[ ] **B.** Acts as an insulator to maintain a constant spinal fluid temperature
[ ] **C.** Acts as a barrier to bacteria
[ ] **D.** Produces cerebral neurotransmitters

Correct answer—A. *Rationales:* CSF is primarily produced in the lateral ventricles of the brain. It acts as a shock absorber and cushions the spinal cord and brain against injury caused by sudden or extreme movement. CSF also functions in the removal of waste products from cerebral tissue. The other options aren't functions of CSF.
Nursing process step: Analysis

52. A client on heparin therapy should be instructed to look for which signs of overdose?
[ ] **A.** Constipation and severe abdominal pain
[ ] **B.** Visual hallucinations and disorientation
[ ] **C.** Hematuria and rectal bleeding
[ ] **D.** Tinnitus and dry mouth

Correct answer—C. *Rationales:* The clinical manifestations of heparin overdose are hematuria, rectal bleeding, epistaxis, petechial formation, and easy bruising. Constipation, severe abdominal pain, visual hallucinations, tinnitus, and dry mouth aren't associated with heparin sodium overdose.
Nursing process step: Assessment

53. Which information is most important to include in the initial history of a client being evaluated for seizures?
[ ] **A.** Recent falls or injury to the head
[ ] **B.** Ethanol use
[ ] **C.** Use of opioids
[ ] **D.** Compliance with taking medications

Correct answer—A. *Rationales:* All of the information listed in the options should be included in the history of a client with seizures; however, a history of falls or head injury, when accompanied by seizures, could indicate severe complications of head injury. These complications may include cerebral irritation or edema, epidural hematoma, and cerebral contusions and may require immediate attention.
Nursing process step: Assessment

54. When administering diazepam (Valium), the nurse should be aware of which life-threatening adverse effect?
[ ] **A.** Respiratory arrest
[ ] **B.** Syncope
[ ] **C.** Hypotension
[ ] **D.** Cardiac arrhythmias

Correct answer—A. *Rationales:* Diazepam is a central nervous system depressant. It should be administered slowly, with periodic reassessment of the client's vital signs, including respiratory status. Syncope, hypotension, and cardiac arrhythmias are adverse effects of diazepam but aren't usually life-threatening.
Nursing process step: Intervention

55. Which of the following should be included in the acute treatment of a cluster headache?
[ ] **A.** Lithium carbonate
[ ] **B.** Oxygen
[ ] **C.** Verapamil (Calan)
[ ] **D.** Topiramate (Topamax)

Correct answer—B. *Rationales:* All the medications listed are appropriate for managing cluster headaches; however, oxygen is the only drug for acute treatment. The other drugs are used to prevent cluster headaches.
Nursing process step: Intervention

56. Diagnostic testing is performed on a client with altered mental status. For which finding would the nurse expect the client to be comatose?

[ ] **A.** Partial pressure of arterial oxygen (PaO_2) between 30 and 50 mm Hg

[ ] **B.** Glasgow Coma Scale score of 9

[ ] **C.** Decerebrate posturing

[ ] **D.** Midposition round pupils

Correct answer—C. *Rationales:* Decerebrate posturing indicates a lesion at the level of the brain stem; this response is usually found in a comatose client. The brain is extremely sensitive to hypoxia, and coma usually results when the PaO_2 falls below 25 mm Hg. A Glasgow Coma Scale score of 7 or lower is associated with comatose states of unconsciousness. Midposition round pupils are a normal finding.

Nursing process step: Assessment

57. Which symptom is associated with a cluster headache?

[ ] **A.** Tearing

[ ] **B.** Fever

[ ] **C.** Aphasia

[ ] **D.** Epistaxis

Correct answer—A. *Rationales:* A cluster headache is characterized by pain episodes that are grouped or clustered together for a few days or a few weeks with long periods of remission. The headache is described as causing unilateral pain behind the eyes or near the temples. Associated symptoms include tearing, rhinorrhea, nasal congestion, and Horner's syndrome. Fever, aphasia, and epistaxis are not associated with cluster headaches.

Nursing process step: Assessment

58. A client who's complaining that he has the worst headache of his life has been vomiting, complaining of photosensitivity, and has difficulty speaking. He's most likely exhibiting symptoms for which condition?

[ ] **A.** Ischemic stroke

[ ] **B.** Ruptured cerebral aneurysm

[ ] **C.** Migraine headaches

[ ] **D.** Acoustic neuroma

Correct answer—B. *Rationales:* Clients with cerebral aneurysms are asymptomatic until the time of bleeding. At the time of rupture, blood is forced into the subarachnoid space, causing symptoms of meningeal irritation, including nausea, vomiting, aphasia, photosensitivity, hypertension, and bradycardia. Symptoms of an ischemic stroke vary, depending on the location of the insult. Contralateral paralysis, aphasia, sensory impairment, and dysphagia commonly occur. Migraine headaches are associated with aura, throbbing sensation, nausea, vomiting, and visual disturbances. Acoustic neuromas can be identified by vertigo, tinnitus, hearing loss, facial weakness, and hoarseness.

Nursing process step: Assessment

59. Nitroprusside (Nitropress) is ordered to treat a client's hypertension. What are the guidelines for administering nitroprusside?

[ ] **A.** Nitroprusside should be reconstituted with normal saline only.

[ ] **B.** Once reconstituted, nitroprusside deteriorates in light.

[ ] **C.** Nitroprusside overdose is treated with acetylcysteine (Acetadote).

[ ] **D.** Nitroprusside should be reconstituted with bacteriostatic water.

Correct answer—B. *Rationales:* Nitroprusside solution should be wrapped in an opaque material promptly to protect it from light, which causes it to deteriorate. Nitroprusside overdose results in cyanide toxicity, which is treated with amyl nitrate inhalations. Nitroprusside should be administered or reconstituted with dextrose in water only.

Nursing process step: Intervention

60. A client has a systolic blood pressure of over 200 mm Hg and a severe headache. The physician orders a nicardipine (Cardene) infusion. What should the nurse explain to the family about the use of this medication?
[ ] **A.** It will relieve the pain of the headache by stimulating endorphins.
[ ] **B.** It will lower the blood pressure by dilating arteries and veins.
[ ] **C.** It will lower the heart rate by blocking calcium channels.
[ ] **D.** It will prevent seizure activity by depressing the central nervous system (CNS).

Correct answer–B. *Rationales:* Intravenous nicardipine is indicated in the treatment of hypertensive emergencies because it lowers the blood pressure by dilating arteries and veins. Nicardipine doesn't relieve headache, lower the heart rate by blocking calcium channels, or prevent seizure activity by depressing the CNS.
Nursing process step: Evaluation

61. Which of the following is the earliest indicator of change in a client's neurologic status?
[ ] **A.** Pupillary reaction
[ ] **B.** Motor response
[ ] **C.** Capillary refill
[ ] **D.** Level of consciousness (LOC)

Correct answer–D. *Rationales:* The earliest indicator of neurologic status is the LOC. A client who exhibits altered mental status or decreased consciousness should be reevaluated by the nursing and medical staff. Changes in the reaction and shape of pupils are late indicators of neurologic problems. Motor response appears as a delayed sign of neurologic status change. Capillary refill is an indicator of circulatory status.
Nursing process step: Assessment

62. What's the purpose of corticosteroid therapy in a client diagnosed with a brain tumor?
[ ] **A.** To control petit mal seizures
[ ] **B.** To relieve symptoms of agitation
[ ] **C.** To reduce cerebral edema
[ ] **D.** To reduce pain

Correct answer–C. *Rationales:* Corticosteroids reduce inflammation and cerebral edema and help prevent an increase in intracranial pressure. Anticonvulsants are used to control petit mal seizures. Antipsychotics and antianxiety drugs may be used sparingly to control agitation. Nonopioids are preferred for use to relieve pain because opioids may make it difficult to assess a client's level of consciousness.
Nursing process step: Intervention

63. Which of the following is a contraindication for lumbar puncture?
[ ] **A.** Increased intracranial pressure (ICP)
[ ] **B.** Fever
[ ] **C.** Elevated white blood cell (WBC) count
[ ] **D.** Positive Kernig's sign

Correct answer–A. *Rationales:* Increased ICP is a contraindication for performing a lumbar puncture because brain stem herniation may result. Fever, elevated WBC, and a positive Kernig's sign are all clinical signs and symptoms of meningitis. Lumbar puncture is indicated for the diagnosis and management of meningitis.
Nursing process step: Analysis

64. A 24-year-old client comes to the emergency department with a severe headache behind the right eye. He has experienced nausea and vomiting for the past 2 hours. Which question is important to ask this client to determine whether the headache is extracranial?
[ ] **A.** "Have you ever had a seizure?"
[ ] **B.** "Have you had a recent earache?"
[ ] **C.** "Do you have a history of hypertension?"
[ ] **D.** "Have you sustained a recent head injury?"

Correct answer–B. *Rationales:* Extracranial causes of headache include ear infection, upper respiratory infection, sinus congestion, and systemic infections. Obtaining a thorough history of recent infections is important to determine whether the headache is extracranial in origin. Key assessment questions related to intracranial causes include a history of seizure disorder, hypertension, and head injury.
Nursing process step: Assessment

65. An 84-year-old client comes to the emergency department with a 28-hour history of garbled speech and progressing hemiplegia. What stroke classification is this?

[ ] **A.** Transient ischemic attack (TIA)
[ ] **B.** Reversible ischemic neurologic deficit
[ ] **C.** Stroke in evolution
[ ] **D.** Completed stroke

Correct answer—C. *Rationales:* The progressive development of deficits described indicates a stroke in evolution. The deficits are more than 24 hours in duration, so the client probably hasn't suffered a TIA. Because the motor symptoms are progressing, it isn't a completed stroke. Reversible ischemic neurologic deficitis unlikely due to the continued progression of both motor and speech deficits.
Nursing process step: Analysis

66. What diagnostic test is used to determine if a stroke is hemorrhagic?

[ ] **A.** Doppler flow studies
[ ] **B.** Computed tomography (CT)
[ ] **C.** EEG
[ ] **D.** Electrocardiogram (ECG)

Correct answer—B. *Rationales:* CT scan is the initial diagnostic test used to determine if a stroke is hemorrhagic. Ischemia may be detected during the early phase, with magnetic resonance imaging. Doppler flow studies may be used later if occlusion is suspected in the carotid or vertebral arteries. EEG is used to determine electrical brain wave activity in unconscious clients. ECG is used to determine electrical and mechanical activity of the heart. Both EEG and ECG may be ordered, but they aren't required to differentiate stroke type.
Nursing process step: Analysis

67. Which of the following is a key indicator of intracranial shunt dysfunction?

[ ] **A.** Inability to look up
[ ] **B.** Increased alertness
[ ] **C.** Agitation
[ ] **D.** Inability to look down

Correct answer—A. *Rationales:* Decreased alertness, decreased intellectual function, and inability to look up are physical examination findings in a client with intracranial shunt dysfunction. Eye position will usually be in the downward, medial gaze station. The client will have decreased alertness without agitation and may become obtunded quickly.
Nursing process step: Assessment

68. When obtaining a medical history on a client presenting with symptoms of Guillain-Barré syndrome, which question is the most important to ask?

[ ] **A.** "Do you have a history of neurologic diseases?"
[ ] **B.** "Have you experienced a recent trauma?"
[ ] **C.** "Have you had an upper respiratory infection or GI disorder within the past month?"
[ ] **D.** "Do you have a history of substance abuse?"

Correct answer—C. *Rationales:* While all the questions listed above are important when Guillain-Barré syndrome is suspected, approximately 50% of all clients with Guillain-Barré syndrome experience a mild febrile illness (upper respiratory infection or GI disorder) 2 to 3 weeks before the onset of symptoms.
Nursing process step: Assessment

69. Which diagnostic test is used to confirm a diagnosis of Guillain-Barré syndrome?

[ ] **A.** Nerve conduction velocity (NCV) test
[ ] **B.** Spinal tap with cerebral spinal fluid (CSF) examination for decreased protein
[ ] **C.** EEG
[ ] **D.** Electrocardiogram (ECG)

Correct answer—A. *Rationales:* Because the signals traveling along the nerves are slower, an NCV test is used as well as a spinal tap for CSF examination. However, the CSF in a client with Guillain-Barré syndrome will have increased protein. EEG and ECG may be ordered, but they don't assist in confirming the diagnosis.
Nursing process step: Analysis

70. Which is the most important neurologic assessment data to collect on a client with suspected dementia?
[ ] **A.** Gait function assessment
[ ] **B.** Mentation assessment
[ ] **C.** Peripheral sensation exam
[ ] **D.** Visual acuity assessment

Correct answer—B. *Rationales:* In clients with dementia, the most commonly lost cognitive ability is memory. Mentation assessment includes memory (recent and remote), problem-solving capability, and calculation exercises. Gait function assessment may indicate other disorders. Although visual acuity and peripheral sensation are part of a comprehensive neurological assessment, they don't provide specific information for clients with dementia.
Nursing process step: Assessment

71. A 70-year-old client presents to the emergency department with a history of hypertension and high cholesterol. He reports that this morning he couldn't move the right side of his body. Currently, the client is able to move all limbs with no detectable weakness. The nurse expects to emergently:
[ ] **A.** transport the client to computed tomography (CT) scan.
[ ] **B.** transport the client to ultrasound.
[ ] **C.** discharge the client to home because his symptoms have resolved.
[ ] **D.** transport the client to X-ray.

Correct answer—A. *Rationales:* A CT scan will be done to evaluate for the presence of bleeding or old infarction. An ultrasound would be done as part of the inpatient workup for carotid artery atherosclerosis. Discharging the patient to home is not an option until further evaluation to determine the cause. X-ray is not indicated for this patient who is experiencing neuro symptoms.
Nursing process step: Intervention

72. Medications that are prescribed for clients with transient ischemic attacks should include:
[ ] **A.** statins.
[ ] **B.** antihypertensive medications.
[ ] **C.** platelet inhibitors.
[ ] **D.** all of the above.

Correct answer—D. *Rationales:* The increased risk of a stroke after a transient ischemic attack can be modified with tight blood pressure control, cholesterol lowering, and initiation of antiplatelet therapy. Two common platelet-inhibiting agents include aspirin and clopidogrel.
Nursing process step: Analysis

73. A client's wife asks the nurse what risks are associated with a transient ischemic attack (TIA). The nurse replies that:
[ ] **A.** there are no additional risks.
[ ] **B.** there's an increased risk of stroke.
[ ] **C.** there's an increased risk of bleeding.
[ ] **D.** there's an increased risk of panic attacks.

Correct answer—B. *Rationales:* Research shows that 10% to 15% of people who have a TIA have a major stroke within 3 months. This information is important to teach families to emphasize the importance of pharmacotherapy adherence and follow-up. Educating the client and family on additional risks is essential. TIAs are not assocaited with increased risk of bleeding or panic attacks.
Nursing process step: Analysis

74. A client presents to the emergency department with complaints of visual field loss. He has a history of transient ischemic attack (TIA) the previous month. The nurse would triage the client as:
[ ] **A.** emergent due to his risk of stroke.
[ ] **B.** emergent due to his risk of retinal detachment.
[ ] **C.** urgent due to his risk of cataracts.
[ ] **D.** urgent due to his risk of glaucoma.

Correct answer—A. *Rationales:* The client who has had a TIA is at increased risk of stroke and should be triaged as emergent. Retinal detachment results in a loss of vision described as a curtain over the eye. Cataracts and glaucoma cause blurred vision and decreased visual acuity, rather than field cuts.
Nursing process step: Assessment

75. A client presents with hemiplegia that started 1 hour before presentation. A computed tomography scan of the head is negative, and the physician has ordered TPA (tissue plasminogen activator). The nurse knows that the maximum dose of TPA is:
[ ] **A.** 100 mg.
[ ] **B.** 80 mg.
[ ] **C.** 90 mg.
[ ] **D.** None of the above; there's no maximum because the dosage is based on weight.

Correct answer–C. *Rationales:* TPA is administered as a weight-based dose of 0.9 mg/kg with a maximum of 90 mg regardless of whether the weight is more than 100 kg.
Nursing process step: Intervention

76. Prior to initiating the TPA (tissue plasminogen activator) infusion for a client who has had an ischemic stroke, the nurse knows that the systolic blood pressure must be:
[ ] **A.** above 120.
[ ] **B.** below 180.
[ ] **C.** above 170.
[ ] **D.** below 205

Correct answer–B. *Rationales:* According to the stroke guidelines for care, a systolic blood pressure above 180 requires treatment prior to the initiation of TPA. A systolic blood pressure that remains above 185 is a contraindication to TPA initiation. Uncontrolled hypertension increases the risk of intracranial bleeding.
Nursing process step: Assessment

77. The physician may order all of the following for blood pressure control prior to and during the ischemic stroke client's TPA (tissue plasminogen activator) infusion except:
[ ] **A.** nicardipine.
[ ] **B.** nitroglycerin.
[ ] **C.** Labetalol.
[ ] **D.** Cardizem.

Correct answer–D. *Rationales:* Cardizem is typically used to treat tachycardia, such as that associated with atrial fibrillation with a fast ventricular rate. Nicardipine, nitroglycerin, and labetalol are all agents used to reduce blood pressure in ischemic stroke.
Nursing process step: Intervention

78. Prior to administering any food or medications to the client who has droop drift and dysarthria associated with an ischemic stroke, the nurse should assess the client's:
[ ] **A.** ability to follow commands.
[ ] **B.** ability to walk.
[ ] **C.** ability to think.
[ ] **D.** ability to swallow.

Correct answer–D. *Rationales:* The client's ability to swallow should be assessed prior to administering anything by mouth when ischemic stroke is diagnosed. This is accomplished first by performing a dysphagia screen. If the dysphagia screen is failed, then the client is kept on nothing-by-mouth status and speech therapy is requested for further testing.
Nursing process step: Assessment

79. If an ischemic stroke client is receiving TPA (tissue plasminogen activator) infusion and starts to vomit bright red blood, the nurse should:
[ ] **A.** notify the physician.
[ ] **B.** place a nasogastric tube.
[ ] **C.** decrease the infusion.
[ ] **D.** stop the infusion.

Correct answer–D. *Rationales:* TPA is a fibrinolytic that decreases the client's ability to clot. The infusion should be stopped immediately. While a client is receiving TPA, all invasive procedures should be avoided due to the increased risk of bleeding. Ninety percent of the infusion infuses over 59 minutes and 10% is given as a bolus over 1 minute.
Nursing process step: Analysis

80. A client who can understand commands but can't speak is described as having:
[ ] **A.** receptive aphasia.
[ ] **B.** expressive aphasia.
[ ] **C.** global aphasia.
[ ] **D.** apraxia.

Correct answer–B. *Rationales:* Expressive aphasia is the inability to speak. Receptive aphasia is the inability to understand, global aphasia is the inability to speak or understand, and apraxia is the inability to remember the purpose or function of an object.
Nursing process step: Analysis

81. The nurse knows that the National Institutes of Health Stroke Scale (NIHSS) can be linked to outcomes. The higher the score, then:

[ ] **A.** the better the outcome.
[ ] **B.** the better the orientation level.
[ ] **C.** the more risk factors for stroke.
[ ] **D.** the poorer the outcome.

Correct answer–D. *Rationales:* The NIHSS assesses the client's level of consciousness, orientation, response to commands, gaze, visual fields, facial movement, motor function, limb ataxia, sensory, language, articulation, and extinction. The higher the score, then the more deficits that are present and the worse the outcome.

Nursing process step: Analysis

82. A 55-year-old client presents complaining of a headache over his left temple area. He also reports that he was unable to comb his hair this morning because the comb hurt his scalp. He has never had a headache like this in the past. He denies recent trauma. The nurse should suspect:

[ ] **A.** cluster headache.
[ ] **B.** migraine.
[ ] **C.** subarachnoid hemorrhage.
[ ] **D.** temporal arteritis.

Correct answer–D. *Rationales:* Based on the American College of Rheumatology guidelines, temporal arteritis usually occurs as a new headache in clients older than age 50 and is accompanied by temporal artery tenderness. The superficial temporal artery supplies the scalp. Cluster headaches are usually chronic. Migraine headaches commonly have associated nausea. Subarachnoid hemorrhage usually follows trauma.

Nursing process step: Analysis

83. A client with temporal arteritis should be prescribed:

[ ] **A.** steroids.
[ ] **B.** anticonvulsants.
[ ] **C.** muscle relaxants.
[ ] **D.** antihistamines.

Correct answer–A. *Rationales:* Oral steroids are an effective treatment for temporal arteritis. If any visual deficits are noted, steroids should be administered I.V. The client will require a thorough physical exam. An erythrocyte sedimentation rate (ESR) may be done and would reveal an ESR greater than 80. The definitive diagnosis is made by temporal artery biopsy.

Nursing process step: Intervention

9 Obstetric emergencies

1. A client complains of abdominal pain. Her last menstrual period was 8 weeks ago. Which type of pain is usually associated with a ruptured ectopic pregnancy?

[ ] **A.** Lower quadrant pain radiating to the shoulder
[ ] **B.** Sharp upper abdominal pain
[ ] **C.** Flank pain
[ ] **D.** Colicky, diffuse abdominal pain

Correct answer—A. *Rationales:* Ectopic pregnancies that are leaking or have ruptured result in referred pain to the shoulder from blood irritating the diaphragm. Sharp upper abdominal pain is too high for pain caused by an ectopic pregnancy. Flank pain may be associated with kidney infection or kidney stones. Colicky, diffuse abdominal pain is commonly associated with intestinal disorders.
Nursing process step: Assessment

2. A client in her 34th week of pregnancy comes to the emergency department and complains of sudden onset of bright red vaginal bleeding. Her uterus is soft, and she's experiencing no pain. Fetal heart tones are 120 beats/minute. Based on this history, the nurse should suspect which condition?

[ ] **A.** Abruptio placentae
[ ] **B.** Preterm labor
[ ] **C.** Placenta previa
[ ] **D.** Threatened abortion

Correct answer—C. *Rationales:* Placenta previa is associated with painless vaginal bleeding that occurs when the placenta, or a portion of the placenta, covers the cervical os. In abruptio placentae, the placenta tears away from the wall of the uterus before delivery; the client usually has pain and a boardlike uterus. Preterm labor is associated with contractions and shouldn't involve bright red bleeding. By definition, threatened abortion occurs during the first 20 weeks of gestation.
Nursing process step: Analysis

3. After a fall down a flight of stairs, a client in her 38th week of pregnancy is brought to the emergency department. Unless contraindicated, she should be placed in which position during assessment?

[ ] **A.** Trendelenburg's
[ ] **B.** Flat on her back
[ ] **C.** Left lateral recumbent
[ ] **D.** Knee-chest

Correct answer—C. *Rationales:* The left lateral recumbent position avoids compression of the inferior vena cava; compressing the vessel may result in decreased uterine blood flow, fetal hypoxia, and maternal hypotension. Trendelenburg's or the flat position would compress this vessel. If a pregnant client must lie flat on a backboard for cervical spine evaluation, a wedge may be placed under the right hip to avoid compressing the vessel. If the umbilical cord is prolapsed, the knee-chest position may be used to avoid compressing the cord.
Nursing process step: Intervention

4. Which intervention is considered inappropriate for a client with placenta previa?

[ ] **A.** Performing a pelvic examination to determine the extent of dilatation

[ ] **B.** Maintaining strict bed rest and observing for further bleeding

[ ] **C.** Monitoring for signs of shock

[ ] **D.** Preparing the client for pelvic ultrasound

Correct answer—A. *Rationales:* A pelvic examination shouldn't be performed on a pregnant client with vaginal bleeding. In cases of placenta previa, the examination could cause further bleeding and damage the placenta. A client with placenta previa should be placed on bed rest and pad count and be monitored for signs of shock if bleeding is heavy and persists. A pelvic ultrasound is useful for detecting placenta previa. The client's bladder should be filled using an indwelling urinary catheter rather than by mouth if cesarean birth is planned or if it's suspected she may require cesarean delivery. In most cases, bed rest and pelvic rest stop the bleeding in a client with placenta previa.

Nursing process step: Intervention

5. A client with pregnancy-associated hypertension probably exhibits which symptoms?

[ ] **A.** Proteinuria, headaches, and vaginal bleeding

[ ] **B.** Headaches, double vision, and vaginal bleeding

[ ] **C.** Proteinuria, headaches, and double vision

[ ] **D.** Proteinuria, double vision, and uterine contractions

Correct answer—C. *Rationales:* A client with pregnancy-associated hypertension complains of headache, double vision, and sudden weight gain. A urine specimen reveals proteinuria. Vaginal bleeding and uterine contractions aren't associated with pregnancy-associated hypertension.

Nursing process step: Assessment

6. A pregnant client arrives in the emergency department and states, "My baby is coming." The nurse sees a portion of the umbilical cord protruding from the vagina. Why should manual pressure be applied to the baby's head?

[ ] **A.** To slow the delivery process

[ ] **B.** To reinsert the umbilical cord

[ ] **C.** To relieve pressure on the umbilical cord

[ ] **D.** To rupture the membranes

Correct answer—C. *Rationales:* Manual pressure is applied to the baby's head by gently pushing up with the fingers to relieve pressure on the umbilical cord. This intervention is effective if the cord begins to pulsate. The mother may also be placed in the knee-chest or Trendelenburg position to ensure blood flow to the baby. Applying manual pressure isn't done to slow the delivery process. A prolapsed cord necessitates an emergency cesarean birth. The nurse shouldn't attempt to reinsert the umbilical cord because this would further compromise blood flow. At this point, the membranes are probably ruptured.

Nursing process step: Evaluation

7. Delivery of an infant is imminent in the emergency department. Meconium is noted in the amniotic fluid. Upon delivery, the neonate is limp and not responding to stimuli. What action should be taken first upon delivery?

[ ] **A.** Stimulation of the neonate

[ ] **B.** Suctioning of the oropharynx and the nasopharynx

[ ] **C.** Endotracheal (ET) intubation with suction applied to the ET tube

[ ] **D.** Placement of an umbilical line

Correct answer—C. *Rationales:* Meconium-stained amniotic fluid can be an emergency for the neonate; therefore, ET intubation with suction applied to the ET tube should be performed. Stimulating the neonate will only cause more amniotic-stained fluid to enter the lungs. It's no longer recommended to routinely perform oropharynx and nasopharynx suctioning for neonates born to mothers with meconium-stained amniotic fluid. Placing an umbilical line isn't necessary at this time.

Nursing process step: Intervention

8. A client in her 34th week of pregnancy presents to the emergency department. Her blood pressure is 180/110 mm Hg, and she complains of headache and blurred vision. During treatment of this client, the nurse should be prepared for which complication?

[ ] **A.** Precipitous delivery
[ ] **B.** Vaginal bleeding
[ ] **C.** Cardiac arrhythmias
[ ] **D.** Seizure activity

Correct answer—D. *Rationales:* These are symptoms of pregnancy-associated hypertension; the client has a potential for seizure activity because of central nervous system irritability. Seizure precautions should be instituted. Precipitous delivery, vaginal bleeding, and cardiac arrhythmias aren't complications of pregnancy-associated hypertension.
Nursing process step: Evaluation

9. Postpartum hemorrhage can occur immediately after delivery or can be delayed as much as 6 weeks. Which of the following is *not* a cause of postpartum hemorrhage?

[ ] **A.** Retained products of conception
[ ] **B.** Vaginal or cervical tear
[ ] **C.** Absent decrease in uterine size
[ ] **D.** Amniotic fluid embolism

Correct answer—D. *Rationales:* Postpartum hemorrhage is defined as blood loss greater than 500 ml and is a common complication of labor and delivery. Amniotic fluid embolism, a complication experienced by the mother, is caused when amniotic fluid leaks into the mother's venous circulation during labor and delivery. It doesn't cause postpartum hemorrhage. Retained products of conception or placental fragments can interfere with involution (absent decrease in the size of the uterus). Vaginal or cervical tears can be a cause of postpartum bleeding.
Nursing process step: Analysis

10. Which of the following indicates imminent delivery?

[ ] **A.** Need to bear down by the mother
[ ] **B.** Rupture of membranes
[ ] **C.** Loss of mucus plug
[ ] **D.** Lengthening of contractions

Correct answer—A. *Rationales:* The desire to bear down or push usually indicates that delivery is near (especially in the multiparous mother). Other signs of imminent delivery are heavy bloody show and a bulging perineum. Rupture of membranes may occur before labor begins. Loss of the mucus plug is likely to occur at the beginning of labor. Lengthening of contractions doesn't necessarily indicate that delivery is imminent.
Nursing process step: Assessment

11. A pregnant trauma client should be assessed for:

[ ] **A.** uterine contractions, vaginal bleeding or ruptured membranes, and fetal heart tones.
[ ] **B.** uterine contractions and vaginal bleeding or ruptured membranes.
[ ] **C.** fetal heart tones and fetal position.
[ ] **D.** uterine contractions, fetal heart tones, and fetal position.

Correct answer—A. *Rationales:* All pregnant trauma clients should be assessed for uterine contractions. A fetal monitor may be applied, or the uterus may be palpated for tone. Observe for vaginal bleeding and ruptured membranes. Fetal heart tones should be part of the vital signs for all pregnant women and may be auscultated with a Doppler stethoscope after about 14 weeks' gestation. Normal fetal heart tones are 120 to 160 beats/minute. It isn't necessary to assess for fetal position at this time.
Nursing process step: Assessment

12. During neonatal resuscitation immediately after delivery, chest compressions should be initiated when the heart rate falls below:

[ ] **A.** 60 beats/minute.
[ ] **B.** 80 beats/minute.
[ ] **C.** 100 beats/minute.
[ ] **D.** 110 beats/minute.

Correct answer—A. *Rationales:* The normal neonatal heart rate is 120 to 160 beats/minute. Heart rates below 60 beats/minute necessitate chest compressions and ventilatory support.
Nursing process step: Intervention

13. The nurse should determine an Apgar score on the neonate at 1 minute and again at 5 minutes. The nurse assesses which parameters?
[ ] **A.** Heart rate, muscle tone, reflexes, respiratory effort, and color
[ ] **B.** Heart rate, temperature, reflexes, respiratory effort, and color
[ ] **C.** Heart rate, muscle tone, weight, respiratory effort, and color
[ ] **D.** Heart rate, muscle tone, reflexes, respiratory effort, and swallowing ability

Correct answer—A. *Rationales:* The Apgar score should be determined at 1 and 5 minutes and should include an assessment of heart rate, muscle tone, reflexes, respiratory effort, and color. A score of 7 to 10 is favorable.
Nursing process step: Assessment

14. What's the most common risk factor for an ectopic pregnancy?
[ ] **A.** Pelvic inflammatory disease (PID)
[ ] **B.** Spontaneous abortion
[ ] **C.** Fertility difficulties
[ ] **D.** Multiple pregnancies

Correct answer—A. *Rationales:* Ectopic pregnancies are typically related to scarring secondary to PID. Spontaneous abortion and multiple pregnancies aren't associated with this condition. Scarring from PID may also result in fertility difficulties.
Nursing process step: Assessment

15. A client in her 36th week of pregnancy arrives in the emergency department complaining of a severe headache. Vital signs are blood pressure, 180/112 mm Hg; pulse, 114 beats/minute; respirations, 22 breaths/minute; and temperature, 98.9° F (37.2° C). The nurse should first prepare for:
[ ] **A.** the possibility of seizure activity.
[ ] **B.** endotracheal (ET) intubation.
[ ] **C.** immediate delivery.
[ ] **D.** emergency cesarean birth.

Correct answer—A. *Rationales:* This client is exhibiting signs and symptoms of pregnancy-associated hypertension, thereby indicating that she's at risk for developing seizure activity. Other manifestations may include proteinuria, edema, epigastric pain, and blurred vision. ET intubation would be needed only if the client developed status epilepticus or became unresponsive. This client isn't about to deliver. A cesarean birth may be indicated if the client is unstable and doesn't quickly respond to treatment. Birth is the definitive treatment for pregnancy-associated hypertension.
Nursing process step: Intervention

16. A client arrives in the emergency department stating, "The baby is coming." Which condition most likely indicates imminent delivery?
[ ] **A.** Ruptured membranes
[ ] **B.** Dilation of the cervix to 7 cm
[ ] **C.** A bulging perineum
[ ] **D.** Braxton Hicks contractions

Correct answer—C. *Rationales:* A bulging perineum indicates that the head is far down into the vagina and delivery is imminent. Ruptured membranes can occur before labor begins. The cervix must be dilated to 10 cm before the client can begin pushing. Braxton Hicks contractions are typically referred to as "false contractions."
Nursing process step: Assessment

17. A client in her 32nd week of pregnancy comes to the emergency department complaining of sudden onset of bright red vaginal bleeding. She isn't complaining of pain. Based on these symptoms, the nurse should suspect:
[ ] **A.** placenta previa.
[ ] **B.** abruptio placentae.
[ ] **C.** preterm labor.
[ ] **D.** threatened abortion.

Correct answer—A. *Rationales:* Painless vaginal bleeding is usually indicative of placenta previa, in which the placenta partially or totally covers the cervical os. In placenta abruptio, the placenta comes away from the wall of the uterus before delivery. With placental abruption, the client usually experiences pain and a boardlike abdomen. Preterm labor may or may not be associated with vaginal bleeding. A client who's 32 weeks' pregnant wouldn't be having a threatened abortion.
Nursing process step: Assessment

18. What should the nurse remember to do when suctioning a neonate's airway at the time of delivery?
[ ] **A.** Use a bulb syringe to suction the nares first.
[ ] **B.** Use a bulb syringe to suction the oral pharynx first.
[ ] **C.** Use a bulb syringe only if the neonate experiences respiratory distress.
[ ] **D.** Lower the neonate's head to assist drainage of fluid.

Correct answer–B. *Rationales:* Suction the mouth first, then the nose. The bulb syringe is used in all instances. The neonate's head should be kept level with the rest of the body.
Nursing process step: Intervention

19. What should the nurse do during delivery of the neonate's head?
[ ] **A.** Instruct the mother to bear down.
[ ] **B.** Instruct the mother to pant and apply gentle pressure to the perineum.
[ ] **C.** Instruct the mother to push for a count of 10.
[ ] **D.** Apply fundal pressure to assist with delivery.

Correct answer–B. *Rationales:* Risk of perineal tears is increased if the mother pushes at the moment of delivery. Having the mother pant while applying gentle pressure to the perineum decreases the risk of tears. Fundal pressure isn't necessary and may cause damage to the uterus.
Nursing process step: Intervention

20. A trauma client who's 36 weeks pregnant is brought to the emergency department in full spinal immobilization. She was involved in a one-car motor vehicle accident. She states that she was wearing her seat belt, and the paramedics who transported her reported minor damage to her car. What should the nurse do next?
[ ] **A.** Place the client in Trendelenburg's position.
[ ] **B.** Remove the client from spinal immobilization.
[ ] **C.** Tilt the client to the left side.
[ ] **D.** Tilt the client to the right side.

Correct answer–C. *Rationales:* The client should be tilted to the left side to relieve pressure on the aorta by the gravid uterus. Trendelenburg's position is contraindicated in this client. Tilting to the right side is preferable to lying flat, but not as beneficial as tilting to the left. It's never appropriate to remove spinal immobilization until the cervical spine has been cleared.
Nursing process step: Intervention

10 Ocular emergencies

1. Conjunctivitis may be caused by bacteria, viruses, allergens, and irritants. Which characteristics differentiate bacterial conjunctivitis from other types?

[ ] **A.** Subacute onset, severe pain, and preauricular adenopathy

[ ] **B.** Recurrent onset without pain with no clear discharge

[ ] **C.** Acute onset, moderate pain, and purulent discharge

[ ] **D.** Acute onset, mild pain, and clear discharge

Correct answer—C. *Rationales:* Bacterial conjunctivitis has an acute onset, moderate pain, copious purulent discharge, and preauricular adenopathy. Viral conjunctivitis has an acute or a subacute onset, mild to moderate pain, and moderate and seropurulent discharge; preauricular adenopathy is common. Allergic conjunctivitis has a recurrent onset, no pain, moderate clear discharge, and no preauricular adenopathy. Irritant conjunctivitis has acute onset, no pain to mild pain, minimal clear discharge, and rarely, preauricular adenopathy.

Nursing process step: Assessment

2. On evaluation of the effectiveness of therapy for conjunctivitis, which finding indicates the need for further treatment?

[ ] **A.** Pain in eye is relieved.

[ ] **B.** Preauricular adenopathy is decreased.

[ ] **C.** Purulent discharge is resolved.

[ ] **D.** Both eyes have purulent discharge.

Correct answer—D. *Rationales:* A client who now has bilateral involvement needs further therapy. After effective treatment for conjunctivitis, eye pain should be relieved, the preauricular adenopathy should be decreased or resolved, and purulent discharge should be absent. Client education on disease transmission and method for cleaning the eye is needed.

Nursing process step: Evaluation

3. Which of the following is the treatment of choice for a client with iritis?

[ ] **A.** Instill topical decongestants, 1 drop three to four times daily.

[ ] **B.** Instill prednisolone (PredForte) and tropicamide (Mydriacyl) to the affected eye.

[ ] **C.** Administer erythromycin (Ilotycin Ophthalmic Ointment).

[ ] **D.** Refer the client immediately to an ophthalmologist.

Correct answer—B. *Rationales:* Iritis is treated with prednisolone to reduce inflammation (five times daily) and tropicamide to reduce ciliary muscle spasm (1 to 2 drops, repeated in 5 minutes if necessary). Topical decongestants and antibiotics are used in the treatment of bacterial conjunctivitis. Referral to an ophthalmologist generally isn't necessary in the treatment of iritis.

Nursing process step: Intervention

4. Central retinal artery occlusion from a blockage of the artery by a thrombus or an embolus is a true ocular emergency. Which of the following is the most definitive assessment finding?

[ ] **A.** Sudden unilateral loss of vision without pain

[ ] **B.** Pupil small but reactive

[ ] **C.** Decreased visual acuity with sudden onset of severe pain

[ ] **D.** Increased intraocular pressure

Correct answer—A. *Rationales:* Central retinal artery occlusion presents with a sudden, painless unilateral loss of vision. Light perception is all that remains in the affected eye. The pupil is dilated and nonreactive. Glaucoma occurs with sudden onset of severe pain, diminished vision, semidilated and nonreactive pupils, and increased intraocular pressure.

Nursing process step: Assessment

5. A 67-year-old man comes to the emergency department with a sudden onset of blindness in his right eye. He denies pain in the affected eye and also reports having similar episodes over the past couple of days; however, in those cases his vision returned. Based on these assessment findings, what would the nurse suspect?

[ ] **A.** Orbital cellulitis
[ ] **B.** Glaucoma
[ ] **C.** Retinal detachment
[ ] **D.** Central retinal artery occlusion

Correct answer—D. *Rationales:* Central retinal artery occlusion results from a sudden painless blindness, usually in one eye. The vision loss may be transient in nature. Orbital cellulitis is an infection of the orbital septum and may cause vision loss but doesn't cause sudden blindness. Glaucoma causes gradual loss of vision, not sudden blindness. Retinal detachment causes a sudden flash of light in one or both eyes or a shadow or curtain over a portion of the visual field but doesn't cause sudden blindness.
Nursing process step: Analysis

6. A client is admitted to the emergency department complaining of pain, photophobia, and blurred vision after falling asleep with his contact lenses in place. Which of the following is the most appropriate intervention?

[ ] **A.** Apply an eye patch.
[ ] **B.** Administer topical anesthetics.
[ ] **C.** Instill nonsteroidal antiinflammatory (NSAID) drops.
[ ] **D.** Instill ophthalmic corticosteroid ointment.

Correct answer—C. *Rationales:* The most appropriate intervention is to instill NSAID drops. The client may require instillation of ophthalmic antibiotic ointment; however, the ointment shouldn't contain a corticosteroid, which would increase the risk of infection. Topical anesthetics may lead to irreversible corneal damage and should never be administered. Studies show that eye patching doesn't speed healing or reduce pain. It may actually increase client discomfort and has been found to interfere with the client's ability to participate in routine activities.
Nursing process step: Intervention

7. Severe cases of corneal abrasion present with which condition?

[ ] **A.** Loss of vision and excessive tearing
[ ] **B.** Corneal surface irregularity and loss of luster
[ ] **C.** Redness and purulent discharge
[ ] **D.** Pupil dilated and nonreactive

Correct answer—B. *Rationales:* Severe corneal abrasions present with corneal surface irregularity and loss of luster. Tearing is common; however, vision is only blurred, not lost. Redness without purulent discharge is also a common finding. The pupils are of normal size and reactivity, unless eyedrops are used for examination and relief of severe pain.
Nursing process step: Assessment

8. A client arrives in the emergency department complaining of pain; he states that something is in his right eye. He had been working under his car. What important information should the nurse obtain before intervention?

[ ] **A.** Allergies to medications
[ ] **B.** Medical history
[ ] **C.** History of diabetes insipitus
[ ] **D.** Surgical history

Correct answer—A. *Rationales:* A client with a lidocaine allergy may be allergic to the medications administered to anesthetize the eye. Many medications have cross-reactivity with drugs commonly used for the examination and treatment of eye injuries. Atropine is also commonly used for eye examination and can worsen glaucoma, not diabetes insipitus. Both a medical and surgical history are necessary, but obtaining information on allergies takes priority.
Nursing process step: Assessment

9. What's the priority in the care of a client with a foreign object in his eye?

[ ] **A.** Irrigate the eye with sterile normal saline.
[ ] **B.** Instill ophthalmic antibiotic ointment.
[ ] **C.** Anesthetize the cornea with proparacaine (Ophthaine).
[ ] **D.** Manually remove foreign bodies before irrigation.

Correct answer—C. *Rationales:* The priority in caring for a client with an extraocular foreign body is to relieve pain with an anesthetic, such as proparacaine or tetracaine solution. Anesthetizing the eye allows for a more comfortable inspection and irrigation with normal saline. Ophthalmic antibiotic ointments are used after the foreign body is removed. If the foreign body isn't removed with irrigation, it should be removed manually.
Nursing process step: Intervention

10. A 58-year-old man was cutting down trees in his yard when a piece of wood flew into his right eye. The eye is red, tearing, and painful. Visual acuity is normal. Upon examination of the eye, small corneal abrasions are noted. What is the priority discharge instruction for this client?

[ ] **A.** Application of topical antibiotics
[ ] **B.** Removal of the wood fragments
[ ] **C.** Eye patch application
[ ] **D.** Routine eye irrigation

Correct answer–A. *Rationales:* The primary discharge instruction for this client is how to apply the topical antibiotics that have been prescribed in order to prevent secondary infection. Eye patch application may also be indicated, but it isn't the primary discharge instruction. Removal of wood fragments and routine eye irrigation should be avoided in order to prevent further damage and irritation.
Nursing process step: Intervention

11. The client is given discharge instructions regarding an extraocular foreign body. Which statement by the client indicates an understanding of the discharge instructions?

[ ] **A.** "I can save the topical anesthetic to use in the future."
[ ] **B.** "I'll wear safety glasses in the future when I am working on my car."
[ ] **C.** "I'll need to see my physician in a week."
[ ] **D.** "I can wear my contact lenses now that the foreign body is removed."

Correct answer–B. *Rationales:* Discharge instructions should include client education regarding prevention and safety issues. Although topical anesthetics effectively eliminate pain, they shouldn't be sent home with a client because they can mask complications of the injury and increase eye damage. Oral analgesia should be prescribed for the client instead. The client should schedule follow-up care with an ophthalmologist within 24 to 48 hours, at which time he can discuss resumption of contact lens use.
Nursing process step: Evaluation

12. Signs and symptoms of retinal detachment include all of the following except:

[ ] **A.** painless decrease in vision.
[ ] **B.** curtain or veil over visual field.
[ ] **C.** increased intraocular pressure.
[ ] **D.** flashing lights.

Correct answer–C. *Rationales:* A client with retinal detachment has a painless decrease in vision and indicates that vision is cloudy or smoky with flashing lights. The client may also indicate that a curtain or veil is over the visual field. Intraocular pressure is normal or low.
Nursing process step: Assessment

13. Which of the following is the primary intervention for a client with retinal detachment?

[ ] **A.** He should be admitted to the hospital on strict bed rest.
[ ] **B.** Both of the client's eyes should be patched.
[ ] **C.** The client should be referred to an ophthalmologist.
[ ] **D.** He should be prepared for emergency surgery.

Correct answer–A. *Rationales:* Immediate bed rest is necessary to prevent further injury. Both eyes may be patched, and the client should receive early referral to an ophthalmologist. If the macula is attached and central visual acuity is normal, the condition should be urgently treated by an ophthalmologist. Retinal reattachment can be accomplished by surgery only. If the macula is detached or threatened, surgery is urgent; prolonged detachment of the macula results in permanent loss of central vision.
Nursing process step: Intervention

14. Which of the following is the initial intervention for a client with a chemical burn of the eye?
[ ] **A.** Patch the affected eye and call the ophthalmologist.
[ ] **B.** Administer a cycloplegic agent to reduce ciliary spasm.
[ ] **C.** Immediately instill a topical anesthetic; then irrigate with copious amounts of normal saline.
[ ] **D.** Administer antibiotics to reduce the chance of infection.

Correct answer–C. *Rationales:* The initial intervention for a chemical burn is to instill a topical anesthetic; immediately, then irrigate the eye with copious amounts of normal saline. Irrigation should be done for at least 15 minutes; then the pH of the eye should be checked. Irrigation should be continued until the pH of the eye reaches 7.0. Double eversion of the eyelids should be performed to look for and remove material lodged in the cul-de-sac. A cycloplegic agent can then be used to reduce ciliary spasm, and an antibiotic ointment can be administered to reduce the risk of infection. Chemical burns are contraindications for patching due to risk that the chemical agent hasn't thoroughly lavaged from the eye. Parenteral narcotic analgesia is usually required for pain relief. An ophthalmologist should also be consulted.
Nursing process step: Intervention

15. Which of the following indicates successful treatment of a chemical burn to the eye?
[ ] **A.** Eye pH of 7.8
[ ] **B.** Evidence of corneal opacity
[ ] **C.** Evidence of decreased visual acuity
[ ] **D.** Relief of pain

Correct answer–D. *Rationales:* Pain is a common complaint with chemical burns to the eye. The client stating that the pain is relieved signifies successful treatment. The normal pH of the eye is 6.9 to 7.2. Improved vision would be indicated by normal visual acuity and no evidence of corneal opacity.
Nursing process step: Evaluation

16. A client is admitted to the emergency department after blunt trauma to the right eye. The client complains of blurred and blood-tinged vision. The nurse's assessment reveals blood in the eye. Which of the following is the most likely type of eye injury?
[ ] **A.** Hyphema
[ ] **B.** Retinal detachment
[ ] **C.** Globe rupture
[ ] **D.** Orbital fracture

Correct answer–A. *Rationales:* The most frequent symptoms of hyphema include impaired visual acuity, blood visualized in the anterior chamber of the eye, and blood tinged vision. Globe ruptures present with decreased visual acuity, shallow anterior chamber, irregularities in pupillary borders, and decreased intraocular pressure. In retinal detachment, the client complains of smoky or cloudy vision, flashing lights, and a curtain or veil over the visual field. Orbital fractures produce alterations in extraocular movement of the affected eye, paresthesia of the lip, crepitus over the fracture site, and periorbital edema.
Nursing process step: Assessment

17. The threat of a secondary bleed occurring in 3 to 5 days is a significant risk in the client with hyphema. Which of the following is an indication of successful prevention of rebleeding?
[ ] **A.** Blood only in the inferior portion of the anterior chamber
[ ] **B.** Improved peripheral vision
[ ] **C.** Blood found only in posterior portion of posterior chamber
[ ] **D.** Blood found only in posterior portion of anterior chamber

Correct answer–A. *Rationales:* Improved visual acuity, decreased blurred vision, and blood found only in the inferior portion of the anterior chamber are signs of improvement. Improved peripheral vision doesn't improve with prevention of rebleeding.
Nursing process step: Evaluation

18. A laceration of the eyelid commonly causes the inability to:
[ ] **A.** raise the upper lid.
[ ] **B.** close the affected eye.
[ ] **C.** look upward or downward with the affected eye.
[ ] **D.** look outward or inward with the affected eye.

Correct answer—A. *Rationales:* A deep laceration to the eyelid usually involves the levator muscle. As a result, the client can't raise the upper lid of the affected eye. In addition, the eye is generally swollen shut, so extraocular movement, which shouldn't be affected, can't be assessed. Orbital fracture can cause loss of extraocular movement and result in an inability to look upward or downward with the affected eye.
Nursing process step: Assessment

19. After blunt trauma to the eye, a client arrives in the emergency department. The client exhibits abnormal extraocular movement, paresthesia of the lip, periorbital edema and ecchymosis, and subconjunctival hemorrhage. Which disorder is most consistent with these assessment findings?
[ ] **A.** Globe rupture
[ ] **B.** Orbital fracture
[ ] **C.** Retinal detachment
[ ] **D.** Eyelid laceration

Correct answer—B. *Rationales:* Orbital fracture occurs after blunt trauma and causes crepitus at the fracture site, paresthesia of the lip, abnormal extraocular movements, subconjunctival hemorrhage, and periorbital edema and ecchymosis. A globe rupture presents with irregularity of pupillary borders, decreased visual acuity, decreased intraocular pressure, and shallow anterior chamber. An eyelid laceration has periorbital edema and bleeding. Retinal detachment has specific visual alterations that include flashes of light, floating black spots, and curtain-like defects that result in decreased peripheral vision.
Nursing process step: Assessment

20. Which intervention is appropriate for a client with an orbital fracture?
[ ] **A.** Heat to the affected eye
[ ] **B.** Analgesics to relieve pain
[ ] **C.** Facial view X-rays
[ ] **D.** I.V. fluids

Correct answer—B. *Rationales:* Ice, not heat, to the affected orbit decreases swelling. Analgesics relieve pain and reduce anxiety. Both orbital and facial view X-rays should be done to verify the extent of fractures. An otolaryngologist and an ophthalmologist should be consulted before the client is discharged from the emergency department (ED). A client with orbital floor or rim fractures with no limitation of ocular mobility and without associated injury of the globe that doesn't require I.V. fluids may be discharged from the ED and referred to an otolaryngologist to be seen in a few days.
Nursing process step: Intervention

21. Which signs or symptoms should the nurse expect to see with a penetrating injury to the eye?
[ ] **A.** Irregular pupillary borders
[ ] **B.** Normal visual acuity
[ ] **C.** Increased intraocular pressure
[ ] **D.** Redness and purulent drainage

Correct answer—A. *Rationales:* A client with a globe rupture has usually had a penetrating injury, and the foreign body can usually be seen in the anterior chamber. The borders of the pupils are irregular. Other signs and symptoms include decreased visual acuity, shallow anterior chamber, and decreased intraocular pressure. Redness and purulent drainage from an eye usually means conjunctivitis.
Nursing process step: Assessment

22. When caring for a client with a penetrating eye injury, the nurse should be sure to perform which intervention?

[ ] **A.** Open the eye to search for a foreign body.
[ ] **B.** Position the client in a supine position.
[ ] **C.** Patch the injured eye lightly.
[ ] **D.** Administer analgesics as prescribed.

Correct answer—D. *Rationales:* If a client is believed to have a globe rupture, the eye shouldn't be opened. The client should be placed in semi-Fowler's position to maintain reduced intraocular pressure. All pressure on or around the injured eye should be avoided to prevent extrusion of intraocular contents. The eye should be protected with a rigid shield. If a shield isn't available, the bottom of a Styrofoam cup works well. Pain can be minimal to severe; therefore, the client should be assessed and analgesics administered as needed. An ophthalmologist should be consulted.
Nursing process step: Intervention

23. Chemical burns constitute a true ocular emergency. Which assessment findings are consistent with a chemical burn?

[ ] **A.** Corneal whitening
[ ] **B.** Dilated, nonreactive pupils
[ ] **C.** Redness and purulent discharge
[ ] **D.** Corneal irregularity and luster

Correct answer—A. *Rationales:* The most significant assessment finding in a chemical burn to the eye, especially an alkaline burn, is corneal whitening. Pain and variable loss of vision also occur. It is also difficult to define specific eye structures. There may be redness but no purulent discharge. A corneal abrasion presents with corneal irregularity and no corneal luster.
Nursing process step: Assessment

24. A client comes to the triage area complaining of a purulent, yellow-green discharge from both eyes. Which disorder is consistent with this complaint?

[ ] **A.** Retinal detachment
[ ] **B.** Subconjunctival hemorrhage
[ ] **C.** Conjunctivitis
[ ] **D.** Hyphema

Correct answer—C. *Rationales:* Conjunctivitis is characterized by purulent, yellow-green discharge from the eyes. Retinal detachment, subconjunctival hemorrhage, and hyphema don't present with drainage from the eye.
Nursing process step: Assessment

25. Which of the following is an important discharge instruction for the client with bacterial conjunctivitis?

[ ] **A.** Correct instillation of a topical anesthetic
[ ] **B.** Detailed instructions on preventing the disease from spreading
[ ] **C.** How to test visual acuity
[ ] **D.** The procedure for irrigation with normal saline

Correct answer—B. *Rationales:* Bacterial conjunctivitis is very contagious, and the client needs to be instructed on hand washing and measures to decrease cross contamination. The client wouldn't be given a topical anesthetic at discharge. Visual acuity is an eye assessment tool performed on all clients with an eye complaint. The client wouldn't be given instructions on normal saline eye irrigation.
Nursing process step: Evaluation

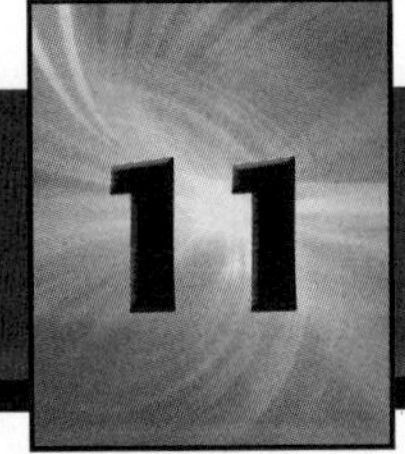

11 Orthopedic emergencies

1. A 16-year-old male is brought to the emergency department with complaints of pain in his right ankle. He states, "I was playing basketball and jumped and landed on the side of my foot." His ankle is discolored and swollen, with limited movement in the affected extremity. Based on these findings, how would this sprain be classified?

[ ] **A.** Mild (first-degree)
[ ] **B.** Moderate (second-degree)
[ ] **C.** Severe (third-degree)
[ ] **D.** Dislocation

Correct answer—C. *Rationales:* Severe sprains involve torn ligaments, which result in pain, swelling, and discoloration. Mild sprains cause only slight pain and swelling. Moderate sprains cause pain, swelling and limited use for a short period of time, and dislocations result in severe swelling and nerve, vein, and artery damage.
Nursing process step: Analysis

2. Which nursing intervention is essential in caring for a client with compartment syndrome?

[ ] **A.** Keeping the affected extremity below the level of the heart
[ ] **B.** Wrapping the affected extremity with a compression dressing to help decrease the swelling
[ ] **C.** Removing all external sources of pressure, such as clothing and jewelry
[ ] **D.** Starting an I.V. line in the affected extremity in anticipation of venogram studies

Correct answer—C. *Rationales:* Nursing measures should include removing all clothing, jewelry, and external forms of pressure (such as pressure dressings or casts) to prevent constriction and additional tissue compromise. The extremity should be maintained at heart level (further elevation may increase circulatory compromise, whereas a dependent position may increase edema). A compression wrap, which increases tissue pressure, could further damage the affected extremity. There's no indication that diagnostic studies would require I.V. access in the affected extremity.
Nursing process step: Intervention

3. Which injury results from excessive stretching or tearing of a ligament?

[ ] **A.** Strain
[ ] **B.** Sprain
[ ] **C.** Fracture
[ ] **D.** Avulsion

Correct answer—B. *Rationales:* A sprain results from excessive stretching or tearing of a ligament. A strain occurs from the overstretching of a tendon or muscle. A fracture is a break in the continuity of the bone as a result of excessive force. An avulsion is a full-thickness separation of the skin.
Nursing process step: Assessment

4. Excessive or continuous stress on a tendon results in which condition?

[ ] **A.** Tinnitus
[ ] **B.** Tendinitis
[ ] **C.** Bursitis
[ ] **D.** Nerve entrapment

Correct answer—B. *Rationales:* Tendinitis is an inflammation of a tendon from excessive or continuous force. It commonly occurs in the shoulder (rotator cuff tendinitis), elbow (tennis elbow), knee (jumper's knee), or heel (Achilles' tendinitis). Tinnitus is ringing in the ears. Bursitis is an inflammation of the bursa, or sac, that covers a bony prominence between bones, muscles, or tendons. Nerve entrapment results from the compression of a nerve, causing ischemia of that nerve.
Nursing process step: Assessment

5. Which intervention should be avoided in a client with a suspected shoulder dislocation?
[ ] **A.** Immobilizing the shoulder to prevent further injury and relieve pain
[ ] **B.** Applying ice
[ ] **C.** Placing the client in a traction splint to eliminate muscle spasms
[ ] **D.** Determining neurovascular status distal to the injury

Correct answer—C. *Rationales:* Traction splints, designed for use on lower extremities, are indicated only for treating femur and proximal tibia fractures; their use in upper-extremity trauma is contraindicated. Immobilizing the shoulder, applying ice, and determining the neurovascular status distal to the injury are all appropriate interventions for a dislocated shoulder.
Nursing process step: Intervention

6. Which of the following isn't indicative of neurovascular compromise in a client with a shoulder dislocation?
[ ] **A.** Intense pain with movement of the joint
[ ] **B.** Numbness of an extremity
[ ] **C.** Inability to move the extremity
[ ] **D.** Paresthesias of the extremity

Correct answer—A. *Rationales:* Clients with a shoulder dislocation have pain with any movement of the joint. When neurovascular compromise has occurred, the client experiences numbness, paresthesia, and the inability to move the extremity.
Nursing process step: Assessment

7. Which of the following isn't an expected outcome for a client with a dislocated shoulder?
[ ] **A.** The client states that the injured shoulder feels better.
[ ] **B.** The client expresses the need to follow-up with an orthopedic surgeon for fixation if the shoulder becomes dislocated again.
[ ] **C.** The client verbalizes activities to avoid to prevent future dislocations.
[ ] **D.** The client's facial expressions and body positioning demonstrate that he is calm and relaxed.

Correct answer—B. *Rationales:* With a history of repetitive dislocation, the client should be evaluated by an orthopedic surgeon for possible joint fixation now, not when it becomes dislocated again. The client should be placed on restricted activity at least until follow-up is complete. The appearance of a calm, relaxed client indicates that interventions of pain control, positioning, and education have been successful.
Nursing process step: Evaluation

8. Which of the following is a primary intervention in a client experiencing fat embolism syndrome?
[ ] **A.** Replacing fluids to maintain cardiac function
[ ] **B.** Administering I.V. corticosteroids
[ ] **C.** Administering high-flow oxygen by way of a nonrebreather mask
[ ] **D.** Providing discharge planning and education

Correct answer—C. *Rationales:* The primary nursing intervention for this syndrome is administering high-flow oxygen. Airway and breathing are always top-priority interventions. After administering oxygen, the primary interventions are mechanical ventilation, if indicated, as well as fluid replacement, administration of I.V. corticosteroids, and client education.
Nursing process step: Intervention

9. After an assault, a client presents to the emergency department complaining of an injury to the left femur. There's an obvious deformity to the middle of the thigh, and bone is protruding. The client's left foot is pale and cool, and palpable pulses are absent. Which of the following is a primary intervention for this client?
[ ] **A.** Applying pneumatic antishock trousers to the client and inflating the left leg compartment
[ ] **B.** Attempting to push the bone back into the wound
[ ] **C.** Administering oxygen at 2 L via nasal cannula
[ ] **D.** Applying firm in-line traction to the left leg, reassessing distal neurovascular status, and anticipating placement of a traction splint

Correct answer—D. *Rationales:* Applying firm in-line traction to the left leg, reassessing the distal neurovascular status, and anticipating the placement of a traction splint are the primary interventions for a client with an open femur fraction. The use of pneumatic antishock trousers is controversial, and their value for stabilizing femur fractures hasn't been established. Protruding bone shouldn't be pushed back into the wound. Administering oxygen to a client with a femur fracture should be done at 10 to 15 L/minute by way of a nonrebreather mask.
Nursing process step: Intervention

10. Which of the following is the primary intervention when caring for an open wound?
[ ] **A.** Cleaning the wound with a solution of Betadine and hydrogen peroxide
[ ] **B.** Covering the wound with a wet sterile dressing
[ ] **C.** Leaving the wound open to air
[ ] **D.** Setting up for immediate wound closure

Correct answer—B. *Rationales:* A break in the skin near the site of a suspected fracture is considered an open fracture until proven otherwise. The proper care for this wound is covering it with a sterile dressing, getting wound cultures, and administering tetanus toxoid and antibiotics as ordered. The wound shouldn't be cleaned or closed by way of a suture until an open fracture is ruled out.
Nursing process step: Intervention

11. An X-ray of the left femur shows a fracture that extends through the midshaft of the bone and multiple splintering fragments. What's this type of fracture called?
[ ] **A.** Compression fracture
[ ] **B.** Greenstick fracture
[ ] **C.** Comminuted fracture
[ ] **D.** Impacted fracture

Correct answer—C. *Rationales:* A comminuted fracture typically is transverse the shaft of the bone and has multiple splintered bone fragments. A closed fracture implies that the skin integrity at or near the point of fracture is intact. A greenstick fracture occurs when the bone buckles or bends and the fracture line doesn't extend through the entire bone. An impacted fracture occurs when the distal and proximal portions of the fracture are wedged into each other. A compression fracture occurs when a severe force presses the bone together on itself.
Nursing process step: Analysis

12. Which of the following *isn't* one of the five Ps for assessing an extremity?
[ ] **A.** Pain
[ ] **B.** Pallor
[ ] **C.** Paresthesia
[ ] **D.** Purulence

Correct answer—D. *Rationales:* The five Ps in the neurovascular assessment of an injured extremity include pain, pallor, paresthesia, pulses, and paralysis. Purulence isn't an assessment of neurovascular status; it's an indication of infection.
Nursing process step: Assessment

13. A client arrives in the emergency department after an industrial accident that resulted in a midforearm amputation. The client has a tourniquet in place, bleeding is minimal, and the amputated part is wrapped in a towel. Which intervention is a priority for this client?
[ ] **A.** Caring for the severed part
[ ] **B.** Removing the tourniquet and controlling bleeding with other methods
[ ] **C.** Preparing the client for reimplantation
[ ] **D.** Obtaining an X-ray of the extremity to rule out a fracture proximal to the point of amputation

Correct answer—B. *Rationales:* A tourniquet is an intervention of last resort to control bleeding. Removing the tourniquet is crucial to preserving as much of the stump as possible for the best therapeutic outcome. Caring for the amputated part, preparing for possible reimplantation, and obtaining X-rays should follow.
Nursing process step: Intervention

14. Which of the following is an appropriate intervention for the preservation of an amputated part?
[ ] **A.** Discard the amputated part if it has been severed longer than 30 minutes.
[ ] **B.** Wrap the amputated part in a towel and moisten with cool tap water.
[ ] **C.** Immerse the amputated part directly into a bath of ice and water.
[ ] **D.** Anticipate the need to X-ray the severed part before reimplantation.

Correct answer—D. *Rationales:* Radiologic examination should be done to rule out fractures and foreign bodies. The severed part can be reimplanted many hours after amputation. It needs to be wrapped in gauze and moistened with sterile normal saline solution. Direct immersion of the amputated part results in tissue damage secondary to thermal injury. The appropriate intervention is to gently clean the amputated part to remove gross debris. Then the part should be wrapped in gauze soaked with normal saline and placed in a plastic bag. The bag should be sealed tightly, placed on ice, and monitored to ensure that the tissue doesn't freeze.
Nursing process step: Intervention

15. Which of the following would be contraindicated in the reimplantation of an amputated body part?
[ ] **A.** Location of the amputation
[ ] **B.** Age of the patient
[ ] **C.** A limb placed in a container of crushed ice and water
[ ] **D.** A limb with excessive bacterial contamination and prolonged time from injury

Correct answer—D. *Rationales:* Amputated parts with excessive bacterial contamination and a prolonged time since the injury are less likely to be reimplanted successfully because of the increased chance of infection and the lowered viability of the limb. Both location and age may affect the outcome of the reimplantation; however, they aren't contraindications. Adequate preservation of the amputated part would increase the success of reimplantation.
Nursing process step: Analysis

16. Which part of the body is most likely to develop compartment syndrome?
[ ] **A.** Upper arm
[ ] **B.** Lower arm
[ ] **C.** Upper leg
[ ] **D.** Joint spaces

Correct answer—B. *Rationales:* Compartment syndrome is most likely to occur in the lower arm, hand, lower leg, and foot. These areas have limited ability to expand with increasing tissue pressures.
Nursing process step: Analysis

17. Which of the following isn't a factor in the development of compartment syndrome?
[ ] **A.** Injury of an extremity
[ ] **B.** Prolonged overuse of an extremity
[ ] **C.** Recent surgery in an extremity
[ ] **D.** Preexisting joint inflammation (arthritis, synovitis)

Correct answer—D. *Rationales:* Common causes of compartment syndrome include:
◆ injury to an extremity.
◆ prolonged overuse of an extremity.
◆ recent extremity surgery.
◆ use of casts, wraps, splints, or pneumatic antishock garments.
◆ circumferential taping of an extremity.
◆ past medical conditions such as hemophilia, nephrotic syndrome, and nerve dysfunctions.

Preexisting joint disease doesn't play a role in the development of compartment syndrome.
Nursing process step: Analysis

18. Which of the following is incorrect regarding a dislocated wrist?
[ ] **A.** It's usually caused by a fall onto outstretched hands.
[ ] **B.** It's frequently associated with sporting mishaps.
[ ] **C.** It may result in median nerve damage.
[ ] **D.** It usually doesn't need casting after it has been relocated.

Correct answer—D. *Rationales:* Casting of the wrist is done after relocation to immobilize the joint and prevent redislocation. Wrist dislocations commonly result from falling onto outstretched hands and frequently are associated with sporting events. Median nerve damage can result from wrist dislocations; therefore, neurovascular assessment distal to the area of injury should be done on all clients who present with an injured extremity.
Nursing process step: Analysis

19. Which surgical intervention is initially used to treat compartment syndrome?
[ ] **A.** Muscle flap
[ ] **B.** Fasciotomy
[ ] **C.** Incision and drainage
[ ] **D.** Amputation

Correct answer—B. *Rationales:* Fasciotomy is a surgical intervention used to treat compartment syndrome. The surgeon makes longitudinal incisions along the affected extremity to relieve tissue pressure and limit compression damage. This procedure should be performed within 8 to 12 hours of the onset, before irreversible damage occurs. A muscle flap and incision and drainage aren't interventions for compartment syndrome. Amputation is the surgical intervention of last resort.
Nursing process step: Intervention

20. Which of the following is the most common site of nerve entrapment syndrome?
[ ] **A.** Arm
[ ] **B.** Leg
[ ] **C.** Thoracic vertebral column
[ ] **D.** Lumbar vertebral column

Correct answer—A. *Rationales:* Nerve entrapment syndrome typically occurs in the arm. The median nerve is involved in pronator syndrome (entrapment occurs at the forearm) and carpal tunnel syndrome (entrapment at the wrist). The ulnar nerve is involved in cubital entrapment syndrome (entrapment at the elbow). The leg, thoracic vertebral column, and lumbar vertebral column aren't involved in nerve entrapment syndromes.
Nursing process step: Analysis

21. Ankle dislocations are commonly associated with which condition?
[ ] **A.** Ligament strain
[ ] **B.** Tendon sprain
[ ] **C.** Bone fracture
[ ] **D.** Muscle strain

Correct answer—C. *Rationales:* Ankle dislocations are commonly associated with fractures. Ligament strains, muscle strains, and tendon sprains don't lead to ankle dislocations.
Nursing process step: Assessment

22. Which statement is appropriate when teaching a client about a strained wrist?
[ ] **A.** "You may resume normal activities on discharge."
[ ] **B.** "Apply heat intermittently for the first 24 to 48 hours; then apply ice up to 72 hours."
[ ] **C.** "Don't use a compression elastic bandage because it may cause compartment syndrome."
[ ] **D.** "Elevate the injured wrist higher than the level of the heart for the first 24 hours to reduce swelling."

Correct answer—D. *Rationales:* Elevating the injury will decrease swelling. The client should be instructed to rest the injured extremity for the first 24 to 48 hours and then gradually increase activity as tolerated. The appropriate intervention is to apply ice for the first 24 hours to reduce swelling, then apply heat. The use of a compression elastic bandage provides support and helps to decrease swelling; it doesn't cause compartment syndrome.
Nursing process step: Evaluation

23. Which of the following interventions would take priority in treating a patient with a pelvic fracture who has a heart rate of 130 beats/minute and a blood pressure of 80/50 mm Hg?

[ ] **A.** Stabilization
[ ] **B.** Fluid resuscitation
[ ] **C.** Pain management
[ ] **D.** Insertion of an indwelling urinary catheter

Correct answer—B. *Rationales*: Because pelvic fractures are associated with large amounts of blood loss, which result in tachycardia and hypotension, fluid resuscitation takes priority in order to prevent hypovolemic shock. Stabilization, pain management and insertion of an indwelling urinary catheter would be indicated after the vital signs are stabilized.
Nursing process step: Intervention

24. Which structure is seldom dislocated?

[ ] **A.** Knee
[ ] **B.** Shoulder
[ ] **C.** Foot
[ ] **D.** Elbow

Correct answer—C. *Rationales:* Dislocations of the foot are rare. Dislocations of the knee, shoulder, and elbow occur in greater frequency than those of the foot.
Nursing process step: Assessment

25. Which intervention is a priority for a client receiving conscious sedation for relocation of a dislocated shoulder?

[ ] **A.** Monitoring the client's respiratory status
[ ] **B.** Assessing the client to determine the need for additional sedation
[ ] **C.** Assessing the extremity's neurovascular status after the relocation is complete
[ ] **D.** Monitoring the client until the level of consciousness (LOC) returns to baseline

Correct answer—A. *Rationales:* When administering conscious sedation, the primary intervention is to monitor the client's respiratory status. Medications given for conscious sedation can cause respiratory depression that may lead to respiratory arrest. Therefore, resuscitation equipment should be readily available. Adequate sedation must be maintained to complete the procedure and provide maximal client comfort. After relocation is complete, the nurse needs to ensure that the neurovascular status is intact. Clients undergoing conscious sedation should be observed until the LOC has returned to baseline.
Nursing process step: Intervention

26. Which statement about obtaining X-rays on a client with an injured extremity is true?

[ ] **A.** Anterior, posterior, and lateral views are the only films needed.
[ ] **B.** X-rays should include the joints immediately above and below the injury.
[ ] **C.** X-rays are indicated only if there's an obvious deformity to the extremity.
[ ] **D.** Open fractures usually don't need X-rays because the location and type of fracture are easily identified based on clinical assessment alone.

Correct answer—B. *Rationales:* X-rays of the injured extremity should include the joints immediately above and below the injured area. The views are necessary to determine whether there are any fractures along the length of the bone or if there's any joint involvement. Anterior, posterior, and lateral views of an injured extremity don't always allow visualization of fractures, so an oblique view may be needed. All extremity injuries involving a suspected fracture must be evaluated by X-ray, regardless of the presence of deformities or degree of integumentary disruption; these indicators don't give insight to the location or severity of the fracture.
Nursing process step: Intervention

27. Which injury to bone *isn't* common in unrestrained front seat passengers involved in motor vehicle crashes?

[ ] **A.** Fractured foot
[ ] **B.** Ankle dislocation
[ ] **C.** Patella dislocation
[ ] **D.** Hip dislocation

Correct answer—A. *Rationales:* Unrestrained front seat passengers may suffer lower-extremity trauma as a result of striking the dashboard with their knees. These injuries include ankle dislocation, knee or patella dislocations, femur fractures, hip fractures or dislocations, and acetabular fractures as a result of the femoral head being pushed through the acetabulum. Patella, ankle, and foot fractures aren't common occurrences in this group of clients.
Nursing process step: Assessment

28. What is the most commonly overlooked injury resulting from a primary blast?
[ ] **A.** Pulmonary barotrauma
[ ] **B.** Rupture of tympanic membranes
[ ] **C.** Intestinal and stomach contusions and rupture
[ ] **D.** Concussion syndrome

Correct answer—D. *Rationales:* Concussions are overlooked most commonly because they typically occur without external signs of trauma. All other choices have apparent signs that are easily recognized, such as shortness of breath and difficulty breathing, pain in the ear or bloody discharge, GI bleeding, and abdominal pain.
Nursing process step: Analysis

29. Which of the following is used for the initial splinting of a pelvic fracture?
[ ] **A.** Long spine board
[ ] **B.** Pneumatic antishock garment
[ ] **C.** Traction splint
[ ] **D.** Bilateral long leg splints

Correct answer—A. *Rationales:* A long spine board is used for the initial splinting of a pelvic fracture. A pneumatic antishock garment may help stabilize a pelvic fracture and tamponade bleeding, but it isn't considered the initial splinting device. Traction splints are indicated for femur and proximal tibial fractures only. Long leg splints aren't indicated for pelvic fractures because they don't stabilize or immobilize the pelvis.
Nursing process step: Intervention

30. Which of the following isn't a type of fracture?
[ ] **A.** Spiral fracture
[ ] **B.** Avulsion fracture
[ ] **C.** Torus fracture
[ ] **D.** Diagonal fracture

Correct answer—D. *Rationales:* A diagonal fracture isn't a type of fracture. A fracture break line does resemble a diagonal line, but it isn't considered a diagonal fracture. An avulsion fracture refers to a bone injury in which a fragment of bone connected to a ligament breaks off from the rest of the bone. A torus fracture, which is a buckling of a bone's surface, is seen in children. A spiral fracture appears to twist with the surface of the affected bone.
Nursing process step: Assessment

31. Which of the following isn't a typical mechanism of injury in the cause of pelvic fractures?
[ ] **A.** Penetrating trauma
[ ] **B.** Falls from a significant height
[ ] **C.** Motor vehicle ejections
[ ] **D.** Pedestrian struck by a motor vehicle

Correct answer—A. *Rationales:* Pelvic fractures commonly result from a client being hit by or thrown from a vehicle or from falling from a significant height. A pelvic fracture may result from penetrating trauma, but this isn't a typical occurrence.
Nursing process step: Assessment

32. Compression fractures most commonly occur in the:
[ ] **A.** femur.
[ ] **B.** vertebrae.
[ ] **C.** humerus.
[ ] **D.** sternum.

Correct answer—B. *Rationales:* The bones of the vertebral column are susceptible to compression fractures. Axial loading forces result in compression of the bones along the vertebral column. The most common type of axial loading occurs with diving accidents and falls.
Nursing process step: Assessment

33. Which factor increases the risk for increased blood loss after a fracture?
[ ] **A.** Extent of fracture
[ ] **B.** Age of client
[ ] **C.** Alcohol abuse
[ ] **D.** Sex of client

Correct answer—C. *Rationales:* Blood disorders, anemia, and alcohol abuse can be contributing factors to increased blood loss after a fracture. The extent of the fracture and the age and sex of the client aren't contributing factors to increased blood loss.
Nursing process step: Assessment

34. The following describes a fracture commonly associated with contact sports: The client presents with the head tilted toward the injured area and the chin directed away from the side of the injury. What's the name of the injury?

[ ] **A.** Shoulder fracture
[ ] **B.** Clavicle fracture
[ ] **C.** Scapular fracture
[ ] **D.** Humerus fracture

Correct answer—B. *Rationales:* The symptoms described are characteristic of a clavicle fracture. Additional symptoms include pain, point tenderness, swelling, crepitus, and deformity to the clavicle. In addition, the client usually can't raise the arm on the affected side. A shoulder fracture is actually a shoulder dislocation with an associated fracture of the proximal humerus. The client complains of pain and the inability to move his shoulder. There may be a disruption of blood flow to the arm. Because of the location of the scapula, it may be fractured in many different areas; however, fractures of this bone are uncommon. Muscles and the ability of the scapula to move along the chest wall protect it from fractures. Great force is required to fracture the scapula.
Nursing process step: Assessment

35. Which of the following isn't an expected outcome in a client with fat embolism syndrome?

[ ] **A.** The client has normal vital signs and cardiac rhythm.
[ ] **B.** The client has good skin color.
[ ] **C.** The client is able to state interventions that might prevent recurrence of the syndrome.
[ ] **D.** The client's arterial blood gas values are within normal limits.

Correct answer—C. *Rationales:* Fat embolism syndrome is an unpredictable complication of trauma to the skeleton, and there are no known self-care interventions that can prevent its occurrence. The expected outcome of treatment is the return of normal vital signs, cardiac rhythm, skin color, and arterial blood gas values.
Nursing process step: Evaluation

36. Elderly clients who fall are most at risk for which injury?

[ ] **A.** Wrist fractures
[ ] **B.** Humerus fractures
[ ] **C.** Pelvic fractures
[ ] **D.** Cervical spine fractures

Correct answer—C. *Rationales:* Elderly clients who fall will usually sustain pelvic and lower-extremity fractures. These injuries are devastating because they can seriously alter an elderly client's lifestyle and reduce functional independence. Wrist fractures usually occur with falls on an outstretched hand or from a direct blow and are commonly found in young men. Humerus fractures and cervical spine fractures aren't age-specific.
Nursing process step: Analysis

37. Which force doesn't play a role in causing fractures?

[ ] **A.** Tension
[ ] **B.** Bending
[ ] **C.** Compression
[ ] **D.** Extension

Correct answer—D. *Rationales:* There's no such force as extension force relative to fractures. The forces that do result in fractures include tension (pulling), compression (longitudinal loading), bending, and torsion (twisting).
Nursing process step: Analysis

38. Which injury is commonly seen in adult pedestrians struck by motor vehicles?

[ ] **A.** Femur fracture
[ ] **B.** Humerus fracture
[ ] **C.** Wrist fracture
[ ] **D.** Forearm fracture

Correct answer—A. *Rationales:* Many adult pedestrians who are struck by cars sustain leg fractures and dislocations. Fractures to the upper extremities aren't typical in pedestrians hit by moving vehicles.
Nursing process step: Assessment

39. Which laboratory study is most relevant to treating a client who has sustained a pelvic fracture?

[ ] **A.** Urine myoglobin
[ ] **B.** Urinalysis
[ ] **C.** Type and crossmatch
[ ] **D.** Serum ethanol

Correct answer—C. *Rationales:* Because of the rich blood supply to the pelvis, fractures to this area can result in significant blood loss. Type and crossmatch is the primary laboratory test in preparing for fluid replacement. Urinalysis and serum ethanol, although part of the trauma workup, don't alter treatment of a pelvic fracture. Urine isn't commonly analyzed for myoglobin with this injury unless the mechanism was a crush injury; even then, urinalysis isn't as high a priority as type and crossmatch.
Nursing process step: Intervention

40. Which of the following is a potential complication of compartment syndrome?

[ ] **A.** Disseminated intravascular coagulation (DIC)
[ ] **B.** Anemia
[ ] **C.** Myoglobinuria
[ ] **D.** Osteomyelitis

Correct answer—C. *Rationales:* Myoglobin may be present in the urine as a result of muscle breakdown. To prevent myoglobin from damaging the renal tubules, the kidneys must be thoroughly flushed. A minimum urine output of 75 to 100 mL/hour needs to be maintained. Sodium bicarbonate can be administered to alkalinize the urine and to decrease precipitation of myoglobin in the renal tubules. Myoglobin in the tubules can lead to renal failure. DIC and anemia aren't complications of compartment syndrome. Osteomyelitis can occur if an infection is present, but it isn't a complication of compartment syndrome.
Nursing process step: Assessment

41. Which of the following is an indication for splint application?

[ ] **A.** To prevent infection
[ ] **B.** To prevent dislocations
[ ] **C.** To prevent damage to blood vessels and nerves
[ ] **D.** To align bones of a comminuted fracture

Correct answer—C. *Rationales:* By immobilizing the injured extremity, the nurse is helping prevent potential damage to nerves and blood vessels. A splint doesn't prevent infections from occurring if the fracture is open. It isn't indicated for dislocation prevention, and it isn't used to align the bones of a comminuted fracture.
Nursing process step: Intervention

42. Which of the following necessitates removal of a cast before the fracture has healed?

[ ] **A.** The client complains of itching under the cast.
[ ] **B.** Pain is still present the day after the injury.
[ ] **C.** It's suspected that the client is developing a pressure ulcer.
[ ] **D.** The client is unable to learn how to use crutches.

Correct answer—C. *Rationales:* If a pressure ulcer is developing, the cast should be removed and the extremity evaluated. Itching is a common complaint and occurs as the skin dries. The client may experience pain during the first 24 hours after the injury. Pain medication and elevation of the injured extremity should help relieve the discomfort. Pain that continues beyond the first 24 hours should be evaluated by the client's health care provider. If using crutches is a problem, the client needs instruction. If inability to use crutches persists, alternate methods may be investigated, such as switching to a walking cast (if the type of fracture permits) or a wheelchair (usually an expensive alternative).
Nursing process step: Evaluation

43. Which of the following isn't appropriate when teaching a client who is using crutches for the first time?

[ ] **A.** Have the client stand and balance on the crutches.

[ ] **B.** Have the client hold the crutches 4 inches to the side and 4 inches in front of the feet.

[ ] **C.** Instruct the client to place all the weight on the axilla when ambulating.

[ ] **D.** Have the client demonstrate a three-point gait.

Correct answer—C. *Rationales:* The client should be instructed not to place any weight on the axilla, not even when resting. Weight on the axilla causes nerve compression and may lead to permanent nerve damage. The hand grips should be positioned to allow a slight bend of the elbows. The weight is distributed to the shoulders, arms, and hands.

Nursing process step: Evaluation

44. Which of the following is an expected outcome for a client with a contusion to the thigh?

[ ] **A.** The client states that the pain has increased.

[ ] **B.** Swelling continues to progress.

[ ] **C.** The client relates understanding of the signs and symptoms that require further evaluation.

[ ] **D.** The client expresses understanding that follow-up care will be needed only if symptoms worsen.

Correct answer—C. *Rationales:* Contusion to the thigh is an injury to the soft tissue caused by blunt force. Hemorrhage into the injured area of the thigh, pain, swelling, and ecchymosis are present, and treatment is aimed at controlling these symptoms. Swelling should begin to decrease if treatment interventions were effective. Interventions should include elevation and the use of cold packs. If the swelling continues, additional interventions will become necessary. Follow-up care is needed regardless of symptoms to ensure resolution of the injury without complications.

Nursing process step: Evaluation

45. When treating a client with a strained knee, "RICE" is recommended. Which of the following isn't an appropriate component of the RICE mnemonic?

[ ] **A.** R—Rest the affected extremity

[ ] **B.** I—Ice application

[ ] **C.** C—Compression with elastic dressing

[ ] **D.** E—Exercise of the affected extremity

Correct answer—D. *Rationales:* The correct mnemonic intervention for the letter E is elevation, which reduces swelling and pain. Exercise should be avoided, and the client should rest the affected extremity. The other options are correct.

Nursing process step: Intervention

46. When does the onset of fat embolism syndrome usually occur?

[ ] **A.** 1 to 2 hours after a traumatic event

[ ] **B.** 4 to 6 hours after a traumatic event

[ ] **C.** 6 to 10 hours after a traumatic event

[ ] **D.** More than 12 hours after a traumatic event

Correct answer—D. *Rationales:* Symptoms of fat embolism syndrome usually occur 12 to 72 hours after a traumatic event, but they may be seen up to 10 days later. All of the other options are incorrect.

Nursing process step: Assessment

47. When splinting the leg of a client with an Achilles tendon rupture, how should the foot be held during splinting?

[ ] **A.** Dorsiflexion

[ ] **B.** Long leg cast

[ ] **C.** Plantar flexion

[ ] **D.** Plantar extension

Correct answer—C. *Rationales*: The client's leg should be placed in plantar flexion position in order to let the tendon rest and prevent further overstretching and injury. The client is usually assigned slow stretching and strengthening exercises. Immobilization initially will allow the tendon to reattach and heal. Both dorsiflexion and plantar extension will result in excess tension on the tendon. An Achilles tendon rupture isn't routinely placed in a cast.

Nursing process step: Intervention

48. Which of the following is the most appropriate intervention to control hemorrhage associated with an extremity injury?

[ ] **A.** Placing a tourniquet 3 to 4 inches above the site of hemorrhage

[ ] **B.** Applying warm compresses to cause vasoconstriction

[ ] **C.** Holding the extremity low and applying pressure

[ ] **D.** Applying a pressure dressing to the site of bleeding

Correct answer—D. *Rationales:* Applying a pressure dressing to the site of bleeding is the first-line intervention for hemorrhage associated with an extremity injury. Applying a tourniquet should be a last resort because it could cause tissue damage. Warmth causes vasodilation and increases bleeding. Holding the extremity below the level of the heart also increases bleeding.

Nursing process step: Intervention

49. Which intervention is appropriate for a client who has a traction splint in place on arrival at the emergency department (ED)?

[ ] **A.** Immediately remove the splint and assess the client's distal neurovascular status.

[ ] **B.** Leave the splint in place and assess the client's distal neurovascular status.

[ ] **C.** Change the traction splint to one that the hospital owns and give the other back to the ambulance crew.

[ ] **D.** Take the splint off if the client's neurovascular status is normal.

Correct answer—B. *Rationales:* If a client arrives in the ED with a traction splint in place, the nurse should ensure that neurovascular status distal to the injury is intact. Next, the nurse should elevate the affected limb. The splint should be left in place until radiographic studies are complete and a fracture is ruled out.

Nursing process step: Intervention

50. Which of the following is a common complication of a pelvic fracture?

[ ] **A.** Urethral injury

[ ] **B.** Muscle spasms

[ ] **C.** Neurovascular compromise

[ ] **D.** Rhabdomyolysis

Correct answer—A. *Rationales:* Urethral injury is a complication of a pelvic fracture. Muscle spasms are common with femur fractures, and neurovascular compromise is seen in extremity trauma. Rhabdomyolysis is defined as the acute destruction of muscle and isn't a complication of a pelvic fracture.

Nursing process step: Evaluation

51. Which of the following indicates an understanding of discharge instructions given after long leg cast placement?

[ ] **A.** The client calls the emergency department (ED) after noticing a foul odor from the cast.

[ ] **B.** After 1 week, the client comes to the ED to have the cast removed.

[ ] **C.** The client verbalizes the need to come to the ED weekly for cast replacement.

[ ] **D.** The client states that he can walk on the cast for short distances and to climb stairs.

Correct answer—A. *Rationales:* A foul-smelling odor coming from the cast may indicate an infection, and the client should return to a heath care professional or the ED. The cast won't be removed after 1 week, nor will it require weekly removal if cared for properly. The client shouldn't ambulate on a long leg cast; doing so stresses the cast and causes damage to the cast and possibly the broken leg.

Nursing process step: Evaluation

52. Which type of splint is used to immobilize a fractured upper extremity?
[ ] **A.** Soft cervical collar
[ ] **B.** Soft splint
[ ] **C.** Long spine board
[ ] **D.** Hard cervical collar

Correct answer–B. *Rationales:* Four basic types of splints are available for immobilizing extremity fractures:
- Soft splints such as a pillow
- Hard splints, which have a firm surface
- Air splints, which are inflatable and provide support
- Traction splints, which provide support and traction.

Long spine boards and soft and hard cervical collars are used to immobilize the spine and aren't indicated for upper-extremity splinting.
Nursing process step: Intervention

53. Uric acid crystals that collect in the synovial fluid of joints can lead to erythema, warmth, and extreme pain. What's this condition called?
[ ] **A.** Bursitis
[ ] **B.** Rheumatoid arthritis
[ ] **C.** Uremia
[ ] **D.** Gout

Correct answer–D. *Rationales:* Gout is caused by urate crystals that collect in the synovial fluid of joints causing rapid inflammation—usually in just a few hours. The pain is severe. Bursitis is the inflammation of the synovial cavities that surround joints; it commonly occurs in the knee or elbow. Rheumatoid arthritis includes joint pain that is typically accompanied by deformity. Uremia is associated with renal insufficiency and is caused by retention of a nitrogenous substance that is normally excreted by the kidneys.
Nursing process step: Assessment

54. In which of the following is replantation unlikely to be successful?
[ ] **A.** Multiple digits
[ ] **B.** The thumb
[ ] **C.** Pediatric extremity amputations
[ ] **D.** Injuries at multiple levels on the same extremity

Correct answer–D. *Rationales:* Injuries at multiple levels on the same extremity make it unlikely that replantation will be successful. Replantation should be considered under the following circumstances:
- Loss of several digits: Hand function would be seriously compromised without them.
- Loss of thumb: It constitutes 40% to 50% of the functional value of the hand because of its role in opposition and grasp, and replantation has a high success rate.
- In children: Their transected nerves regenerate well, and they readily adapt to using a replanted part.

Nursing process step: Evaluation

55. Which symptom constitutes a medical emergency in a client with acute lower back pain with suspected herniated lumbar disc?
[ ] **A.** Pain radiating down one or both legs
[ ] **B.** Paresthesia
[ ] **C.** Back pain with sneezing
[ ] **D.** Incontinence

Correct answer–D. *Rationales:* Incontinence is a medical emergency, possibly indicative of cauda equina syndrome, and should be evaluated immediately. Pain, paresthesia, and back pain with sneezing are all symptoms of nonemergency herniated lumbar disc.
Nursing process step: Assessment

56. A client who's receiving muscle relaxants as part of his discharge instructions asks about adverse effects. The most common adverse effect of muscle relaxants is:
[ ] **A.** anxiety.
[ ] **B.** drowsiness.
[ ] **C.** increased alertness.
[ ] **D.** nausea and vomiting.

Correct answer–B. *Rationales:* Drowsiness is the most common adverse effect experienced. Nausea and vomiting can occur with any medication but aren't usual adverse effects of muscle relaxants. Anxiety and alertness aren't usual adverse effects of muscle relaxants.
Nursing process step: Intervention

57. Treatment for carpal tunnel syndrome (CTS) sometimes involves surgical decompression of the nerve. The nerve usually responsible for the CTS symptoms is the:

[ ] **A.** radial nerve.
[ ] **B.** ulnar nerve.
[ ] **C.** median nerve.
[ ] **D.** spinal accessory nerve.

Correct answer—C. *Rationales:* The median nerve, which serves sensation in the palm of the hand and movement of the small muscles of the hand, is the nerve involved in CTS. Ulnar and radial nerves can be involved but aren't the cause. The spinal accessory nerve is responsible for shoulder muscle strength.
Nursing process step: Analysis

58. A client comes to the emergency department after a motor vehicle collision. The client was the driver and had his seat belt fastened. There's no evidence of cervical spine or head injury; however, the client complains of right knee pain. On exam, he has pain with range of motion, and severe swelling of the knee. X-rays show a distal femur fracture. What's the most likely finding in the aspiration fluid?

[ ] **A.** Blood
[ ] **B.** Pus
[ ] **C.** Urate crystals
[ ] **D.** Lymph

Correct answer—A. *Rationales:* Blood is the most likely fluid to be aspirated in the setting of a severe trauma femur fracture with knee swelling and pain. Pus would be seen if infection were present. Urate crystals are seen in gout, and lymph isn't usually seen in the knee joint.
Nursing process step: Analysis

59. A 35-year-old female comes to the emergency department with a 5-day history of migratory polyarthralgia involving the wrist, elbow, and knee, and a recent skin rash involving necrotic pustules over her extremities (mainly feet and soles). The likely diagnosis is:

[ ] **A.** early-stage syphilis.
[ ] **B.** mononucleosis.
[ ] **C.** rheumatoid arthritis.
[ ] **D.** gonococcal arthritis.

Correct answer—D. *Rationales:* This is a typical presentation for gonococcal arthritis, which is more common in women under age 40 during menses or pregnancy. Genitourinary symptoms are seen in about 25% of clients; fever, in about 50% of clients. Syphilis presents with a chancre in early stages and causes a salmon-colored maculopapular rash usually appearing on the palms and soles, but it isn't necrotic in appearance. Polyarthralgia may be seen in secondary syphilis. Mononucleosis presents with a high fever, a severe sore throat, and swollen glands and tonsils. Rheumatoid arthritis doesn't involve rash.
Nursing process step: Analysis

60. Ligamentous injuries of the knee may include:

[ ] **A.** medial meniscus, posterior cruciate ligament, and anterior cruciate ligament.
[ ] **B.** medial collateral ligament, lateral collateral ligament, and anterior cruciate ligament.
[ ] **C.** medial collateral ligament, deltoid ligament, and anterior cruciate ligament.
[ ] **D.** deltoid ligament, anterior talofibular ligament, and anterior cruciate ligament.

Correct answer—B. *Rationales:* The medial meniscus isn't a ligament. The deltoid and anterior talofibular ligaments are located at the ankle joint. The medial and lateral collateral ligaments and the anterior and posterior cruciate ligaments comprise the ligaments of the knee joint.
Nursing process step: Assessment

61. Which of the following about costochondritis is true?
[ ] **A.** It's a chronic inflammation of the cervical vertebrae.
[ ] **B.** Inflammation may be due to a recent injury.
[ ] **C.** The pain is similar to that of a rib fracture.
[ ] **D.** It's seen most commonly in people older than age 20.

Correct answer—C. *Rationales:* The pain of costochondritis is similar to that of a rib fracture; however, any client presenting with chest pain who is at risk for myocardial ischemia must have a thorough cardiac evaluation before the symptoms can be considered musculoskeletal in origin. Costochondritis is an acute inflammation of the rib and sternal junction and may involve one or several junctions. Inflammation can be due to physical exertion or repetitive movements, not a recent injury. Costochondritis is seen most commonly in people older than age 40.
Nursing process step: Analysis

62. Which of the following interventions is most appropriate for costochondritis?
[ ] **A.** Medications and exercise to strengthen muscles
[ ] **B.** Rest, deep breathing, and medications
[ ] **C.** Deep breathing alone
[ ] **D.** Medications alone

Correct answer—B. *Rationales*: Rest, deep breathing, and taking medications as prescribed are indicated. Clients should be instructed to avoid exertional activities that may exacerbate symptoms. Medications and deep breathing alone aren't appropriate interventions.
Nursing process step: Intervention

63. What's the most common causative organism in osteomyelitis?
[ ] **A.** *Escherichia coli*
[ ] **B.** *Streptococcus agalactiae*
[ ] **C.** *Serratia marcescens*
[ ] **D.** *Staphylococcus aureus*

Correct answer—D. *Rationales*: Osteomyelitis is an infection of the bone, most commonly a result of direct contamination from open fractures, penetrating wounds, or surgical procedures. *S. aureus* is a common organism found on human skin and therefore is the main cause of the infection. Both *E. coli* and *S. agalactiae* are commonly found in the GI tract; *S. marcescens* is found in water.
Nursing process step: Analysis

64. Which of the following foreign bodies can be difficult to visualize on X-ray and may require a computed tomography (CT) scan?
[ ] **A.** Glass
[ ] **B.** Metal
[ ] **C.** Rubber
[ ] **D.** Vegetative foreign bodies

Correct answer—D. *Rationales:* Vegetative foreign bodies, such as thorns and wood, generally aren't visible on X-ray unless they're very large. Therefore, a CT scan would be indicated. Glass, metal, and rubber are all radio-opaque and can be visualized on X-ray.
Nursing process step: Analysis

65. What are the four mechanisms that affect individuals who are involved in a blast situation?
[ ] **A.** Primary, secondary, pattern of Injury, and miscellaneous
[ ] **B.** Primary, secondary, tertiary, and miscellaneous
[ ] **C.** Primary, secondary, projectiles, and explosives
[ ] **D.** Primary, secondary, tertiary, and projectiles

Correct answer—B. *Rationales:* Primary is the initial blast or air wave. Secondary is the flying debris, the pieces of which act as projectiles. Tertiary is the distance an individual's body travels from the blast and where it has impact. Miscellaneous is the inhalation of dust or toxic gases, thermal burns, radiation, and so forth. The other options don't meet all the criteria for the mechanism of a blast situation.
Nursing process step: Analysis

66. Which of the following interventions is *not* indicated in removing a foreign body?
[ ] **A.** Cleanse the area around the entry site thoroughly with mild antiseptic solution.
[ ] **B.** Soak the part of the body containing a wooden splinter to soften its removal.
[ ] **C.** Apply gentle, careful traction with small forceps to remove objects that lie close to or protrude through the skin.
[ ] **D.** Administer antibiotics, if ordered.

Correct answer—B. *Rationales:* Don't soak the part of the body containing a wooden splinter because wood absorbs liquid and disintegrates during removal. All of the other interventions are appropriate when attempting to remove a foreign body.
Nursing process step: Intervention

67. What are the signs and symptoms of possible joint effusion?
[ ] **A.** Warmth and pain with limited range of motion
[ ] **B.** Redness and ecchymosis
[ ] **C.** Warmth and pain with full range of motion
[ ] **D.** Ecchymosis and tenderness

Correct answer—A. *Rationales*: The inflammatory process will cause pain and redness and the joint will be warm to touch. The limited range of motion is caused by pain and swelling. Ecchymosis doesn't occur with joint effusion.
Nursing process step: Assessment

68. Achilles tendon rupture is an injury that occurs most commonly during stop-and-start sports. Which of the following would you expect to find in a client with a suspected Achilles tendon rupture?
[ ] **A.** Palpable deformity along the tendon
[ ] **B.** Sharp pain in the lower foot
[ ] **C.** Ability to stand up on the toes
[ ] **D.** Ambulation despite pain

Correct answer—A. *Rationales:* The Achilles tendon, the longest tendon in the body, is a fibrous cord connected to the bone located on the posterior portion of the foot. Complete tears of the tendon cause a severe, sharp pain in the back of the ankle or lower calf, not in the foot. An Achilles tendon rupture also results in an inability to stand up on the toes on the injured leg. Injuries to the Achilles tendon lead to difficulty when ambulating.
Nursing process step: Assessment

12 Mental health emergencies

1. After being struck by a car, a 3-year-old child is brought to the emergency department by paramedics. The parents arrive shortly afterward and are informed by the physician that their child is dead. The mother becomes hysterical, throws herself on the floor, and begins screaming. Which intervention is the most appropriate for the mother at this time?

[ ] **A.** Support and encourage the mother's expression of grief and provide her with privacy.

[ ] **B.** Tell her to get off the floor. Her behavior is inappropriate.

[ ] **C.** Obtain a physician's order and administer diazepam (Valium) by mouth.

[ ] **D.** Provide the family with accurate information regarding the incident.

Correct answer—A. *Rationales:* Families need to be encouraged to express grief in whatever way they desire, as long as they don't harm themselves or others. The nurse's role is to help families focus on the grief, not to alleviate it. Families need accurate information to deal with the death of a loved one. However, they must be able to listen at the time the information is given. Diazepam may cloud or even delay the grieving process.

Nursing process step: Intervention

2. When communicating with a grieving family, the nurse should:

[ ] **A.** use words such as *dead, died*, or *death.*

[ ] **B.** tell the family, "Everything will be all right."

[ ] **C.** tell the family, "It was for the best."

[ ] **D.** tell the family that the client didn't suffer.

Correct answer—A. *Rationales:* Using words such as *dead, died*, or *death* reinforces reality, prevents denial, and supports the grief process. Telling the family that "everything will be all right" or that "it was for the best" only minimizes their feelings. Telling the family that the client didn't suffer is helpful but should be stated only if it's true.

Nursing process step: Implementation

3. What's a realistic short-term goal for a mother whose child has just died?

[ ] **A.** Making funeral arrangements

[ ] **B.** Sharing her feelings with the nurse

[ ] **C.** Cleaning out the child's closet

[ ] **D.** Leaving the emergency department (ED) just after learning about the death

Correct answer—B. *Rationales:* By being able to share her feelings, the mother is acknowledging the death and beginning the work of grief. This step should begin in the ED. Making funeral arrangements and cleaning out the child's closet aren't short-term goals and aren't realistic in the initial stages of grief. It isn't desirable for the mother to leave the ED until she has had time to ask questions and to process and accept the information.

Nursing process step: Evaluation

4. Which of the following is the priority when assessing a client who has ingested a handful of unknown pills?
[ ] **A.** Determine whether the client was trying to harm himself or herself
[ ] **B.** Determine whether the client has a support system
[ ] **C.** Determine whether the client has any life-threatening conditions
[ ] **D.** Determine whether the client has a history of suicide attempts

Correct answer—C. *Rationales:* If the client's physical condition is life-threatening, the priority is to treat the medical condition. Any compromise in the client's airway, breathing, or circulation must be addressed immediately. It's also imperative to determine the time of ingestion because it may affect treatment. The psychiatric evaluation, which includes intent to harm oneself, existence of an adequate support system, and client history, can be done after the client is medically stable.
Nursing process step: Assessment

5. When providing notification of a client's death to a family in the emergency department, what is most important for the nurse to keep in mind?
[ ] **A.** Use medical terminology to provide distance and professionalism.
[ ] **B.** Avoid giving specific facts about the victim and the death.
[ ] **C.** Remember that responses to grief vary.
[ ] **D.** Prevent the survivors from viewing the body.

Correct answer—C. *Rationales:* The responses of survivors are diverse, unpredictable, and variable depending on multiple factors. Medical jargon can be confusing, especially to a family in crisis. Speak in clear language that's easy to understand. Providing details (such as chronology of events, circumstances of death, and treatment) can provide comfort to survivors. Whenever possible, family members should be given the option to be present during resuscitation. After efforts are ceased, the family should be allowed to view the body.
Nursing process step: Intervention

6. Initial interventions for the client with acute anxiety include all of the following *except*:
[ ] **A.** providing the client with a safe, quiet, and private place.
[ ] **B.** encouraging the client to verbalize feelings and concerns.
[ ] **C.** approaching the client in a calm, confident manner.
[ ] **D.** touching the client in an attempt to comfort.

Correct answer—D. *Rationales:* The nurse must establish rapport and trust with the anxious client before using therapeutic touch because touching an anxious client may actually increase anxiety. Trust can be established by approaching the client in a calm and confident manner, providing a place that is quiet, safe, and private, and encouraging the client to verbalize feelings and concerns.
Nursing process step: Intervention

7. A 25-year-old man on a psychiatric hold is brought to the emergency department (ED) by police. He's in four-point restraints. The client was reportedly observed running through the street naked, smashing windows, and screaming. He's now calm, nonverbal, and diaphoretic and has both vertical and horizontal nystagmus. He's noted to have a 2″ (5 cm) laceration to his right arm.Which of the following is the priority when assessing this client?
[ ] **A.** Evaluating his mental status and obtaining a full set of vital signs
[ ] **B.** Performing a primary assessment quickly and ruling out other signs of trauma
[ ] **C.** Determining whether the client can cooperate so that the restraints can be removed
[ ] **D.** Sending a urine specimen for toxicology screening

Correct answer—B. *Rationales:* A quick primary assessment is indicated on all clients in the ED. This client is a danger to himself and may have sustained other life-threatening injuries not noted by the police. The mental status examination and vital signs need to be done but aren't the priority. Removing the restraints before fully examining the client may place both the client and the ED staff at great risk. Obtaining a urine specimen for toxicology screening takes time and shouldn't determine the initial care.
Nursing process step: Assessment

8. Which of the following is the most appropriate immediate intervention for a client who is in four-point restraints and has vertical and horizontal nystagmus and a 2″ (5 cm) laceration on his arm?
[ ] **A.** Suturing his arm laceration
[ ] **B.** Obtaining an order and administering haloperidol (Haldol) I.M. or I.V.
[ ] **C.** Leaving him in restraints
[ ] **D.** Obtaining a psychiatric consult

Correct answer—C. *Rationales:* Ensuring the safety of the client and staff is a top priority. A client with a history of violence in the prehospital setting is at risk for violence in the emergency department. The client should be fully evaluated before restraints are removed. Suturing can be done later, and a psychiatric consult isn't indicated until the client is medically stable. Haloperidol may be ordered after an evaluation by the physician.
Nursing process step: Intervention

9. Which of the following is important when restraining a violent client?
[ ] **A.** Have three staff members present: one for each side of the body and one for the head.
[ ] **B.** Always tie restraints to side rails.
[ ] **C.** Have an organized, efficient team approach after the decision is made to restrain the client.
[ ] **D.** Secure restraints to the gurney with knots to prevent escape.

Correct answer—C. *Rationales:* Emergency department personnel should use an organized, team approach when restraining violent clients so that no one is injured in the process. The leader, located at the client's head, should take charge; four staff members are required to hold and restrain the limbs. For safety reasons, restraints should be fastened to the bed frame instead of the side rails. For quick release, loops should be used instead of knots.
Nursing process step: Implementation

10. Which of the following medications would the nurse expect to administer to reverse a dystonic reaction?
[ ] **A.** Prochlorperazine
[ ] **B.** Diphenhydramine (Benadryl)
[ ] **C.** Haloperidol (Haldol)
[ ] **D.** Midazolam

Correct answer—B. *Rationales:* Diphenhydramine I.M. or I.V. can quickly reverse this condition. Prochlorperazine and haloperidol are both capable of causing dystonia, not reversing it. Midazolam would make the client drowsy.
Nursing process step: Intervention

11. Which of the following is a potential risk factor for violence in the emergency department (ED)?
[ ] **A.** A relief float nurse to provide breaks
[ ] **B.** Long waits for service
[ ] **C.** A buddy system for client transports
[ ] **D.** Restricting visitors into the department

Correct answer—B. *Rationales:* Long wait times, as well as overcrowding, can increase the risk of violence in the ED. Working understaffed (especially during meal times) and transporting clients alone can put the staff at risk for violence. It's important to set clear visitor policies and enforce them consistently.
Nursing process step: Analysis

12. The nurse determines that a suicidal client is a danger to himself. Appropriate nursing interventions include all of the following *except*:
[ ] **A.** communicating with the family regarding the care plan.
[ ] **B.** ensuring that a psychiatric consult is obtained.
[ ] **C.** ensuring that a psychiatric hold is written and placed on the medical record.
[ ] **D.** allowing the client to ambulate around the emergency department (ED) to work off his nervous energy.

Correct answer—D. *Rationales:* It's the nurse's responsibility to protect the suicidal client by providing a safe environment. Thus, suicidal clients must remain under close observation at all times. It isn't appropriate for suicidal clients to wander around the ED alone. The nurse must ensure that a psychiatric consultation is obtained so that the client can be placed on a psychiatric hold and detained for further psychiatric evaluation. Communicating with the client and family regarding the care plan and expectations is also essential.
Nursing process step: Intervention

13. Victims of domestic violence should be assessed for what important information while they're in the emergency department?
[ ] **A.** The reasons they stay in abusive relationships (for example, lack of financial autonomy and isolation)
[ ] **B.** Readiness to leave the perpetrator and knowledge of resources
[ ] **C.** The use of drugs or alcohol
[ ] **D.** A history of previous victimization

Correct answer—B. *Rationales:* Victims of domestic violence must be assessed for their readiness to leave the perpetrator and their knowledge of the resources available to them. Nurses can then provide the victims with information and options to enable them to leave when they're ready. The reasons they stay in the relationship are complex and can be explored at a later time. The use of drugs or alcohol is irrelevant. There's no evidence to suggest that previous victimization results in a person's seeking or causing abusive relationships.
Nursing process step: Assessment

14. A 27-year-old male is brought to the emergency department with seizure-like activity. He's currently unresponsive, his tongue is protruding, and he's having muscle spasms of the face and hands. His family states that he has been using drugs lately but they're not sure what type. What should the nurse expect is happening to the client?
[ ] **A.** Status epileptic seizures
[ ] **B.** Neuroleptic malignant syndrome
[ ] **C.** Dystonic reaction
[ ] **D.** Conversion disorder

Correct answer—C. *Rationales:* These symptoms are classic symptoms of a dystonic reaction. Dystonic reactions (that is, dyskinesias) are characterized by involuntary movements of the tongue, lips, face, trunk, and extremities. Status epileptic seizures occur in greater intensity and are longer and life-threatening. Neuroleptic malignant syndrome is a rare but life-threatening reaction that involves muscle rigidity, fever, and altered mental status. Conversion disorder is the presence of physiological symptoms that have no medical explanation and are caused by a psychological conflict.
Nursing process step: Analysis

15. Which of the following is a recommended guideline for universal screening for domestic violence?
[ ] **A.** The screening should take place in front of a friend or family member the client trusts.
[ ] **B.** The screening should be limited to a yes-or-no question on the medical history questionnaire.
[ ] **C.** The screening should include indirect questions.
[ ] **D.** The screening should be conducted in the client's primary language.

Correct answer—D. *Rationales:* A certified interpreter should be used if needed to conduct the interview in the client's primary language. The encounter should be done while the client is alone, away from friends and family. A question about domestic violence can be asked on a medical history questionnaire, along with a face-to-face encounter. Questions should be direct and nonjudgmental.
Nursing process step: Intervention

16. In a toddler, which injury is probably the result of child abuse?
[ ] **A.** A hematoma on the occipital region of the head
[ ] **B.** A 1″ (2.5 cm) forehead laceration
[ ] **C.** Several small, dime-sized circular burns on the child's back
[ ] **D.** A small isolated bruise on the right lower extremity

Correct answer—C. *Rationales:* Small circular burns on a child's back are no accident and may be from cigarettes. Toddlers are injury prone because of their developmental stage, and falls are frequent because of their unsteady gait. Therefore, head injuries aren't uncommon. A small area of ecchymosis isn't suspicious in this age-group.
Nursing process step: Assessment

17. Which statement would be most appropriate or therapeutic when the nurse suspects domestic violence?
[ ] **A.** Ask directly, "Is someone hurting you at home?"
[ ] **B.** Comment, "This doesn't look like you fell. Is there something else you want to tell me?"
[ ] **C.** Tell her, "You should leave him. You don't deserve this!" Call the police and encourage her to press charges.
[ ] **D.** State, "Wow, you're really injury prone."

Correct answer–A. *Rationales:* Victims of domestic violence want to be asked directly. It's important to let them know that help is available when they're ready and that they aren't alone. They should be given the resources to leave when it's safe for them to do so. The statements in options B and D are indirect and imply that the nurse really doesn't want to know. The statement in option C is judgmental.
Nursing process step: Intervention

18. Which intervention is inappropriate for a suspected sexual assault victim?
[ ] **A.** Emphasize that you're there to help and that she's safe.
[ ] **B.** Allow the client to verbalize her feelings.
[ ] **C.** Provide the client with privacy (by leaving her alone) until she's ready to talk.
[ ] **D.** Offer to call friends or family for her when she's ready.

Correct answer–C. *Rationales:* Never leave a rape victim alone because doing so increases feelings of isolation, fear, and anxiety. Emphasizing that you're there to help and that she's safe establishes rapport and trust. Encouraging a client to talk helps her sort through her thoughts and feelings and lowers her anxiety level. Friends and family can provide a feeling of safety when the client is ready.
Nursing process step: Intervention

19. Which group of characteristics would the nurse expect to see in the schizophrenic client?
[ ] **A.** Disheveled appearance, flight of ideas, grandiose delusions, and auditory hallucinations
[ ] **B.** Periods of hyperactivity and irritability alternating with depression
[ ] **C.** Delusions of jealousy and persecution, paranoia, and mistrust
[ ] **D.** Sadness, apathy, feelings of worthlessness, anorexia, and weight loss

Correct answer–A. *Rationales:* A disheveled appearance, flight of ideas, grandiose delusions, and auditory hallucinations are all characteristic of the classic schizophrenic client. These clients aren't able to care for their physical appearance. They frequently hear voices telling them to do something either to themselves or to others. Additionally, they verbally ramble from one topic to the next. Periods of hyperactivity and irritability alternating with depression is characteristic of bipolar or manic disease. Delusions of jealousy and persecution, paranoia, and mistrust are characteristics of paranoid disorders. Sadness, apathy, feelings of worthlessness, anorexia, and weight loss are characteristics of depression.
Nursing process step: Assessment

20. Which statement about child abuse *isn't* true?
[ ] **A.** Nurses are required by law to report only actual cases of child abuse, not cases of suspected abuse.
[ ] **B.** Nurses should be direct and nonjudgmental when communicating with parents who are suspected of abusing their children.
[ ] **C.** It should be documented on the medical record that a report was made to the Child Protective Agency.
[ ] **D.** Documentation should be objective and should use quotes when documenting what the patient says.

Correct answer–A. *Rationales:* Nurses are required by law to report both actual and suspected cases of child abuse. Nurses should be direct and nonjudgmental when communicating with parents who are suspected of abusing their children. The medical record should show documentation that the Child Protective Agency was notified of the case. Documentation should reflect exactly what is being communicated by the patient.
Nursing process step: Intervention

21. Which medication would probably be ordered for a schizophrenic client?
[ ] **A.** Ziprasidone (Geodon)
[ ] **B.** Haloperidol (Haldol)
[ ] **C.** Lithium
[ ] **D.** Clomipramine (Anafranil)

Correct answer—B. *Rationales:* Haloperidol I.M. or I.V. is the drug of choice for acute psychotic behavior. Ziprasidone is also an antipsychotic drug; however, it takes longer to produce sedation than haloperidol. Lithium is useful in bipolar or manic disorder, and clomipramine is used for depression.
Nursing process step: Intervention

22. Sudden infant death syndrome (SIDS) is one of the most common causes of death in infants. At what age is the diagnosis of SIDS most likely?
[ ] **A.** At age 6 to 8 weeks
[ ] **B.** At age 1 week to 1 year, peaking at age 2 to 4 months
[ ] **C.** At age 6 months to 1 year, peaking at age 10 months
[ ] **D.** At age 1 to 2 years

Correct answer—B. *Rationales:* SIDS can occur any time between age 1 week and 1 year but is most common among infant ages 2 to 4 months.
Nursing process step: Assessment

23. When interviewing the parents of an injured child, which of the following is the strongest indicator that child abuse may be a problem?
[ ] **A.** The injury isn't consistent with the history or the child's age.
[ ] **B.** The mother and father tell different stories regarding what happened.
[ ] **C.** The family is poor.
[ ] **D.** The parents are argumentative and demanding with emergency department personnel.

Correct answer—A. *Rationales:* When the child's injuries are inconsistent with the history given or impossible because of the child's age and developmental stage, the nurse should be suspicious that child abuse is occurring. The parents may tell different stories because their perception may be different regarding what happened. Changing their stories when different health care workers ask the same question is an indication that child abuse may be a problem. Child abuse occurs in all socioeconomic groups. Parents may argue and be demanding because of the stress of having an injured child.
Nursing process step: Assessment

24. When communicating with the grieving family after a sudden infant death syndrome (SIDS) death, it's most important that the nurse:
[ ] **A.** stress that the death isn't the parents' fault, that it was unpreventable and unpredictable.
[ ] **B.** stress that an autopsy must be done to confirm the diagnosis.
[ ] **C.** stress that the parents are still young and can have more children.
[ ] **D.** instruct the parents to place other infants on their backs to sleep.

Correct answer—A. *Rationales:* SIDS deaths are unexpected and sudden, and their cause is unclear. It's important that the parents don't believe that the death is their fault or that they could have prevented it. Although it's important to inform the parents that an autopsy needs to be performed, it is secondary. Stressing that they're still young and can have more children minimizes their feelings of grief. Instructing the parents to place other infants on their backs to sleep implies that the parents did something to cause the death.
Nursing process step: Intervention

25. When discharging a client after treatment for a dystonic reaction, it's most important that the nurse ensures that the client understands which of the following?

[ ] **A.** Results of treatment are rapid and dramatic but may not last.

[ ] **B.** Although uncomfortable, this reaction isn't serious.

[ ] **C.** The client shouldn't buy drugs on the street again.

[ ] **D.** The client must continue to take diphenhydramine (Benadryl) for the next 2 to 3 days to prevent a return of symptoms.

Correct answer—D. *Rationales:* Phenothiazines have a half-life of 24 hours; therefore, oral diphenhydramine must be continued for the next 2 days to prevent the return of symptoms. Results of treatment are rapid and dramatic and will last if the client receives and understands appropriate discharge instructions. Dystonic reactions can be life-threatening when airway patency is compromised. Lecturing the client about buying drugs on the street isn't appropriate.
Nursing process step: Evaluation

26. Which history is most consistent with the diagnosis of sudden infant death syndrome (SIDS)?

[ ] **A.** The child had been physically abused and was found in the evening.

[ ] **B.** The infant was considered ill and had many medical problems.

[ ] **C.** The infant was healthy and was found dead shortly after being put down to sleep.

[ ] **D.** The child is usually described as lethargic, irritable, and feeding poorly.

Correct answer—C. *Rationales:* Children who are diagnosed with SIDS are typically healthy with no previous medical problems. They're usually found dead sometime after being put down to sleep. Depending on how long the infant has been dead, a SIDS baby may have a mottled complexion with extreme cyanosis of the lips and fingertips, or pooling of blood in the legs and feet that may be mistaken for bruises.
Nursing process step: Assessment

27. A middle-age woman brings her mother to the emergency department. The mother has multiple bruises and skin breakdown. The woman states that her mother is confused and falls all the time. When eliciting a history from the daughter, it's most important that the nurse:

[ ] **A.** agree with the daughter that older people do fall all the time and that it's impossible to prevent them from getting skin breakdown from immobility.

[ ] **B.** ask specifically if the daughter is experiencing great stress and frustration caring for her mother at home, whether she has multiple demands, and if she has any resources available to her.

[ ] **C.** determine whether there's a history of family violence, including domestic violence and child abuse.

[ ] **D.** inquire about a history of alcoholism.

Correct answer—B. *Rationales:* Elder abuse is typically rooted in frustration and stress on the part of the abuser. The family member caring for the parent may feel overburdened and exhausted and may need support. Asking the family member about the stress and frustration associated with caring for a parent demonstrates concern and appreciation for the situation. Nurses can then help families mobilize community resources. That older people fall a lot is a misconception that contributes to the underdetection of elder abuse. Determining if there's a history of family violence or alcoholism is important. Clients and their families may not offer this information freely, and it isn't as important as determining the caretaker's stressors.
Nursing process step: Assessment

28. What's the best approach for the nurse to take when an elderly client doesn't acknowledge the abuse and wants to stay in the home?
[ ] **A.** Provide the client and family with appropriate resources and report the abuse as required by state law.
[ ] **B.** Call the police and have the client removed from the home.
[ ] **C.** Arrange for a visiting nurse to make home visits.
[ ] **D.** Insist that the client confront the situation so that a crisis intervention plan can be initiated.

Correct answer—A. *Rationales:* When the client is alert and oriented, she should be offered choices and the nurse should respect whatever decision she makes. Nurses must report elder abuse as required by their state law. Forcefully removing a client from the home isn't advisable. Clients have the right to stay in the abusive relationship if they choose to do so. A visiting nurse is only one resource available to family members, and they should be provided with several options. Insisting that the client confront the situation isn't appropriate. The client may not have the required coping mechanisms and may not be ready to confront the situation at this time.
Nursing process step: Intervention

29. A 40-year-old executive who was laid off from work unexpectedly 2 days earlier comes to the emergency department complaining of fatigue and an inability to cope. He admits drinking excessively over the past 48 hours. This is an example of:
[ ] **A.** alcoholism.
[ ] **B.** a manic episode.
[ ] **C.** situational crisis.
[ ] **D.** depression.

Correct answer—C. *Rationales:* A situational crisis results from a specific event in a person's life. The person is overwhelmed by the situation and reacts emotionally. Fatigue, insomnia, and inability to make a decision are common. The situational crisis may precipitate behavior that in turn causes a crisis (alcohol or drug abuse). The information provided is insufficient to label this client an alcoholic. A manic episode is characterized by euphoria and labile affect. Symptoms of depression are usually present for 2 or more weeks.
Nursing process step: Assessment

30. Victims of sexual assault can experience posttraumatic stress reactions after the attack. Which statement does this include?
[ ] **A.** Denial of the event
[ ] **B.** Anger, guilt, and humiliation
[ ] **C.** Fatigue and self-blame
[ ] **D.** Flashbacks, recurring dreams, and numbness

Correct answer—D. *Rationales:* Posttraumatic stress involves recurring dreams about the event or flashbacks to the event. The victims feel a general sense of numbness and estrangement from others. Emotional reactions such as denial of the event, anger, guilt, humiliation, fatigue, and self-blame are all normal feelings after rape but aren't consistent with posttraumatic stress.
Nursing process step: Assessment

31. Which of the following is an expected outcome for a violent client in the emergency department (ED)?
[ ] **A.** The client and staff aren't injured.
[ ] **B.** The client demonstrates his frustration.
[ ] **C.** The client agrees to therapy.
[ ] **D.** The client's family agrees to family counseling.

Correct answer—A. *Rationales:* Avoiding injury to the staff and client, allowing the client to verbalize feelings of frustration, and avoiding further demonstrations of aggressive behavior are expected outcomes for a violent client in the ED. It's important for the client to agree to therapy, but that doesn't guarantee elimination of violence now. The client's family going to counseling won't eliminate violence.
Nursing process step: Evaluation

32. Which of the following isn't true about sudden cardiac death syndrome survivors?
[ ] **A.** Their usual coping behaviors may be inadequate.
[ ] **B.** The event represents a threat to their survival.
[ ] **C.** The person is physiologically stable on arrival at the emergency department (ED).
[ ] **D.** Loss and grief reactions may occur.

Correct answer—C. *Rationales:* The survivor of sudden cardiac death is physiologically unstable either before arrival or on arrival at the ED. These people have survived resuscitation and experienced a close brush with death. Their usual coping mechanisms may not be adequate, and both loss and grief reactions may occur.
Nursing process step: Assessment

33. Which of the following is important to remember when caring for a client in restraints or seclusion?
[ ] **A.** Monitor individuals in restraints every hour.
[ ] **B.** Inform the client of behavioral criteria that will lead to discontinuation of the restraints or seclusion.
[ ] **C.** Physical restraints should be used as a first-line therapy for clients at risk for medical therapy interruption.
[ ] **D.** Adults placed in restraints must have an order within 24 hours.

Correct answer—B. *Rationales:* Behavioral criteria that will lead to discontinuation of restraints or seclusion must be established and communicated. Individuals in restraints or seclusion require continuous monitoring as well as a careful assessment every 15 minutes. Staff should be trained in the use of de-escalation techniques, mediation, and self-protection to avoid the use of restraints or seclusion. All individuals placed in restraints or seclusion, regardless of age, must have an order for restraints and seclusion issued by a licensed independent practitioner within 1 hour of the initiation of the restraints or seclusion.
Nursing process step: Intervention

34. A client presents to the emergency department (ED) with signs of ineffective coping. What's the most realistic nursing goal for this client?
[ ] **A.** To help the client improve coping skills
[ ] **B.** To help the client develop a plan for better communication
[ ] **C.** To help the client identify the precipitating event and select realistic options
[ ] **D.** To help the client develop a plan to deal with stress more effectively

Correct answer—C. *Rationales:* In the ED, it's realistic for the nurse to help the client identify the precipitating event and possible options. It isn't realistic to strive for improvement in coping skills, better communication, or dealing with stress more effectively. These goals require long-term planning that can't be done in the ED.
Nursing process step: Evaluation

35. Which of the following is an appropriate nursing intervention for the client with bipolar disorder?
[ ] **A.** Obtaining a lithium (Lithonate) level and urine toxicology screen for drugs
[ ] **B.** Orienting the client to current reality (person, place, and time) if delusional
[ ] **C.** Restraining the client as needed for safety
[ ] **D.** All of the above

Correct answer—D. *Rationales:* All answer options are appropriate interventions. Lithium is the drug of choice for bipolar disorder, and drug levels should be measured. A toxicology screen is important to rule out substance toxicity, which can mimic psychiatric illness. Delusional clients should be reoriented to reality. If mania isn't controlled, the client is at risk for harming himself and others. Restraints may be necessary.
Nursing process step: Implementation

36. Which of the following is an appropriate nursing intervention for a client experiencing an anxiety attack?
[ ] **A.** Place the client with another client in order to stimulate the client.
[ ] **B.** Physically restrain the client.
[ ] **C.** Place the client in a calm, quiet environment.
[ ] **D.** Allow the family to remain with the client.

Correct answer—C. *Rationales:* A client who is experiencing a panic attack should be placed in a calm, quiet environment to minimize sensory overload. Placing the family with another client and allowing the family to remain with the client may contribute to an increased anxiety level. Restraining the client will further increase the client's anxiety.
Nursing process step: Intervention

37. For which reasons are antidepressants not usually prescribed for a depressed client being discharged from the emergency department?
[ ] **A.** Therapeutic response is usually immediate.
[ ] **B.** Overdoses are rare.
[ ] **C.** The client needs to return for appropriate psychiatric follow-up, and he might not comply if he's given the medication.
[ ] **D.** Medication can take the place of therapy.

Correct answer—C. *Rationales*: The client who's depressed needs to receive psychiatric follow-up and not simply be given antidepressants. A client taking antidepressants needs to be followed carefully because therapeutic response may not be seen for several weeks to months and overdoses of the drugs can be lethal. Medication should never be given alone.
Nursing process step: Intervention

38. Which of the following is an appropriate intervention for a client who has been sexually assaulted?
[ ] **A.** If the client must be undressed, have her place each article of clothing in a plastic bag for evidence.
[ ] **B.** Have the client collect a clean-catch urine specimen.
[ ] **C.** Obtain a meal and drink for the client.
[ ] **D.** Explain to the client that reporting to law enforcement is mandatory.

Correct answer—D. *Rationales:* Although it's the client's choice whether to be interviewed by law enforcement, health care workers are required to report the assault to law enforcement. Articles of clothing should be placed in paper evidence bags. If the client must urinate before the nurse examiner arrives, have her collect a random first-catch specimen. The client should be kept on nothing-by-mouth status until the nurse examiner has collected oral evidence.
Nursing process step: Intervention

39. A dystonic reaction can be caused by which of the following medications?
[ ] **A.** Diazepam (Valium)
[ ] **B.** Haloperidol (Haldol)
[ ] **C.** Clomipramine (Anafranil)
[ ] **D.** Clonazepam (Klonopin)

Correct answer—B. *Rationales*: Haloperidol is a phenothiazine and is capable of causing dystonic reactions. Diazepam and clonazepam are benzodiazepines, and amitriptyline is a tricyclic antidepressant. Benzodiazepines and tricyclic antidepressants don't cause dystonic reactions. Benzodiazepines can cause drowsiness, lethargy, and hypotension. Tricyclics can cause a decreased level of consciousness, tachycardia, dry mouth, and dilated pupils.
Nursing process step: Implementation

40. A 43-year-old woman comes to the emergency department complaining her heart is "beating too hard" and she's frightened she might be having a heart attack. As you gather more information, you learn that she constantly worries about her safety and has "this feeling" that some sort of natural disaster is imminent. In addition, she has had difficulty sleeping and has felt constantly "on edge" for the last 4 months. Based on the assessment findings and history provided, which of the following might the nurse suspect?
[ ] **A.** She may be demonstrating signs of early Alzheimer's.
[ ] **B.** Her behavior suggests possible drug abuse.
[ ] **C.** She's exhibiting symptoms of anxiety or panic.
[ ] **D.** She's malingering and seeking attention.

Correct answer—C. *Rationales:* The client presents with excessive worry and anxiety about several life circumstances that have no factual or logical basis. This anxiety has persisted for 4 months and she's also demonstrating signs of autonomic hyperactivity as revealed by the heart palpitations and sleep difficulty. Alzheimer's results in forgetfulness, not anxiety. Findings are not consistent with drug abuse or seeking attention.
Nursing process step: Assessment

41. Which short-term intervention is appropriate for a client with acute anxiety and possible panic attacks?
[ ] **A.** Refer her to the medical social worker for an evaluation.
[ ] **B.** Assist in making a referral to a physician for a medication consultation.
[ ] **C.** Develop behavioral and cognitive strategies to reduce or eliminate irrational anxiety.
[ ] **D.** Suggest greater involvement in group and community service activities.

Correct answer—B. *Rationales:* A full medication evaluation should be done as soon as possible so she can obtain proper pharmacological support to address the immediate impact of her condition. After the primary symptoms are addressed, other treatment strategies can then be implemented.
Nursing process step: Intervention

42. A 22-year-old law student comes into the emergency department feeling despondent. He can't concentrate, has been sleeping poorly, and his grades have dropped dramatically in the last 3 months. When further questioned, he relates that he's afraid to disappoint his father, who's a well-known attorney in the community. He states that he sees no way out and wishes he were dead. What's the nurse's priority in treating this client?

[ ] **A.** Suggest the client drop out of law school and pursue the career he has always wanted.

[ ] **B.** Recommend that the father be notified and a collaborative meeting be set up with the client, his family, the physician, and the nurse to discuss the issues.

[ ] **C.** Ask the client if he has a specific plan to harm himself. If he says yes, he should immediately be placed on suicide precautions.

[ ] **D.** Suggest the client join a support group with others who have had similar suicidal feelings.

Correct answer—C. *Rationales:* Suicidal ideation is a sign of acute crises, and immediate steps must be taken to evaluate and ensure his safety. The client has indicated that he has the intent, plan, and means to hurt himself; therefore, action must be taken without hesitation. He should be hospitalized and monitored on a one-to-one basis until a psychiatrist can do a full evaluation and make appropriate treatment recommendations. Since the client is experiencing suicidal ideations, it is not appropriate to suggest dropping out or joining a support group. Notification without the clients permission is a HIPAA violation.

Nursing process step: Intervention

43. Which of the following is the appropriate tool to use in the emergency department when assessing a suicidal client?

[ ] **A.** F.A.S.T

[ ] **B.** SAS

[ ] **C.** FACES

[ ] **D.** SADD PERSONS

Correct answer—D. *Rationales:* The SADD PERSONS scale is a tool to provide a consistent approach in the suicidal client. The F.A.S.T. is a neurological assessment tool, SAS is a sedation-level assessment tool to monitor the effectiveness of sedation, and the FACES is a pain-scale tool for children.

Nursing process step: Assessment

44. A client becomes agitated and violent in group therapy. He screams obscenities, shoves a nurse to the floor, and attempts to leave the hospital. He has a history of violent behavior and is in treatment for alcoholism. The nurse should:

[ ] **A.** attempt to physically intervene and restrain the client from leaving.

[ ] **B.** immediately call a security alert to assemble a group as a show of force in order to safely restrain the client from harming others.

[ ] **C.** attempt to calm the client by soothing words and gentle touch for reassurance.

[ ] **D.** attend to the person who was shoved on the floor.

Correct answer—B. *Rationales:* A show of force with a number of people present is useful in restraining violent behavior. If necessary, security or other persons properly trained in the use of physical restraint may need to actively intervene per hospital protocol. The client should then be contained to protect others. If the physician deems it appropriate, pharmacologic intervention may be necessary.

Nursing process step: Intervention

45. What is a priority assessment for a patient with a suspected eating disorder?

[ ] **A.** Cardiac rhythm

[ ] **B.** Appetite and weight changes

[ ] **C.** History of psychological illness

[ ] **D.** Skin turgor

Correct answer—A. *Rationales:* Patients with eating disorders may experience changes in their cardiac rhythm due to electrolyte imbalances. These imbalances can lead to potentially fatal cardiac arrhythmias. All of the other options are relevant but do not take priority.

Nursing process step: Assessment

13 Client care management

1. A client comes to the emergency department with ventricular tachycardia at a rate of 170 beats/minute and blood pressure is 90/60 mm Hg. The client is awake and oriented and has substernal chest pain. During synchronized cardioversion, the client becomes unconscious and his cardiac rhythm changes to ventricular fibrillation. Which of the following is the nurse's priority?

[ ] **A.** Administer amiodarone (Cordarone) by I.V. bolus.
[ ] **B.** Administer bretylium by I.V. bolus.
[ ] **C.** Administer synchronized countershock at 300 joules.
[ ] **D.** Defibrillate at 200 joules.

Correct answer—D. *Rationales:* According to the standards of the American Heart Association, the client should be defibrillated, then given epinephrine. Clients in ventricular fibrillation can't be cardioverted using the synchronization mode. Although amiodarone may be used in the treatment of ventricular fibrillation, they aren't considered first-line pharmacologic agents.
Nursing process step: Intervention

2. Which physiologic abnormalities can occur as a result of multiple packed red blood cell transfusions?

[ ] **A.** Hypocalcemia and hypothermia
[ ] **B.** Hypochloremic acidosis and hypothermia
[ ] **C.** Hyponatremia and hypothermia
[ ] **D.** Hypercalcemia and hypothermia

Correct answer—D. *Rationales:* Hypercalcemia can occur after massive blood transfusion because of the presence of the preservative EDTA. Hypernatremia and hyperchloremic acidosis can also occur.
Nursing process step: Assessment

3. Why should topical nitroglycerin agents be removed from the chest before defibrillation?

[ ] **A.** Massive drug administration
[ ] **B.** Deactivation of the drug
[ ] **C.** Electrical arcing
[ ] **D.** Reflex tachycardia

Correct answer—C. *Rationales:* These agents should be removed or wiped off before defibrillation because electrical arcing can occur when topical medications are present. Defibrillation has no effect on administration or deactivation of topical nitroglycerin. Nitroglycerin in combination with defibrillation doesn't cause reflex tachycardia.
Nursing process step: Intervention

4. Which agent is used in the treatment of organophosphate poisoning?

[ ] **A.** Naltrexone (ReVia)
[ ] **B.** Atropine
[ ] **C.** Activated charcoal
[ ] **D.** Flumazenil (Romazicon)

Correct answer—B. *Rationales:* Organophosphate insecticides (cholinesterase inhibitors) bind to prevent the breakdown of acetylcholine, resulting in pulmonary edema and excessive oral secretions. Atropine (an anticholinergic agent) promotes drying of pulmonary secretions and is considered an end point in treatment. Flumazenil is used in the treatment of barbiturate overdose; naltrexone is used in the treatment of opioid toxicity; and activated charcoal is used to facilitate binding of the ingested toxic substance and to promote excretion of the substance through the GI tract.
Nursing process step: Intervention

5. When administering agents by way of an endotracheal (ET) tube, the nurse should:
[ ] **A.** stop cardiopulmonary resuscitation, administer the agent, and hyperventilate the client.
[ ] **B.** continue cardiopulmonary resuscitation, administer the agent, and resume normal ventilations.
[ ] **C.** continue cardiopulmonary resuscitation, administer the agent, and flush with sterile water.
[ ] **D.** place the syringe needle deep into the ET tube and vigorously instill the agent.

Correct answer—A. *Rationales:* Medication administration by way of an ET tube requires momentary cessation of cardiopulmonary resuscitation, followed by hyperventilation to nebulize the medication. Needles should never be placed in the ET tube. Resuming normal ventilations doesn't propel the drug into the lungs or clear the tube of any remaining drug. Flushing the tube with sterile water places excess fluid in the lungs, further compromising the client's oxygenation.
Nursing process step: Implementation

6. In which of the following is cardioversion contraindicated?
[ ] **A.** Methemoglobinemia
[ ] **B.** Cyanide toxicity
[ ] **C.** Hypermagnesemia
[ ] **D.** Digoxin toxicity

Correct answer—D. *Rationales:* Elective cardioversion should be avoided in the presence of digoxin toxicity because there's a likelihood of arrhythmogenesis. Cardioversion can be safely used with methemoglobinemia, cyanide toxicity, and hypermagnesemia.
Nursing process step: Analysis

7. Four clients come to triage at the same time. The first client is a 7-year-old with a history of asthma who was wheezing before coming to the emergency department; according to the child's mother, the wheezing has decreased. The second client is a 33-year-old male with sickle cell anemia who complains of pain in his joints and lower back. The third client is a 12-year-old with a 1″ (2.5 cm) laceration on his foot. The area isn't bleeding at this time. The fourth client is a 16-year-old soccer player with a tibia-fibula deformity. You suspect a closed fracture. Which of these clients should come back to the treatment area first?
[ ] **A.** The 7-year-old with asthma
[ ] **B.** The 33-year-old with sickle cell anemia
[ ] **C.** The 12-year-old with a foot laceration
[ ] **D.** The 16-year-old with a possible closed fracture

Correct answer—A. *Rationales:* The asthma client may not exhibit wheezing as air movement significantly decreases, but any problems in airway and breathing are considered life-threatening and should be seen immediately. In most cases, a sickle cell anemia client is considered stable but urgent; this client would be seen second. The 12-year-old with a foot laceration would most likely be seen third and the closed fracture fourth. Closed fractures and lacerations are considered stable and nonurgent as long as no neurovascular compromise is noted.
Nursing process step: Assessment

8. A client presenting to the emergency department has a narrow complex tachycardia at a rate of 160 beats/minute and is unresponsive. Blood pressure is 70/50 mm Hg. Which of the following is the highest treatment priority?
[ ] **A.** Administer synchronized cardioversion.
[ ] **B.** Administer oxygen at 100% by way of a nonrebreather mask.
[ ] **C.** Administer adenosine I.V. push.
[ ] **D.** Administer asynchronized cardioversion.

Correct answer—B. *Rationales:* Airway and breathing are always the first priority of assessment and intervention. Because the client is unresponsive, supplemental oxygen is the first priority. Next comes synchronized cardioversion, which is the treatment of choice in clients with symptomatic narrow complex tachycardia. Asynchronized cardioversion is indicated in pulseless ventricular tachycardia or ventricular fibrillation.
Nursing process step: Intervention

9. Metastatic disease is an absolute contraindication for all of the following *except*:
[ ] **A.** heart valve donation.
[ ] **B.** eye (cornea) donation.
[ ] **C.** saphenous vein donation.
[ ] **D.** bone donation.

Correct answer—B. *Rationales:* Transmissibility of malignant cells is possible with heart valve, saphenous vein, and bone donation because of the vascularity of these tissues. The cornea isn't vascular, thus eliminating the possibility of disease transmission.
Nursing process step: Analysis

10. Which drug is used to treat symptomatic bradycardia in a client who has had a heart transplant?
[ ] **A.** Epinephrine
[ ] **B.** Atropine
[ ] **C.** Isoproterenol (Isuprel)
[ ] **D.** Adenosine (Adenocard)

Correct answer—C. *Rationales:* Isoproterenol is the drug of choice in the treatment of symptomatic bradycardia after heart transplantation because of its potent beta-adrenergic effect in clients without intact vagal innervation. In cardiac transplantation, the vagus nerve isn't attached to the transplanted heart. Adenosine slows electrical conduction through the atrioventricular node and is used to treat symptomatic supraventricular tachycardia. Atropine is an anticholinergic agent used in the treatment of symptomatic bradycardia in clients with intact vagal innervation. Epinephrine is a potent sympathomimetic agent that mimics the sympathetic nervous system.
Nursing process step: Intervention

11. Which of the following is a normal systolic blood pressure for a 3-year-old child?
[ ] **A.** 60 mm Hg
[ ] **B.** 86 mm Hg
[ ] **C.** 100 mm Hg
[ ] **D.** 120 mm Hg

Correct answer—B. *Rationales:* Using the formula: systolic blood pressure = 80 + age in years × 2, the estimated normal blood pressure for a 3-year-old child is 80 (3 × 2) = 86.
Nursing process step: Assessment

12. Which of the following is the most common cause of trauma death in children?
[ ] **A.** Homicide
[ ] **B.** Drowning
[ ] **C.** Motor vehicle collisions
[ ] **D.** Fires and burn injuries

Correct answer—C. *Rationales:* According to the Centers for Disease Control and Prevention, motor vehicle collisions are the number one cause of pediatric deaths, followed by homicide, suicide, drowning, pedestrian injuries, fires, and burns.
Nursing process step: Evaluation

13. To decrease the likelihood of bradyarrhythmias in children during endotracheal intubation, succinylcholine (Anectine) is used with:
[ ] **A.** epinephrine.
[ ] **B.** isoproterenol (Isuprel).
[ ] **C.** atropine.
[ ] **D.** lidocaine (Xylocaine).

Correct answer—C. *Rationales:* Succinylcholine is an ultra-short-acting depolarizing agent used for rapid-sequence intubation and may cause bradycardia, especially in children. Atropine is the drug of choice in treating succinylcholine-induced bradycardia. Lidocaine is used in adults only. Epinephrine bolus and isoproterenol aren't used in rapid-sequence intubation because of their profound cardiac effects.
Nursing process step: Intervention

14. Which agent can't be administered by intraosseous infusion?
[ ] **A.** Sodium bicarbonate
[ ] **B.** Dopamine
[ ] **C.** Calcium chloride
[ ] **D.** Isoproterenol (Isuprel)

Correct answer—D. *Rationales:* The following agents can be safely administered by intraosseous infusion: blood, bretylium, calcium, chloride, colloids, crystalloids, dobutamine, dopamine, epinephrine, glucose, and sodium bicarbonate.

Isoproterenol, which doesn't fall into any of the above categories, can't be administered by the intraosseous route.
Nursing process step: Intervention

15. Which of the following is the circulating blood volume in a 20-kg child?
[ ] **A.** 1,500 mL
[ ] **B.** 1,600 mL
[ ] **C.** 1,700 mL
[ ] **D.** 1,800 mL

Correct answer—B. *Rationales:* Children have a circulating blood volume of 80 mL/kg. Therefore, a 20-kg child has a circulating blood volume of 1,600 mL.
Nursing process step: Analysis

16. When assessing an elderly client with upper GI bleeding, the nurse should determine that which of the following isn't a risk factor?
[ ] **A.** Nonsteroidal anti-inflammatory drug use
[ ] **B.** Gender
[ ] **C.** *Helicobacter pylori* infection
[ ] **D.** Smoking

Correct answer—B. *Rationales:* Gender hasn't been identified as a risk factor in upper GI bleeding. Cigarette smoking, use of nonsteroidal anti-inflammatory drugs, and *H. pylori* infection have been implicated as major risk factors.
Nursing process step: Assessment

17. Which of the following would not be seen in a client who is brain dead?
[ ] **A.** Neurogenic pulmonary edema
[ ] **B.** Neurogenic hyperthermia
[ ] **C.** Neurogenic diabetes insipidus
[ ] **D.** Neurogenic shock

Correct answer—B. *Rationales:* After permanent interruption of cerebral circulation (brain death), the client frequently experiences pulmonary edema, diabetes insipidus, or neurogenic shock. Loss of thermoregulatory mechanisms results in hypothermia.
Nursing process step: Assessment

18. A medical examiner's case may include all of the following *except*:
[ ] **A.** homicide or suspicion of homicide.
[ ] **B.** unwitnessed cardiac arrest.
[ ] **C.** traumatic death.
[ ] **D.** poisoning.

Correct answer—B. *Rationales:* Forensic examination of a client after death is common when the cause of death is suspected of being unnatural. Homicide or suspected homicide, death after traumatic injury, and poisoning may be attributed to malicious acts or product failure involving others. Further investigation is required in these cases. Unwitnessed cardiac arrest isn't considered unnatural.
Nursing process step: Analysis

19. Management of the potential organ donor includes:
[ ] **A.** maintaining urine output above 100 mL/hour.
[ ] **B.** maintaining hematocrit (HCT) below 30%.
[ ] **C.** manipulating the ventilatory settings to maintain partial pressure of oxygen of 60 mm Hg.
[ ] **D.** maintaining central venous pressure less than 2 mm Hg.
Nursing process step: Intervention

Correct answer—A. *Rationales:* Maintaining urine output above 100 mL/hour in a potential organ donor ensures adequate perfusion of the renal glomeruli. Systolic blood pressure should be maintained above 100 mm Hg. Central venous pressure should be maintained within normal limits to prevent neurogenic pulmonary edema. HCT should be maintained above 30% to ensure adequate intravascular fluid volume. Oxygen and carbon dioxide levels are maintained within normal limits to ensure organ and tissue oxygenation.
Nursing process step: Intervention

20. Which site is the most reliable in assessing the pulse of a hemodynamically unstable adult?

[ ] **A.** Radial

[ ] **B.** Popliteal

[ ] **C.** Carotid

[ ] **D.** Dorsalis pedis

Correct answer—C. *Rationales:* Because of sympathetic nervous system influences resulting in peripheral vasoconstriction, the central carotid pulse is the most reliable site in assessing pulse quality in the hemodynamically unstable adult. Radial, dorsalis pedis, and popliteal pulses are generally palpable in clients with a systolic pressure greater than 80 mm Hg. Femoral pulses are palpable in clients with a systolic pressure greater than 70 mm Hg, and carotid pulses are palpable in clients with a systolic pressure greater than 60 mm Hg.

Nursing process step: Assessment

21. Why might a client with diabetes who also has myocardial ischemia not have classic chest pain?

[ ] **A.** Aspartame (Nutra-Sweet) use

[ ] **B.** Insulin use

[ ] **C.** Sulfonylurea agent use

[ ] **D.** Chronic neuropathy

Correct answer—D. *Rationales:* Chronic neuropathy, commonly seen in a client with diabetes mellitus, interferes with the transmission of pain impulses. A client with diabetes who has myocardial ischemia may be pain free. Careful history combined with subjective findings should be used in diagnosing cardiac emergencies in a client with diabetes. The use of aspartame, sulfonylurea agents, or insulin doesn't interfere with pain impulse transmission to the brain.

Nursing process step: Assessment

22. The nurse would expect to see respiratory acidosis as a result of:

[ ] **A.** salicylate toxicity.

[ ] **B.** aldosteronism.

[ ] **C.** severe scoliosis.

[ ] **D.** high altitudes.

Correct answer—C. *Rationales:* Scoliosis prevents the thoracic cage from expanding and, therefore, decreases tidal volumes. Respiratory acidosis occurs in severe cases of scoliosis. High altitudes, aldosteronism, and salicylate toxicity produce respiratory alkalosis.

Nursing process step: Assessment

23. Encouraging fantasy, play, and participation in their care is a useful developmental approach for which pediatric age-group?

[ ] **A.** Preschool (ages 3 to 5)

[ ] **B.** Adolescence (ages 10 to 19)

[ ] **C.** School-age (ages 5 to 10)

[ ] **D.** Toddler (ages 1 to 3)

Correct answer—A. *Rationales:* A child in the preschool age-group has a rich fantasy life. Combined with his strong concept of self, fantasy play and participation in care can minimize the trauma of being in the emergency department. An adolescent should be allowed choices and control. A school-age child is modest and needs to have his privacy respected; in addition, procedures should be explained to him. A toddler should be examined in the presence of his parents because he fears separation. Offer choices when possible.

Nursing process step: Intervention

24. After any type of traumatic injury, a child may experience:

[ ] **A.** bradycardia.

[ ] **B.** aerophagia.

[ ] **C.** hypothermia.

[ ] **D.** Cushing's phenomenon.

Correct answer—B. *Rationales:* Swallowing of air (aerophagia) occurs in children, causing gastric dilatation that impedes diaphragmatic expansion. Cushing's phenomenon is bradycardia in the presence of increasing blood pressure; it's associated with an increase in intracranial pressure. Hypothermia is seen when the child's clothing is removed and the child is exposed to the ambient environment.

Nursing process step: Assessment

25. Which of the following is an ominous sign of impending cardiac arrest in children?
[ ] **A.** Tachycardia
[ ] **B.** Increased peripheral vascular resistance
[ ] **C.** Tachypnea
[ ] **D.** Bradycardia

Correct answer—D. *Rationales:* Bradycardia is an ominous sign of cardiac arrest in children and should be considered the result of hypoxia until proven otherwise. Tachypnea is indicative of respiratory distress or anxiety; tachycardia is seen with febrile illness. Increased peripheral resistance isn't a common finding in children and is associated with ingestion of pharmacologic agents.
Nursing process step: Assessment

26. Which of the following is a late sign of hypovolemic shock in a child?
[ ] **A.** Absence of bilateral breath sounds
[ ] **B.** Presence of hypotension
[ ] **C.** Presence of flushing of the skin
[ ] **D.** Presence of tachycardia

Correct answer—B. *Rationales:* Because a child can compensate for blood loss by increasing his intrinsic heart rate and peripheral vascular resistance, up to 33% of blood volume may be lost before a change in blood pressure. Capillary refill is a sensitive indicator of perfusion in the pediatric client. Absence of breath sounds is commonly seen in a client with pneumothorax. Tachycardia is commonly seen with anxiety or febrile illness. Flushing of the skin is seen with toxic ingestion.
Nursing process step: Assessment

27. Which medication can't be administered using an endotracheal (ET) tube?
[ ] **A.** Naltraxone (ReVia)
[ ] **B.** Amiodarone
[ ] **C.** Epinephrine
[ ] **D.** Atropine

Correct answer—B. *Rationales:* Naltraxone, atropine, diazepam, epinephrine, and lidocaine are the five agents that can be administered using an ET tube.
Nursing process step: Intervention

28. Which statement about adenosine (Adenocard) administration is correct?
[ ] **A.** Adenosine should be given by I.V. push over 1 to 3 minutes.
[ ] **B.** Adenosine should be given by continuous I.V. infusion over 20 to 30 minutes.
[ ] **C.** Adenosine should be given by deep I.M. injection.
[ ] **D.** Adenosine should be given by I.V. push over 1 to 3 seconds, followed by a 10-mL flush with normal saline.

Correct answer—D. *Rationales:* The half-life of adenosine is 10 seconds; therefore, it requires rapid I.V. push administration, followed by a 10-mL infusion with normal saline.
Nursing process step: Evaluation

29. A client is chosen as a match for a donor heart based on:
[ ] **A.** blood type only.
[ ] **B.** blood type and donor-recipient weight compatibility.
[ ] **C.** HLA crossmatch compatibility only.
[ ] **D.** donor-recipient age compatibility.

Correct answer—B. *Rationales:* A client is compatible with a donor heart if ABO type and body weight are compatible. HLA-antigen typing may be used for high-risk clients. Age, HLA crossmatch compatibility, and ABO type aren't used in determining allocation independent of one another.
Nursing process step: Assessment

30. Anencephalics can't become organ donors for which reason?
[ ] **A.** They don't fully meet the criteria for brain death.
[ ] **B.** They have multiple congenital anomalies that preclude transplantation.
[ ] **C.** They are medical examiner cases that require autopsy.
[ ] **D.** It's recommended that families not be approached about donation after the loss of an anencephalic infant.

Correct answer—A. *Rationales:* Organ donation in the United States occurs after the determination of death using neurologic criteria (brain death). The Uniform Determination of Death Act states that death is determined when there's irreversible damage to the entire brain. Because anencephalics are born without a cerebrum, they can't fulfill this criterion. Anencephalics commonly have multiple congenital anomalies, although these aren't what exclude them from donation. Organ donation can occur in medical examiner cases. Federal law requires that all families be approached with the option of organ or tissue donation after the loss of a loved one, unless prior documentation indicates that this isn't their wish.
Nursing process step: Analysis

31. Which of the following is true about critical incident stress?
[ ] **A.** Defined by each individual
[ ] **B.** Seen frequently throughout the career of emergency providers
[ ] **C.** Seen as occupation-related stress
[ ] **D.** Seen only in the direct caregiver

Correct answer—A. *Rationales:* There's no exact definition for critical incident stress—it's a personally defined term. What one person determines as critical incident stress may have no significant impact on another person. Therefore, all individuals should be evaluated based on their perception versus that of the examiner. Comparisons between involved individuals may obscure the diagnosis. Critical incident stress doesn't happen frequently, and it may be occupation-related stress. It can involve on-scene and off-scene personnel.
Nursing process step: Analysis

32. Dopamine is ordered for administration to a client with hypotension. Which agent is used to counteract soft-tissue necrosis after extravasation?
[ ] **A.** Sodium bicarbonate
[ ] **B.** Phentolamine (Regitine)
[ ] **C.** Naloxone
[ ] **D.** Ranitidine (Zantac)

Correct answer—B. *Rationales:* Phentolamine is used both prophylactically and in the treatment of dopamine extravasation to prevent tissue sloughing and necrosis. Sodium bicarbonate promotes further tissue damage. Naloxone is used to reverse the effects of opioid analgesics. Ranitidine is used as a prophylactic histamine-2 blocking agent.
Nursing process step: Intervention

33. A kidney transplant recipient verbalizes an understanding of discharge teaching when he states:
[ ] **A.** "I should take acetaminophen (Tylenol) if I have a fever."
[ ] **B.** "I should have flank pain for a few weeks postoperatively."
[ ] **C.** "I should notify the physician immediately if I develop flank pain, fever, or weakness."
[ ] **D.** "I can stop taking my immunosuppressant drugs when I begin to feel better."

Correct answer—C. *Rationales:* Successful discharge teaching should show evidence that the client can identify signs and symptoms of rejection. These symptoms include fever, malaise, flank pain or tenderness, and a decrease in urine output. Once these symptoms are identified, the client should understand the importance of reporting them to the physician immediately so that immunosuppressive therapy can be increased. The client should also understand that immunosuppressive therapy must continue for life.
Nursing process step: Evaluation

34. Dopamine is inappropriate for a client with:
[ ] **A.** hypotension secondary to tachyarrhythmias.
[ ] **B.** euvolemic hypotension.
[ ] **C.** continued hypovolemic hypotension after fluid resuscitation.
[ ] **D.** concomitant dobutamine infusion.

Correct answer—A. *Rationales:* Dopamine is a potent alpha, beta, and dopaminergic receptor-stimulating agent used in the treatment of hypotension after correction of hypovolemia. Tachycardia is a common adverse effect of dopamine at high doses; therefore, it's contraindicated in the treatment of tachyarrhythmia-induced hypotension. Dopamine is indicated for treating euvolemic hypotension and continued hypovolemic hypotension after fluid resuscitation combined with surgical intervention. It's also used concomitantly with dobutamine to increase systemic blood pressure and cardiac output.
Nursing process step: Evaluation

35. Which cadaveric tissues can't be banked for future transplantation?
[ ] **A.** Heart valves
[ ] **B.** Bone marrow
[ ] **C.** Meniscus and cartilage
[ ] **D.** Saphenous veins

Correct answer—B. *Rationales:* Bone marrow can't be stored—it must be transplanted shortly after procurement. Heart valves, saphenous veins, and meniscus and cartilage can be cryopreserved for later transplantation.
Nursing process step: Analysis

36. The physician orders a continuous infusion of lidocaine (Xylocaine) at 3 mg/minute for the treatment of premature ventricular complexes after a lidocaine bolus administration. Lidocaine is mixed in a concentration of 1 g in 250 mL of dextrose 5% in water by way of an infusion pump. What's the infusion rate in milliliters per hour (assuming the use of microdrip 60-gtt/mL tubing)?
[ ] **A.** 15 mL/hour
[ ] **B.** 30 mL/hour
[ ] **C.** 45 mL/hour
[ ] **D.** 75 mL/hour

Correct answer—C. *Rationales:* First, determine the concentration of the lidocaine by changing 1 g to 1,000 mg. Then divide 1,000 mg by 250 mL, which is 4 mg/mL. So, the concentration of the lidocaine is 4 mg/mL. Then use the following formula: dosage in milligrams per minute multiplied by 60 minutes divided by the concentration in milligrams per milliliter equals the pump setting in milliliters per hour.
3 mg/minute $\times$ 60 = (180) divided by 4 = 45 mL/hour.
Nursing process step: Intervention

37. What's the most commonly reported emotional change resulting from critical incident stress?
[ ] **A.** Panic
[ ] **B.** Euphoria
[ ] **C.** Hebephrenia
[ ] **D.** Depression

Correct answer—A. *Rationales:* Panic is the most commonly reported emotional change. Euphoria, hebephrenia, and depression aren't seen after critical incident stress and are attributed to other mental illnesses.
Nursing process step: Assessment

38. Which test would best detect signs of rejection in a client who has received a liver transplant?
[ ] **A.** Blood culture
[ ] **B.** White blood cell (WBC) count
[ ] **C.** Liver biopsy
[ ] **D.** Decreased partial thromboplastin time (PTT)

Correct answer—C. *Rationales:* After liver transplantation, a liver biopsy is primarily used to monitor clients for rejection. Positive blood cultures in the liver transplant client indicate infection. The client's WBC count probably wouldn't be elevated, due to the immunosuppressive therapy used to prevent rejection. The client's PTT would probably be increased because the liver isn't functioning properly.
Nursing process step: Evaluation

39. The physician orders a continuous infusion of dopamine 400 mg in 250 mL of dextrose 5% in water at 10 mcg/kg/minute by way of an infusion pump in a 70-kg client. Which of the following is the infusion rate in milliliters/hour (assuming the use of microdrip 60-gtt/mL tubing).

[ ] **A.** 26 mL/hour
[ ] **B.** 30 mL/hour
[ ] **C.** 36 mL/hour
[ ] **D.** 40 mL/hour

Correct answer—A. *Rationales:* The concentration of dopamine is 1,600 mcg/mL (change 400 mg to 400,000 mcg and then 400,000 mcg divided by 250 mL = 1,600 mcg/mL). To infuse 10 mcg/kg/minute, the nurse should infuse 26 mL/hour. Use the following formula: Dosage in microgram per kilogram per minute multiplied by the client's weight in kilograms, multiplied by 60 minutes, divided by the drug concentration in micrograms per milliliter. 10 mcg/kg/minute × 70 kg = (700) × 60 minutes = (42,000) divided by 1,600 mcg/mL = 26 mL/hour.
Nursing process step: Intervention

40. What is the role of the National Disaster Medical System (NDMS)?

[ ] **A.** To support local and regional medical assistance teams and assist with evacuations during a disaster
[ ] **B.** To help equip local and state emergency preparedness agencies for their preparation and response during a disaster
[ ] **C.** To take over state health operations after a disaster
[ ] **D.** To provide supplemental medical insurance to victims of a disaster

Correct answer—A. *Rationales:* The NDMS is a federally funded and coordinated system that augments the nation's medical response capability and assists local or regional authorities in dealing with the medical impacts of disasters. This includes providing medical assistance in the form of personnel, teams, supplies, and equipment as well as assisting with evacuation of victims and helping coordinate treatment for victims at definitive-care facilities in unaffected areas. NDMS does not take over state health operations or provide supplemental medical insurance. The Federal Emergency Management Agency is responsible for working with state and regional emergency preparedness agencies for their preparation during a disaster and for providing insurance or financial assistance to victims of a disaster.
Nursing process step: Analysis

41. Administration of nitroglycerin (Tridil) is ordered at 50 mcg/minute by way of an infusion pump. The infusion is prepared as nitroglycerin 100 mg in 250 mL of dextrose 5% in water. What's the infusion rate in milliliters/hour (assuming the use of microdrip 60-gtt/mL tubing)?

[ ] **A.** 6 mL/hour
[ ] **B.** 8 mL/hour
[ ] **C.** 10 mL/hour
[ ] **D.** 12 mL/hour

Correct answer—B. *Rationales:* The concentration of nitroglycerin is 0.04 mg/mL or 400 mcg/mL (100 mg divided by 250 mL = 0.04 mg/mL). To infuse 20 mcg/minute, the nurse should infuse 8 mL/hour. Use the following formula: Dosage in micrograms per minute multiplied by 60 minutes, divided by the concentration of drug = pump setting. 50 mcg/minute × 60 minutes = (3,000) divided by 400 mcg/mL = 7.5 or 8 mL/hour.
Nursing process step: Intervention

42. Administration of dobutamine (Dobutrex) is ordered at 6 mcg/kg/minute by way of an infusion pump in a 75-kg client. The concentration is 500 mg in 250 mL of dextrose 5% in water. What's the infusion rate in milliliters/hour (assuming the use of 60-gtt/mL tubing)?

[ ] **A.** 11 mL/hour
[ ] **B.** 12 mL/hour
[ ] **C.** 14 mL/hour
[ ] **D.** 15 mL/hour

Correct answer—C. *Rationales:* The concentration of dobutamine is 2 mg/mL or 2,000 mcg/mL (500 mg divided by 250 mL = 2 mg/mL). To infuse 6 mcg/kg/minute, the nurse should infuse 14 mL/hour. Use the following formula: Dosage in micrograms per kilogram per minute multiplied by the client's weight in kilograms, multiplied by 60 minutes, divided by the concentration of drug in micrograms per milliliter. 6 mcg/kg/minute × 75 kg = (450) × 60 minutes = (27,000) divided by 2,000 mcg/mL = 13.5 or 14 mL/hour.
Nursing process step: Intervention

43. Where is the best place to hear a vesicular breath sound?
[ ] **A.** During expiration in a patient with pulmonary edema
[ ] **B.** During inspiration in a patient with a pneumothorax
[ ] **C.** During inspiration in a patient with normal pulmonary physiology
[ ] **D.** During expiration in a patient with partial airway obstruction

Correct answer—C. *Rationales:* Vesicular breath sounds are the normal breath sounds heard over the peripheral lung fields (alveoli) primarily during inspiration. Vesicular sounds are commonly described as soft, blowing, or rustling sounds. Crackles or rales would be heard with pulmonary edema. Diminished or absent breath sounds would be heard with a pneumothorax, and stridor may be heard with airway obstruction.
Nursing process step: Assessment

44. Which statement about administering nitrous oxide-oxygen 50:50 mixture is true?
[ ] **A.** It's safe for use in the first and second trimesters of pregnancy.
[ ] **B.** The client self-administers the drug until pain is relieved.
[ ] **C.** Prolonged use may produce tachypnea.
[ ] **D.** It may be beneficial in relieving pain from pneumothorax or abdominal obstruction.

Correct answer—B. *Rationales:* Nitrous oxide is self-administered by the client until adequate analgesia is obtained. Nitrous oxide use is safe only in the third trimester of pregnancy, and it may worsen pneumothorax or intestinal obstruction. Prolonged use of nitrous oxide doesn't result in tachypnea.
Nursing process step: Evaluation

45. Which of the following is a necessary coenzyme in the metabolism of glucose?
[ ] **A.** Thiamine (vitamin B_1)
[ ] **B.** Protamine
[ ] **C.** Aspartame
[ ] **D.** Levothyroxine (Synthroid)

Correct answer—A. *Rationales:* Thiamine is a water-soluble vitamin that is a necessary coenzyme in most human metabolic processes, especially carbohydrate (glucose) metabolism. Protamine is used to reverse the effects of heparin sodium. Aspartame is an artificial sweetener that has no medicinal value. Levothyroxine is used for treating hypothyroidism.
Nursing process step: Analysis

46. Which of the following best defines magnesium sulfate?
[ ] **A.** Stimulates the central nervous system (CNS)
[ ] **B.** Depresses the CNS
[ ] **C.** Used in the treatment of atrioventricular block
[ ] **D.** Used to promote diuresis in clients with renal disease

Correct answer—B. *Rationales:* Magnesium sulfate depresses smooth, cardiac, and skeletal muscle in addition to depressing the CNS. It's commonly used to treat ventricular arrhythmia, torsades de pointes, and hypomagnesemia. It's also used in the postpartum management of preeclampsia and eclampsia. Magnesium sulfate is contraindicated in clients with preexisting renal disease and atrioventricular block.
Nursing process step: Analysis

47. A client will receive a kidney-pancreas transplant based on:
[ ] **A.** blood type only.
[ ] **B.** blood type and donor-recipient weight compatibility.
[ ] **C.** blood type and HLA compatibility.
[ ] **D.** HLA compatibility only.

Correct answer—C. *Rationales:* Allocation of a combined cadaver kidney-pancreas for transplantation is based on donor-recipient ABO type and HLA compatibility. ABO type, donor-recipient weight compatibility, and HLA compatibility aren't used independently of one another in determining pancreas allocation.
Nursing process step: Assessment

48. While assessing a client in triage, the nurse notices that the client is dyspneic and short of breath. These signs and symptoms are usually associated with:
[ ] **A.** bradycardia.
[ ] **B.** eupnea.
[ ] **C.** tachycardia.
[ ] **D.** bradypnea.

Correct answer—C. *Rationales:* Dyspnea and shortness of breath stimulate the sympathetic nervous system, causing catecholamine release, and result in tachycardia. Bradycardia is seen with vagal stimulation. Eupnea is a normal finding. When a client is short of breath, his respiratory rate increases, thereby eliminating bradypnea as a possible choice.
Nursing process step: Assessment

49. Increased cardiac responsiveness to catecholamines is the desired effect of which drug?
[ ] **A.** Epinephrine
[ ] **B.** Dopamine
[ ] **C.** Sodium bicarbonate
[ ] **D.** Atropine

Correct answer—C. *Rationales:* Sodium bicarbonate stabilizes ion balance and potentiates the effects of sympathomimetic (catecholamine) agents such as dopamine. Epinephrine is used in the treatment of ventricular arrhythmias; atropine is used in the treatment of bradyarrhythmias.
Nursing process step: Evaluation

50. When communicating with someone whose primary language isn't English, it's best to:
[ ] **A.** use slang or jargon instead of actual terms.
[ ] **B.** avoid use of the word "not."
[ ] **C.** use the passive voice instead of the active voice.
[ ] **D.** repeat misunderstood statements using the same words.

Correct answer—B. *Rationales:* The nurse should avoid using the word "not"; it can become lost in a sentence and create the opposite meaning. Likewise, active voice should be used in communication. Jargon and slang aren't readily translatable across languages or dialects. When statements are misunderstood, they should be repeated using different words.
Nursing process step: Intervention

51. Which statement about a continuous I.V. infusion of nitroglycerin is correct?
[ ] **A.** The I.V. bag is wrapped in aluminum foil to prevent exposure to light.
[ ] **B.** Filtered I.V. tubing is used.
[ ] **C.** Polyvinyl chloride tubing is used.
[ ] **D.** The infusion is diluted in dextrose 5% in water (D_5W) in a glass bottle.

Correct answer—D. *Rationales:* Nitroglycerin must be mixed in D_5W in a glass bottle and administered by way of nonfiltered, nonpolyvinyl chloride (plastic) tubing. A plastic container or tubing will absorb up to 80% of diluted nitroglycerin. Aluminum foil is wrapped around the I.V. bag when administering nitroprusside (Nitropress).
Nursing process step: Evaluation

52. Teaching is effective when the client receiving a monoamine oxidase (MAO) inhibitor states:
[ ] **A.** "I should avoid using antihistamines."
[ ] **B.** "I can no longer eat bread."
[ ] **C.** "I must avoid decaffeinated cola."
[ ] **D.** "I must refrain from eating ham and pork."

Correct answer—A. *Rationales:* When taking an MAO inhibitor, the client must avoid using antihistamines, which can potentiate the MAO inhibitor's effects and result in acute hypertensive crisis. The client should also avoid foods that contain tryptophan or tyramine. If the client requires elective surgery with general anesthesia or a local anesthetic that contains sympathomimetic vasoconstrictors, the MAO inhibitor should be discontinued within 10 days of the surgery.
Nursing process step: Evaluation

53. Anticholinergic crisis (toxicity) after antihistamine overdose is treated with:
[ ] **A.** pralidoxime.
[ ] **B.** naloxone.
[ ] **C.** dopamine.
[ ] **D.** physostigmine.

Correct answer—D. *Rationales:* Anticholinergic crisis may be caused by various medications and plant alkaloids. It produces hypertension, tachycardia, mydriasis, decreased bowel sounds, urine retention, and dry skin. The treatment is support of airway and breathing. Activated charcoal should be administered if the ingestion is within 1 hour of presentation. Physostigmine is the antidote; it inhibits acetylcholinesterase and can be used in conjunction with benzodiazepines to control delirium and seizures. Pralidoximine is the antidote for organophosphates that cause a cholinergic crisis. Naloxone is used to reverse the effects of opioid analgesics. Dopamine is used to increase systemic blood pressure and cardiac output.
Nursing process step: Intervention

54. Continuous I.V. nitroglycerin (Tridil) infusion in a client with acute myocardial infarction (MI) is effective when what happens?
[ ] **A.** Pain and ventricular preload are reduced.
[ ] **B.** Pain and ventricular afterload are reduced.
[ ] **C.** Pain is reduced and ventricular afterload is increased.
[ ] **D.** Pain is reduced and ventricular preload is increased.

Correct answer—A. *Rationales:* Nitroglycerin is a potent preload reducer. It's used after an acute MI to relieve pain and to decrease atrial and ventricular preload to minimize myocardial oxygen consumption and ischemia.
Nursing process step: Evaluation

55. The triage nurse should give highest priority to which client?
[ ] **A.** The client with crushing chest pain
[ ] **B.** The client with seizures
[ ] **C.** The client with severe abdominal pain
[ ] **D.** The client with heart failure

Correct answer—A. *Rationales:* The client with crushing chest pain is probably presenting with an acute myocardial infarction and should be seen immediately. The client with seizures, who isn't in status epilepticus, can be seen within 30 to 60 minutes of arrival at the emergency department. The client with abdominal pain, who doesn't present with signs of shock, and the client with heart failure, who isn't in acute distress, can also be seen within 30 to 60 minutes of arrival.
Nursing process step: Assessment

56. A multiple-trauma client with a hemothorax arrives in the emergency department. A chest tube is placed. Initially, 500 mL of blood drains from the tube. The client's vital signs are blood pressure, 146/74 mm Hg, and heart rate, 138 beats/minute. Respirations are controlled by mechanical ventilation at a rate of 16 breaths/minute. Which assessment parameter should be closely monitored over the next hour?
[ ] **A.** Vital signs
[ ] **B.** Central venous pressure
[ ] **C.** Chest tube drainage
[ ] **D.** Urine output

Correct answer—C. *Rationales*: The chest tube drainage should be monitored closely because the initial drainage was 500 mL. If the client continues to lose blood at a rate of 200 mL/hour or more, he may require surgical intervention to identify and repair the source of bleeding. Monitoring vital signs, central venous pressure, and urine output are all important in assessing fluid status, but monitoring chest drainage is the highest priority.
Nursing process step: Assessment

57. A child with a history of varicella and aspirin intake is brought to the emergency department. The nurse suspects Reye's syndrome. Which assessment findings are consistent with this syndrome?

[ ] **A.** Vomiting, decreased level of consciousness (LOC), and impaired liver function

[ ] **B.** Joint inflammation, red macular rash with a clear center, and low-grade fever

[ ] **C.** Peripheral edema, fever for 5 or more days, and "strawberry tongue"

[ ] **D.** Red, raised "bull's eye"–shaped rash, malaise, and joint pain

Correct answer—A. *Rationales:* Reye's syndrome occurs in children with a history of a viral infection, varicella, or influenza. It's usually associated with the administration of aspirin. The child presents with severe vomiting, dehydration, and decreased LOC, which can lead to coma and death. As the disease progresses, the child also develops impaired liver function. A child with joint pain, a red macular rash with a clear center, and a low-grade fever probably has rheumatic fever. The child presenting with peripheral edema, fever for more than 5 days, and a "strawberry tongue" probably has Kawasaki disease. The child with a red, raised "bull's eye" rash, malaise, and joint pain should be tested for Lyme disease.

Nursing process step: Assessment

58. The nurse is working triage on a busy Sunday. One half hour ago, the nurse triaged a 34-year-old client with lower back pain. He was assigned to level 4 based on his vital signs and history. The client returns to the nurse to complain about the wait. Several level 2 and 3 clients are still awaiting beds as well as clients waiting to be assessed. The nurse's next action should be to:

[ ] **A.** reassure the client that he's okay to wait and will be seen soon.

[ ] **B.** medicate the client with hydrocodone to make him more comfortable during his wait.

[ ] **C.** tell the client that it's a very busy day, and if he goes home and takes some ibuprofen, he can come back tomorrow if his back still hurts.

[ ] **D.** reassess the client for any change in his signs or symptoms.

Correct answer—D. *Rationales:* The client should be reassessed for any change in his signs or symptoms to rule out the evolution of a more emergent problem. A client's condition may change while awaiting treatment, thus moving him from one triage level to another. Reassuring the client that he's okay without reexamining him places the nurse at legal risk should an emergency condition have emerged. Although some institutions have standing orders to medicate with acetaminophen or ibuprofen for pain or fever, opioids shouldn't be given until the client receives his screening examination and an emergency medical condition is ruled out. Telling the client to go home could be construed as an EMTALA violation because he hasn't had his screening examination.

Nursing process step: Evaluation

59. During reexamination, the client with lower back pain relates new weakness in his legs and confesses in a whisper that he doesn't seem to be able to control his bowels. To what triage level should the nurse assign him now?

[ ] **A.** Upgrade to level 2; the additional symptoms indicate a more emergent process is occurring.

[ ] **B.** Remain at level 4; he's just "working the system" to get in faster.

[ ] **C.** Upgrade to level 3 because the client's pain is worse than first estimated.

[ ] **D.** Downgrade to level 5; the additional symptoms indicate that the pain medication is beginning to work.

Correct answer—A. *Rationales:* Upgrade to level 2 because the additional symptoms indicate a more emergent process is occurring. Back pain with the emergence of leg weakness and bowel incontinence is indicative of increasing pressure on the lower spinal cord, such as cauda equina syndrome, which is a high-risk condition that can have devastating results if left untreated. Level 3 isn't appropriate because it's for stable, low-risk clients. Likewise, the symptoms can't be attributed to any medication. Leaving him at level 4 is incorrect as well because this category is for clients with minor injuries or medical problems, who have a very low probability of deterioration.

Nursing process step: Assessment

14 Respiratory emergencies

1. An unrestrained passenger is thrown 20′ (6 m) from a car that hit an embankment. On admittance to the emergency department, the client is conscious; his vital signs are blood pressure, 90/60 mm Hg; pulse, 130 beats/minute with weak radial pulses; and respirations, 26 breaths/minute and shallow. Capillary refill is delayed. The lungs are clear bilaterally with diminished breath sounds on the right. Paradoxical chest movement is noted on the right side. Arterial blood gas analysis shows increased pH, decreased $PaCO_2$, and diminished PaO_2. A chest X-ray shows a right pneumothorax and multiple rib fractures on the right (4th to 7th). The client's skin is pale and cool, and he's confused and restless. What's the most likely diagnosis for this client?

[ ] **A.** Tension pneumothorax
[ ] **B.** Flail chest
[ ] **C.** Ruptured diaphragm
[ ] **D.** Massive hemothorax

Correct answer—B. *Rationales:* The client's multiple rib fractures caused a flail chest. Signs include:

- bruised skin.
- extreme pain.
- paradoxical chest movements.
- rapid and shallow respirations.
- tachycardia.
- hypotension.
- respiratory acidosis.
- cyanosis.

Flail chest can also cause tension pneumothorax, a condition in which air enters the chest but can't be ejected during exhalation. Classic signs are tracheal deviation (away from the affected side), cyanosis, severe dyspnea, absent breath sounds on the affected side, distended jugular veins, and shock. The client with a ruptured diaphragm presents with hyperresonance on percussion, hypotension, dyspnea, dysphagia, shifted heart sounds, and bowel sounds in the lower to middle chest. A client with massive hemothorax shows signs of shock (tachycardia, hypotension), dullness on percussion on the injured side, decreased breath sounds on the injured side, respiratory distress and, possibly, mediastinal shift.

Nursing process step: Assessment

2. What's the definition of flail chest?

[ ] **A.** An unstable segment of the chest wall that moves paradoxically with respirations
[ ] **B.** A compressed rib cage with open chest wound
[ ] **C.** A fracture of two adjacent ribs, bilaterally
[ ] **D.** A fracture of two or more ribs in two or more places

Correct answer—D. *Rationales:* Flail chest is a fracture of two or more ribs in two or more places, resulting in a free-floating segment of the chest wall. Paradoxical chest movement is commonly a sign of flail chest; however, until the chest muscles relax or pain relief is achieved, paradoxical movements are unlikely to be seen. Flail chest is usually a closed injury. Bilateral injury isn't required in flail chest. If bilateral injury is present, the risk of mortality increases drastically.

Nursing process step: Assessment

3. Which of the following assessment findings wouldn't indicate a flail chest?

[ ] **A.** Paradoxical movement of the chest wall
[ ] **B.** Sucking chest wound
[ ] **C.** Respiratory distress
[ ] **D.** Pulmonary contusion

Correct answer—B. *Rationales:* A sucking chest wound is indicative of an open pneumothorax. All other findings are associated with flail chest.

Nursing process step: Assessment

4. What's the most likely laboratory finding in a client with acute respiratory distress syndrome (ARDS)?
[ ] **A.** Elevated carboxyhemoglobin level
[ ] **B.** Decreased PaO_2
[ ] **C.** Elevated $PaCO_2$
[ ] **D.** Decreased HCO_3^-

Correct answer—B. *Rationales:* Hypoxemia is a universal finding in ARDS. The $PaCO_2$ is low early in the disease because of hyperventilation, and it rises later in the disease because of fatigue and worsening clinical status. The bicarbonate level may be low in ARDS and is related to reduced tissue oxygenation. Reduced oxygenation leads to anaerobic metabolism and accumulating lactate. HCO_3^- in the serum combines with the lactate, reducing circulating HCO_3^- levels. The carboxyhemoglobin level is increased in a client with an inhalation injury, which commonly progresses to ARDS; however, this isn't a common cause of ARDS.
Nursing process step: Assessment

5. What's the most appropriate intervention for a client with chronic obstructive pulmonary disease (COPD)?
[ ] **A.** Administer 100% oxygen by way of a nonrebreather mask.
[ ] **B.** Obtain and monitor arterial blood gas (ABG) levels.
[ ] **C.** Restrict fluids.
[ ] **D.** Place the client in a supine position.

Correct answer—B. *Rationales:* The client with COPD has abnormal ABG levels, which may predispose him to respiratory distress. The client is hypoxemic with hypercapnia. Oxygen should be administered at low concentrations to maintain hypoxic drive. If the PaO_2 remains inadequate at low dose, the nurse should increase the oxygen while continuously monitoring the client's respiratory status. A client with COPD usually benefits from adequate hydration to liquefy secretions. Allow the client to assume a position that facilitates ventilation, usually a forward-leaning high Fowler's position.
Nursing process step: Intervention

6. Impaired pulmonary capillary permeability, high positive end-expiratory pressure (PEEP) on a ventilator, and an inability to maintain adequate oxygen saturation are signs of which of the following?
[ ] **A.** Emphysema
[ ] **B.** Pulmonary effusion
[ ] **C.** Chronic bronchitis
[ ] **D.** Acute respiratory distress syndrome (ARDS)

Correct answer—D. *Rationales:* Acute respiratory distress syndrome (ARDS) is an acute physiologic syndrome characterized by noncardiac pulmonary edema caused by increased pulmonary capillary permeability, high PEEP, and low oxygen saturation despite the use of supplemental oxygen. Emphysema is a permanent condition that's caused by alveolar destruction. Pulmonary effusion is caused by excessive fluid accumulation in the pleura, and chronic bronchitis is a narrowing of the airway passages and an increase in mucus production.
Nursing process step: Assessment

7. A client with chronic obstructive pulmonary disease (COPD) is given discharge instructions regarding nutritional support. Which statement indicates the need for further teaching?
[ ] **A.** "I should eat five or six small meals each day."
[ ] **B.** "I will limit my fluid intake at mealtime."
[ ] **C.** "I should select most of my foods from the carbohydrate group."
[ ] **D.** "I should rest for 30 minutes before each meal."

Correct answer—C. *Rationales:* The client with COPD has a markedly increased need for protein and calories to maintain an adequate nutritional status. The client's diet should be high in both protein and calories and should be divided into five or six small meals per day. Fluid intake should be maintained at 3 L/day unless contraindicated. Fluids should be taken between meals to reduce gastric distention and pressure on the diaphragm. The client with COPD should rest for 30 minutes before each meal to conserve energy and decrease dyspnea. The client should also avoid exercise and breathing treatments for at least 1 hour before and after eating.
Nursing process step: Evaluation

8. Right-sided heart failure can occur secondary to pulmonary embolus. Which finding is consistent with this development?
[ ] **A.** Physiologic S_2 split heart sound
[ ] **B.** Peaked P wave on electrocardiogram (ECG)
[ ] **C.** Expiratory wheeze
[ ] **D.** Pericardial friction rub

Correct answer—B. *Rationales:* Elevated pulmonary pressures resulting from pulmonary emboli can lead to dysfunction of the right heart, which in turn can lead to an increase in right atrial volume, showing an altered P wave on the ECG. The lead to monitor for this finding is lead II. In this lead, the P wave is taller and more peaked than a normal P wave. A physiologic S_2 split is normal. When pulmonary pressures become severely elevated, the split becomes pathologic. Breath sounds are generally clear in a client with pulmonary emboli, although a pleural friction rub may be heard.
Nursing process step: Assessment

9. Air trapping, inflammation of smooth muscles, and mucus secretion are classical signs of what respiratory illness?
[ ] **A.** Pulmonary effusion
[ ] **B.** Asthma
[ ] **C.** Chronic bronchitis
[ ] **D.** Acute respiratory distress syndrome (ARDS)

Correct answer—B. *Rationales:* Inflammation of smooth muscle leading to constriction and mucus production results in air trapping, respiratory acidosis, and hypoxemia, the classic definition of asthma. Pulmonary effusion is caused by excessive fluid accumulation in the pleura. Chronic bronchitis is a narrowing of the airway passages and an increase in mucus production, but it doesn't produce air trapping. ARDS is an acute physiologic syndrome characterized by noncardiac pulmonary edema caused by increased pulmonary capillary permeability, high PEEP, and low oxygen saturation despite the use of supplemental oxygen.
Nursing process step: Assessment

10. Which diagnostic study most accurately identifies the presence of a pulmonary embolus?
[ ] **A.** Bronchoscopy
[ ] **B.** Chest X-ray
[ ] **C.** Ventilation/perfusion ($\dot{V}/\dot{Q}$) scan
[ ] **D.** Pulmonary angiography

Correct answer—D. *Rationales:* Although riskier than a $\dot{V}/\dot{Q}$ scan, pulmonary angiography confirms the presence of a pulmonary embolus. Bronchoscopy is typically used in differential diagnosis of pneumonia. A chest X-ray is usually done to rule out other pulmonary problems, such as pneumonia and atelectasis. A $\dot{V}/\dot{Q}$ scan is used to locate the inadequately perfused area; however, results aren't definitive.
Nursing process step: Assessment

11. Which drug is safe for administration to the client with asthma?
[ ] **A.** Beta-adrenergic blockers
[ ] **B.** Beta$_2$-agonists
[ ] **C.** Aspirin
[ ] **D.** Nonsteroidal anti-inflammatory drugs (NSAIDs)

Correct answer—B. *Rationales:* Beta$_2$-agonists are the first-line drugs of choice for the client with asthma. They relax bronchial smooth muscle and enhance mucociliary clearance. Beta-adrenergic blockers, aspirin, and NSAIDs all worsen asthma.
Nursing process step: Analysis

12. Which finding is consistent with blood loss greater than 1,500 mL in a client with a hemothorax?
[ ] **A.** Mediastinal shift
[ ] **B.** Blood pressure more than 80 mm Hg systolic
[ ] **C.** Capillary refill greater than 2 seconds
[ ] **D.** Increased urinary output

Correct answer—A. *Rationales:* A mediastinal shift, systolic blood pressure less than 80 mm Hg, and a capillary refill greater than 4 seconds can all be associated with a hemothorax greater than 1,500 mL. The client with a massive hemothorax has mediastinal shift, blood pressure depicting decompensation, diminished peripheral blood flow, decreased urine output, and respiratory distress.
Nursing process step: Assessment

13. After teaching the client with asthma about inhalers, which statement indicates the need for further instruction?
[ ] **A.** "I should hold the inhaler upright and shake it well."
[ ] **B.** "I should hold my breath for 5 to 10 seconds after each puff."
[ ] **C.** "I should hold the inhaler in my mouth and make sure I have a good seal with my lips."
[ ] **D.** "I should hold my head back and forcefully exhale."

Correct answer—D. *Rationales:* If the client states "I should hold my head back and forcefully exhale," further teaching is necessary. The correct technique for using an inhaler is as follows: The inhaler must be mixed thoroughly before administration. The client should hold his breath for 5 to 10 seconds to allow the medication to reach as far as possible into the lungs. If the client has difficulty with this technique, a spacer device may be added to the inhaler. A forced exhalation isn't recommended because coughing, small-airway closure, and air trapping may result.
Nursing process step: Evaluation

14. The first priority for a client with pulmonary embolus is:
[ ] **A.** correcting the hypoxia with oxygen by way of a face mask.
[ ] **B.** administering heparin.
[ ] **C.** considering thrombolytic therapy.
[ ] **D.** administering morphine to treat pain.

Correct answer—A. *Rationales:* The priority is always airway, breathing, and circulation. Provide oxygen by face mask. If hypocapnia is present on admission, arterial blood gas (ABG) analysis should be repeated within 15 to 20 minutes. Worsening hypocapnia with progressive obtundation is an indication for emergency intubation. A loading dose of heparin should be administered, followed by a continuous drip. The heparin should be titrated to an activated partial thromboplastin time 1½ to 2 times the control. Heparin therapy is sufficient treatment for most clients with pulmonary emboli. For clients who present with significant hemodynamic compromise, streptokinase (Streptase) and tissue plasminogen activator (alteplase [Activase]) have been approved for use in pulmonary emboli. Pain increases oxygen demand and anxiety, and it should be treated with morphine or meperidine (Demerol). The nurse should monitor ABG levels carefully to prevent carbon dioxide retention.
Nursing process step: Analysis

15. Measuring lung function by determining the client's peak expiratory flow rate (PEFR) is an important step in determining the success of asthma management. What's the optimal PEFR?
[ ] **A.** PEFR greater than 80% of predicted or personal best
[ ] **B.** PEFR variability 20% to 30%
[ ] **C.** PEFR less than 50% of predicted or personal best
[ ] **D.** PEFR variability less than 30%

Correct answer—A. *Rationales:* The optimal PEFR is greater than 80% of predicted or personal best with a variability of less than 20%. Monitoring PEFR helps assess the severity of obstruction. The nurse should evaluate the client's response to treatment and detect changes in airflow. If PEFR is increasing and subjective symptoms are decreasing, medication or dosage needn't be changed. If PEFR is decreasing and symptoms are increasing, the client can better judge his status and adjust medications appropriately.
Nursing process step: Evaluation

16. What's the most likely finding on a lateral neck X-ray in a child with epiglottiditis?
[ ] **A.** Supraglottic narrowing
[ ] **B.** Steeple sign
[ ] **C.** Thickened mass
[ ] **D.** Subglottic narrowing

Correct answer—C. *Rationales:* X-ray assessment of the lateral neck assists in diagnosing common respiratory emergencies in children. The lateral neck X-ray of a child with epiglottiditis shows a thickened mass. The steeple sign is found in the client with viral croup syndrome. Subglottic narrowing with membranous tracheal exudate is found in bacterial tracheitis. Supraglottic narrowing isn't a diagnostic indicator.
Nursing process step: Assessment

17. Which intervention would be *least* effective for a client who's breathing deeply and coughing productively?
[ ] **A.** Incentive spirometry every 2 hours
[ ] **B.** Sitting in a chair at the bedside three times per day
[ ] **C.** Splinting the abdomen when coughing
[ ] **D.** Suctioning the client every 2 hours and when necessary

Correct answer—D. *Rationales:* If the client is effectively removing secretions, suctioning can be harmful. Suctioning can cause mucosal trauma, hypoxemia, and even pulmonary infection. Incentive spirometry every 2 hours, sitting in a chair at bedside three times per day, and splinting the abdomen to facilitate coughing are all measures to prevent pneumonia.
Nursing process step: Evaluation

18. Diagnostic tests that might be helpful in supporting a diagnosis of pneumonia include:
[ ] **A.** complete blood count (CBC) and chest X-ray.
[ ] **B.** CBC, chest X-ray, and lumbar puncture.
[ ] **C.** chest X-ray and sedimentation rate.
[ ] **D.** CBC with differential and electrolytes.

Correct answer—A. *Rationales:* A CBC is helpful in determining the presence of infection and identifying the microbial (viral, bacterial, fungal) agent. A chest X-ray can identify the location of the pneumonia. Sedimentation rate, electrolytes, and lumbar puncture don't assist in the differential diagnosis of pneumonia.
Nursing process step: Assessment

19. What's the priority intervention for a child with epiglottiditis?
[ ] **A.** Administering oxygen by face mask
[ ] **B.** Administering parenteral antibiotics
[ ] **C.** Assisting with intubation
[ ] **D.** Monitoring the electrocardiogram for arrhythmias

Correct answer—C. *Rationales:* Because children are at high risk for developing abrupt airway obstruction, the most important intervention for a child with epiglottiditis is airway management. Intubation should be performed as soon as possible in a controlled environment. Children need supplemental oxygen, but most are so anxious that they won't allow a mask to stay in place. Provide humidified "blow-by" oxygen administered by the parent, if possible. The child needs parenteral antibiotics; however, the priority is airway management. The most common rhythm in this client is sinus tachycardia related to compensation.
Nursing process step: Analysis

20. A client was admitted to the emergency department after being involved in a single-car collision. On inspection, the nurse finds tachypnea, bulging of the intercostal spaces on the left side, labored breathing with accessory muscle use, and jugular vein distention. There is hyperresonance on the left side and absent breath sounds on the left. What's the most likely diagnosis, based on the findings described above?
[ ] **A.** Tension pneumothorax
[ ] **B.** Flail chest
[ ] **C.** Ruptured diaphragm
[ ] **D.** Massive hemothorax

Correct answer—A. *Rationales:* Tension pneumothorax presents with severe respiratory distress, hypotension, diminished breath sounds over the affected area, hyperresonance, jugular vein distention and, eventually, tracheal shift. A finding of multiple rib fractures in a client with respiratory distress verifies a diagnosis of flail chest. A client with a ruptured diaphragm presents with hyperresonance on percussion, hypotension, dyspnea, dysphagia, shifted heart sounds, and bowel sounds in the lower to middle chest.
A client with massive hemothorax shows signs of shock (tachycardia, hypotension), dullness on percussion on the injured side, decreased breath sounds on the injured side, respiratory distress, and possibly, mediastinal shift.
Nursing process step: Assessment

21. What's the most common cause of traumatic pneumothorax?
[ ] **A.** Broken ribs
[ ] **B.** Gunshot wound
[ ] **C.** Barotrauma
[ ] **D.** Central line insertion

Correct answer—A. *Rationales:* The most common cause of traumatic pneumothorax is broken ribs. Other common causes include penetrating trauma (gunshot or knife wound), insertion of a central venous pressure catheter, barotrauma in mechanically ventilated clients, and closed pleural biopsy.
Nursing process step: Assessment

22. Which finding indicates that a chest tube isn't effective in the management of a pneumothorax?
[ ] **A.** Client resting, respirations 12 breaths/minute
[ ] **B.** Breath sounds equal bilaterally, equal chest excursion
[ ] **C.** Client anxious, respirations 36 breaths/minute, with cyanosis
[ ] **D.** Trachea midline, jugular veins not distended

Correct answer—C. *Rationales:* After chest tube insertion, the client should be calm. A client who's anxious with cyanosis and rapid respirations is showing signs of respiratory distress. If the chest tube is effective, respirations should be within normal limits for the age of the client. Breath sounds should be heard in all lobes bilaterally with equal excursion of chest. The trachea should be midline without jugular vein distention.
Nursing process step: Evaluation

23. What's the primary goal in the treatment of a client with acute respiratory distress syndrome (ARDS)?
[ ] **A.** Identifying and treating the underlying condition
[ ] **B.** Maintaining nutritional requirements
[ ] **C.** Maintaining adequate tissue oxygenation
[ ] **D.** Preventing secondary infection

Correct answer—A. *Rationales:* Identifying and treating the underlying condition is the primary goal. If the condition causing ARDS isn't treated, injury to the lung continues, preventing adequate tissue oxygenation and predisposing the client to secondary infection. The nurse should also provide adequate nutritional support in the form of increased protein and calories and limited carbohydrate intake.
Nursing process step: Analysis

24. A 24-year-old male is transported via EMS to the emergency department after having fallen from a roof. Upon assessing, the nurse notes lack of breath sounds on the left side. A chest tube is inserted in the left chest, but instead of releasing air, the catheter expels blood. What might be the reason for this?
[ ] **A.** Tension pneumothorax
[ ] **B.** Pulmonary artery perforation
[ ] **C.** Hemothorax
[ ] **D.** Simple pneumothorax

Correct answer—C. *Rationales:* Hemothorax is caused by free blood in the pleural space, usually caused by trauma, which will result in diminished or absent breath sounds on the affected side. Pulmonary artery perforation will result in the loss of a large amount of blood and can lead to shock. A tension pneumothorax is a life-threatening condition caused by an accumulation of air in the pleural space. A simple pneumothorax doesn't require chest decompression.
Nursing process step: Assessment

25. What's the most appropriate bronchodilator for a client who's taking a nonselective beta-adrenergic blocker?
[ ] **A.** Ephedrine
[ ] **B.** Epinephrine
[ ] **C.** Metaproterenol
[ ] **D.** Theophylline

Correct answer—C. *Rationales:* The use of a beta$_2$-agonist bronchodilator, such as metaproterenol, would be most effective. Nonselective beta-adrenergic blockers interfere with the bronchodilating effects of ephedrine, theophylline, and epinephrine. The beta-adrenergic effects of epinephrine remain unblocked, increasing systemic vasoconstriction.
Nursing process step: Intervention

26. What's the definitive therapy for a client with a massive hemothorax?

[ ] **A.** Emergency thoracotomy
[ ] **B.** Chest tube insertion
[ ] **C.** Fluid resuscitation
[ ] **D.** Supplemental oxygenation

Correct answer—A. *Rationales:* The definitive treatment for a client with a massive hemothorax is emergency thoracotomy. It's imperative to identify and repair the source of bleeding. Temporary measures to stabilize the client include chest tube insertion and, possibly, autotransfusion, fluid resuscitation (crystalloids and colloids), and supplemental oxygenation.
Nursing process step: Intervention

27. What's the most serious injury associated with a fracture of the first or second rib?

[ ] **A.** Cervical spine injury
[ ] **B.** Aortic rupture
[ ] **C.** Tracheal tear
[ ] **D.** Clavicular fracture

Correct answer—B. *Rationales:* Although a cervical spine injury, tracheal tear, or clavicular fracture can be associated with a fracture of the first or second rib, the most serious injury is aortic rupture, which often results in immediate death from severe hemodynamic compromise. Suspect an aortic rupture in a trauma client with motor, sensory, or pulse deficits in the lower extremities. Such deficits usually result from disruption of blood flow to the spinal cord. Other symptoms include unexplained hypotension and chest or back pain. A cervical spine injury can also be serious, especially if it involves a C3, C4, or higher lesion, which can result in respiratory depression. Tracheal tears lead to pneumomediastinum and have the potential for tension pneumothorax if undetected. Clavicular fractures cause great pain; however, they seldom cause more severe consequences.
Nursing process step: Assessment

28. What's the most important treatment for the client with tension pneumothorax?

[ ] **A.** Elevate the head of the client's bed.
[ ] **B.** Administer 100% oxygen by way of a nonrebreather mask.
[ ] **C.** Infuse normal saline solution at a keep-vein-open rate.
[ ] **D.** Assist with needle decompression.

Correct answer—D. *Rationales:* All of the options listed are important in the treatment of tension pneumothorax, but the most important is needle decompression. A 14G needle is inserted into the second intercostal space at the midclavicular line on the affected side. A chest tube insertion should follow needle decompression.
Nursing process step: Intervention

29. What's the most appropriate position to facilitate oxygen exchange in the client with acute respiratory distress syndrome (ARDS)?

[ ] **A.** Side-lying position with the right lung down
[ ] **B.** Side-lying position with the left lung down
[ ] **C.** Prone position slightly on the right side
[ ] **D.** Semi-Fowler's position lying on the left side

Correct answer—C. *Rationales:* Research has shown that improved oxygenation parameters are seen when a client with ARDS is placed in the prone position. In ARDS, neither lung is functioning properly; therefore, the good lung down doesn't help determine positioning. Changing the client's position at least every 2 hours is important. The right lung down usually produces the next best oxygenation parameters. This lung has three lobes and isn't compressed by the heart. The nurse should allow 15 minutes after each turn for stabilization of parameters. If they don't improve, the client should be turned to a more functional position.
Nursing process step: Intervention

30. Which finding is commonly associated with a poor outcome in a client with a pulmonary contusion?
[ ] **A.** Temperature of 100.4° F (38° C)
[ ] **B.** Crackles in the bases
[ ] **C.** Hemoptysis
[ ] **D.** White blood cell count of 30,000 μL

Correct answer—B. *Rationales:* Fluid overload, as evidenced by crackles in the bases, is consistently associated with a poor outcome in clients with pulmonary contusions. A pulmonary contusion causes an inflammatory response that results in an increase in temperature and white blood cells; however, the levels aren't elevated as high as those seen in options A and D. The client with pulmonary contusion is expected to have hemoptysis. The blood may be expectorated or suctioned from the endotracheal tube, if the client is intubated. Restriction of fluids, meticulous monitoring of intake and output, and monitoring of central venous pressure are appropriate interventions.
Nursing process step: Assessment

31. Which intervention is most appropriate for a client with a pulmonary contusion?
[ ] **A.** Restrict fluid administration if there are no signs of shock.
[ ] **B.** Provide supplemental humidified oxygen.
[ ] **C.** Position the client to facilitate breathing.
[ ] **D.** Assist with removal of secretions.

Correct answer—A. *Rationales:* The intervention identified with the best outcome for a client with a pulmonary contusion is restricted fluid administration during initial care. If the client isn't exhibiting symptoms of hypovolemic shock, fluids should be kept at a keep-veinopen rate. Providing supplemental oxygen, positioning the client to facilitate breathing, and assisting with removal of secretions are all treatments for pulmonary contusion.
Nursing process step: Intervention

32. Effective treatment of a client with pulmonary contusion is best identified by:
[ ] **A.** diminished breath sounds in right lower lobe.
[ ] **B.** increased respiratory rate and effort.
[ ] **C.** decreased complaints of pain.
[ ] **D.** respiratory acidosis with hypoxemia.

Correct answer—C. *Rationales:* Effective treatment of a client with pulmonary contusion is evidenced by:
- equal bilateral breath sounds.
- improved respiratory rate, rhythm, depth, and effort.
- vital signs within normal limits.
- arterial blood gases within acceptable limits.
- decreased complaints of pain.
- improved skin and mucous membrane color.

Nursing process step: Evaluation

33. Treatment of a client with a rib fracture includes:
[ ] **A.** placing the client in the supine position.
[ ] **B.** taping the chest circumferentially to relieve pain.
[ ] **C.** controlling pain to assist with breathing.
[ ] **D.** forcing fluids to prevent dehydration.

Correct answer—C. *Rationales:* Pain control for a client with rib fractures is a priority to ensure adequate expansion of lung tissue and to facilitate turning, coughing, and deep breathing. The client should be placed in high Fowler's position to facilitate gas exchange and breathing. Avoid circumferential taping of the chest because it predisposes the client to atelectasis. The lung directly below the fractured rib is often bruised (pulmonary contusion). Fluids should be monitored closely to decrease the risk of pulmonary edema.
Nursing process step: Intervention

34. A client presents with a history of mild respiratory infection and a dry cough for the past week. The client has recently developed a loose, productive cough. He is afebrile, appears nontoxic, and has had no difficulty eating or drinking. What's the most likely diagnosis for this client?

[ ] **A.** Acute asthma

[ ] **B.** Acute bronchitis

[ ] **C.** Pneumonia

[ ] **D.** Chronic obstructive pulmonary disease (COPD)

Correct answer—B. *Rationales:* Clients with acute bronchitis initially have dry coughs that become more productive; they usually appear nontoxic. Most clients with asthma have exposure to allergens as an important history finding. A client with pneumonia usually has an elevated temperature, productive cough, and coarse crackles. A client with COPD has a chronic productive cough, exercise intolerance, and increased anteroposterior diameter of the chest. Infection is the most common cause of acute respiratory arrest in clients with asthma who appear toxic on admission.

Nursing process step: Assessment

35. What's the most appropriate treatment for a client with bronchitis?

[ ] **A.** Antibiotic therapy for 7 to 10 days

[ ] **B.** Supportive care, including increased fluids, rest, and humidity

[ ] **C.** Expectorants every 4 to 6 hours during the day and cough suppressants at night

[ ] **D.** Beta$_2$-agonist inhaler (two puffs every 6 hours)

Correct answer—B. *Rationales:* Therapy for a client with acute bronchitis includes humidified air, increased fluids, and rest. The most likely medications are bronchodilators, corticosteroids, and antianxiety drugs. These clients need a calm environment and benefit from postural drainage. Cough suppressants may help at night.

Nursing process step: Intervention

36. Which statement indicates successful education of a client with acute bronchitis?

[ ] **A.** "As long as I limit my fluid intake, I shouldn't have further symptoms."

[ ] **B.** "I can continue smoking as long as I don't smoke in a closed area."

[ ] **C.** "I should wear a mask when around people with a cold."

[ ] **D.** "I should use my bronchodilator to reduce symptoms."

Correct answer—D. *Rationales:* The medications prescribed for acute bronchitis may include bronchodilators, corticosteroids, expectorants, and antianxiety drugs. The client must increase fluid intake to liquefy secretions. Bronchitis is an inflammation resulting from irritation of the bronchial mucosa by pollen, smoking, or inhalation of irritating substances. The environmental irritant must be removed. A cold doesn't cause acute bronchitis.

Nursing process step: Evaluation

37. The client with acute bronchitis requires careful monitoring when receiving which treatment?

[ ] **A.** Oxygen therapy

[ ] **B.** Fluid resuscitation

[ ] **C.** Humidified air

[ ] **D.** Postural drainage

Correct answer—A. *Rationales:* The client should be monitored closely when given low-flow oxygen to decrease chances of depressing the respiratory drive. Increasing fluids to liquefy secretions, humidifying the air, and performing postural drainage are also important therapy for a client with acute bronchitis.

Nursing process step: Evaluation

38. What's the most common cause of chest trauma–related deaths?

[ ] **A.** Falls

[ ] **B.** Assaults

[ ] **C.** Firearms

[ ] **D.** Motor vehicle accidents

Correct answer—D. *Rationales:* Motor vehicle accidents account for two-thirds of all chest trauma–related deaths. Other causes of thoracic injuries are falls, assaults, firearms, stabbings, crush injuries, and motor vehicle–pedestrian accidents.

Nursing process step: Assessment

39. Which respiratory sound is most commonly associated with laryngotracheobronchitis (croup)?
[ ] **A.** Crackles
[ ] **B.** Barking cough
[ ] **C.** Rales
[ ] **D.** Wheezing

Correct answer—B. *Rationales:* A barking cough occurs most commonly with croup; coughing frequency increases at night. Crackles, or rales, are popping noises heard most often during inspiration. They indicate that fluid, pus, or mucus is in the smaller airways. When heard, the nurse should instruct the client to cough and breathe deeply; the nurse should then auscultate again. The sounds may have cleared. Wheezing is a high-pitched musical sound. It can be heard during inspiration and expiration and usually accompanies an asthma attack or bronchospasm.
Nursing process step: Assessment

40. High levels of oxygen in a client with chronic obstructive pulmonary disease (COPD) can result in which condition?
[ ] **A.** Increased ventilatory drive
[ ] **B.** Diminished ventilatory drive
[ ] **C.** Ventilation/perfusion mismatch
[ ] **D.** Profound decrease in Pco_2

Correct answer—B. *Rationales:* A client with COPD has had an elevated carbon dioxide level for a prolonged time and no longer depends on carbon dioxide level changes to regulate ventilations. The client depends on hypoxia or lower PaO_2 level changes to regulate ventilations. If high levels of oxygen are administered, the client will lose the hypoxic respiratory drive and respirations will decrease or even stop. As respirations decrease, Pco_2 levels rise, not decrease. COPD leads to a ventilation/perfusion mismatch. The alveoli enlarge and overdistend, thereby decreasing the surface area of alveoli to capillary. Increasing the oxygen level doesn't increase the ventilation/perfusion mismatch.
Nursing process step: Evaluation

41. The presence of a barrel chest and cyanosis are indicative of what respiratory pathology?
[ ] **A.** Pulmonary edema
[ ] **B.** Chronic bronchitis
[ ] **C.** Cystic fibrosis
[ ] **D.** Pulmonary fibrosis

Correct answer—B. *Rationales:* The barrel chest is a hallmark sign of an obstructive pulmonary disease, such as chronic bronchitis or and emphysema, because of the abnormal permanent enlargement of the air spaces distal to the terminal bronchioles. Barrel chest isn't indicative of pulmonary edema, cystic fibrosis, or pulmonary fibrosis.
Nursing process step: Assessment

42. Which finding is consistent with a diagnosis of hyperventilation?
[ ] **A.** Increased mental acuity
[ ] **B.** Respiratory acidosis
[ ] **C.** Left arm pain
[ ] **D.** Carpopedal spasms

Correct answer—D. *Rationales:* Clients with hyperventilation exhibit carpopedal spasms, anxiety, jaw pain, tachypnea, diffuse chest pain, confusion, diaphoresis, and headache. They exhibit respiratory alkalosis, not acidosis.
Nursing process step: Assessment

43. What's a life-threatening condition that occurs with penetrating chest wounds and results in impaired gas exchange and risk for deficient fluid volume?
[ ] **A.** Pneumothorax
[ ] **B.** Cardiac contusion
[ ] **C.** Open pneumothorax
[ ] **D.** Ruptured esophagus

Correct answer—C. *Rationales:* An open pneumothorax, which causes equalization of atmospheric and intrathoracic pressures, leads to lung collapse and impaired gas exchange. A hemothorax is commonly associated with an open pneumothorax and results in a risk of fluid volume deficit. Cardiac contusion usually results from blunt trauma. A ruptured esophagus does have the risk of fluid volume deficit; however, the most serious complications result from infection.
Nursing process step: Assessment

44. The nurse is caring for a client who has an endotracheal (ET) tube and is on mechanical ventilation for respiratory failure. The ventilator's high-pressure alarm begins to sound. The nurse knows that the high-pressure alarm will sound for which of the following reasons?

[ ] **A.** Obstruction of the circuit tubing
[ ] **B.** The ventilator becoming disconnected from the ET tube
[ ] **C.** The ET tube becoming displaced because it wasn't properly secured
[ ] **D.** None of the above

Correct answer—A. *Rationales:* Obstruction of the ventilator circuit tubing, obstruction of the ET (from biting the ET when not properly sedated), or higher intrathoracic pressure will increase the expiratory pressure, which will sound the alarm. An interruption of the circuit from the ETT tube will prevent the client from being ventilated, and the client's oxygenation and SpO_2 will drop.
Nursing process step: Assessment

45. What's the most appropriate treatment for a client with a stable open pneumothorax?

[ ] **A.** Chest tube insertion
[ ] **B.** Emergency thoracotomy
[ ] **C.** Autotransfusion
[ ] **D.** I.V. infusion of dextrose 5% in water

Correct answer—A. *Rationales:* If the client's vital signs are stable with no signs of shock, the most appropriate intervention is chest tube insertion for reexpansion of the lung. If the client is unstable, an emergency thoracotomy is the definitive therapy. Autotransfusion may be used to stabilize the client until transportation to surgery. Lactated Ringer's solution and normal saline are the only crystalloids acceptable for administration in traumatic emergencies.
Nursing process step: Intervention

46. A client with an open pneumothorax is admitted to the emergency department. A nonporous dressing was placed in the field. Which finding suggests worsening of the client's condition?

[ ] **A.** Respiratory rate within normal limits
[ ] **B.** Decreased breath sounds on the affected side
[ ] **C.** Tracheal shift with jugular vein distention (JVD)
[ ] **D.** Blood pressure 120/80 mm Hg

Correct answer—C. *Rationales:* The finding that suggests a worsening of the client's condition is a tracheal shift with JVD, which indicates tension pneumothorax. The respiratory rate within normal limits and blood pressure 120/80 mm Hg are acceptable outcomes. The client will have decreased breath sounds until reexpansion of the lung has been achieved.
Nursing process step: Evaluation

47. What's the definitive diagnostic study for a client with suspected esophageal disruption?

[ ] **A.** Chest X-ray
[ ] **B.** Complete blood count (CBC) with differential
[ ] **C.** Esophagography
[ ] **D.** Esophagoscopy

Correct answer—D. *Rationales:* The most definitive study is esophagoscopy, used in a client who has a negative esophagogram but is suspected of having esophageal disruption. Chest X-rays often show mediastinal widening, which occurs in aortic and tracheobronchial ruptures. A CBC with differential won't assist with an esophageal rupture.
Nursing process step: Assessment

48. What's the treatment of choice for a client with pneumothorax?

[ ] **A.** Chest tube insertion
[ ] **B.** Emergency thoracotomy
[ ] **C.** Needle thoracostomy
[ ] **D.** Emergent intubation

Correct answer—A. *Rationales:* Pneumothorax is treated with the insertion of a chest tube connected to an underwater seal; the tube remains in place until reexpansion of the lung is achieved. An emergency thoracotomy is reserved for a hemodynamically unstable client. Needle thoracostomy is used in the treatment of tension pneumothorax. Most clients with pneumothorax don't require emergent intubation.
Nursing process step: Intervention

49. What's the most likely intervention for a client with a suspected diaphragmatic rupture?
[ ] **A.** Needle thoracostomy
[ ] **B.** Rapid infusion of I.V. fluids
[ ] **C.** Preparation for surgical intervention
[ ] **D.** Transfer to unit for observation

Correct answer—C. *Rationales:* Preparing a client for surgical intervention is the most important intervention. Needle thoracostomy is contraindicated in this client because of the risk of puncturing the bowel and releasing its contents into the chest cavity. The potential for serious complications contraindicates transfer for observation. I.V. fluids may be necessary if the bowel compresses large vessels, causing a decrease in preload. A gastric tube should also be inserted.
Nursing process step: Intervention

50. A client who has sustained chest trauma and is suspected of having rib involvement will be hospitalized if which condition exists?
[ ] **A.** The client is a child.
[ ] **B.** There's one rib fracture.
[ ] **C.** Rib one or two has been fractured.
[ ] **D.** The client has asthma.

Correct answer—C. *Rationales:* Admission to the hospital for clients with rib fractures is based on the location of the fracture (first or second rib) and fractures of more than three ribs. Elderly, rather than young clients, are hospitalized. Clients with asthma generally aren't hospitalized with rib fractures unless they meet the above criteria.
Nursing process step: Analysis

51. What's the initial treatment for a client with a tracheobronchial injury?
[ ] **A.** Suctioning to maintain airway patency
[ ] **B.** Preparing for chest tube insertion
[ ] **C.** Intubating and providing mechanical ventilation
[ ] **D.** Preparing for surgical intervention

Correct answer—A. *Rationales:* The priority intervention is to maintain airway patency, which is accomplished by suctioning. Chest tube insertion and surgical intervention will be necessary after the client is stabilized. If the client is intubated, the end of the endotracheal tube must be positioned distal to the injury. It's also advisable to monitor for possible pneumothorax.
Nursing process step: Intervention

52. Emergency medical service transports a 52-year-old male in respiratory distress. The client's respiratory rate is 40 beats/minute, and his oxygen saturation is 86% on 10 L of oxygen/minute on a partial-rebreather mask. He can't speak full sentences, but the nurse determines that he has had previous visits to the emergency department because of hypoxemia and hypercarbia. Auscultation reveals rhonchi, and his secretions are thin and scant. Based on these assessment findings, what should the nurse determine is the cause of this client's symptoms?
[ ] **A.** The client is in acute respiratory distress syndrome (ARDS).
[ ] **B.** The client is having an exacerbation of emphysema.
[ ] **C.** The client is having an exacerbation of asthma.
[ ] **D.** The client is in heart failure.

Correct answer—B. *Rationales:* This client is having an exacerbation of emphysema. The hallmark pathophysiology of emphysema and chronic bronchitis is hypoxemia and hypercarbia. Secretions, particularly thick secretions, are noted in a client with bronchitis, not emphysema. White or pink, blood-tinged phlegm or frothy secretions are more indicative of heart failure.
Nursing process step: Assessment

53. Which finding indicates effective treatment of a tracheobronchial injury?
[ ] **A.** Respiratory rate of 36 breaths/minute
[ ] **B.** Tracheal shift
[ ] **C.** Jugular vein distention (JVD)
[ ] **D.** Improved arterial blood gas (ABG) levels

Correct answer—D. *Rationales:* Findings consistent with improved status after tracheobronchial injury include vital signs within normal limits, decreased air leak, improved ABG levels, improved tissue perfusion, and no increase in subcutaneous emphysema. Tachypnea and tracheal shift with JVD suggest tension pneumothorax, a possible complication of tracheobronchial injury.
Nursing process step: Evaluation

54. Which of the following laboratory tests would the physician order for a client suspected of pneumonia?
[ ] **A.** Blood cultures
[ ] **B.** D-dimer
[ ] **C.** Prothrombin time and partial thromboplastin time (PT/PTT)
[ ] **D.** Sputum culture

Correct answer—A. *Rationales:* Blood cultures are considered the gold standard laboratory test to assess for specificity of organism-causing pneumonia, although a sputum culture may be ordered. A D-dimer assesses for protein fragments in the blood after blood clots are dissolved by fibrinolysis, and PT/PTT assesses for clotting times.
Nursing process step: Assessment

55. Which of the following isn't a common sign or symptom of a pulmonary embolus (PE)?
[ ] **A.** Acute onset of unexplained respiratory distress
[ ] **B.** Cough
[ ] **C.** Bradycardia with heart block
[ ] **D.** Chest pain

Correct answer—C. *Rationales:* All of the answers are signs and symptoms of a PE except for bradycardia. Rather, one would expect to see tachycardia as a result of a PE.
Nursing process step: Assessment

56. A client has a history of heart failure and has recently been hospitalized for pneumonia. He has audible, adventitious lung sounds. Which of the following lung sounds would the nurse not expect to hear?
[ ] **A.** Stridor
[ ] **B.** Crackles
[ ] **C.** Wheezing
[ ] **D.** Rhonchi

Correct answer—A. *Rationales:* Crackles, wheezing, and rhonchi are all possible with a client experiencing an exacerbation of heart failure or pneumonia. Stridor, however, is located in the upper airway and is a result of partial obstruction of the larynx or trachea.
Nursing process step: Assessment

57. A 19-year-old client has extensive burns to his head, face, neck, and chest with much of his hair, including his eyebrows, burned off from an ignited flammable liquid. He is conscious, breathing, and in significant pain. He's noted to have a mildly hoarse voice. A baseline physical assessment has been completed. The most reliable additional assessment of the client's breathing status would include:
[ ] **A.** arterial blood gases (ABG).
[ ] **B.** complete blood count (CBC).
[ ] **C.** mixed venous gases.
[ ] **D.** oxygen saturation monitoring.

Correct answer—A. *Rationales:* Any client involved in a fire in an enclosed space may have inhaled several of many products of incomplete combustion including carbon monoxide, cyanide containing compounds, and other toxic compounds. Many of these substances, carbon monoxide being especially important, bind to hemoglobin and will give a false saturation reading. An oxygen saturation monitor doesn't differentiate among oxygen, carbon monoxide, or any other toxic substance bound to the hemoglobin. Arterial blood gases give a specific value for the PaO_2, a much more reliable number to ascertain oxygenation status. Mixed venous gases don't yield as useful information as an ABG. A CBC will give the hemoglobin value important in oxygen transport; however, the hemoglobin is usually reported in the ABG results.
Nursing process step: Assessment

58. Priority nursing management of this client's airway after burn inhalation would include:
[ ] **A.** delivering high-flow oxygen by rebreather mask.
[ ] **B.** monitoring for stridor, increasing hoarseness of voice, and decrease in oxygen saturation.
[ ] **C.** preparing for emergent intubation.
[ ] **D.** preparing for emergency cricothyrotomy.

Correct answer—C. *Rationales:* Burns of the face may indicate burns to the large and small airways. Though they initially appear stable, a burn will quickly swell and loss of the airway can occur rapidly. The priority for inhalation burn injury is to secure the airway with intubation. Waiting for the situation to worsen may delay intubation to the point at which intubation or even emergency cricothyrotomy is very difficult or impossible. Delivery of high-flow oxygen is appropriate but a rebreather mask doesn't secure an airway.
Nursing process step: Analysis

59. Other signs consistent with burn inhalation injury include:
[ ] **A.** rapid easing of the work of respiration.
[ ] **B.** carbonaceous or black-tinged sputum.
[ ] **C.** persistent wet and productive cough.
[ ] **D.** moist mucous membranes.

Correct answer—B. *Rationales:* Black-tinged (carbon-aceous) sputum from smoke generated in the fire is a hallmark sign of inhalation injury. Respiration may become increasingly difficult as the injury matures. The mucous membranes of the burn-injured client are commonly dry. The client may have rales and rhonchi on auscultation but the cough is dry and generally nonproductive.
Nursing process step: Assessment

60. When deciding interventions for clients exposed to carbon dioxide (CO_2), ethane, methane, propane, or other fuel gases, the emergency nurse bases her interventions on the knowledge that:
[ ] **A.** these gases bind to hemoglobin and require high-flow oxygen and occasionally hyperbaric treatment.
[ ] **B.** these gases don't bind to hemoglobin and often only require "fresh air" and supplemental oxygen.
[ ] **C.** each gas has an individual treatment and antidote.
[ ] **D.** exposure to these gases is benign, requiring no treatment.

Correct answer—B. *Rationales:* Methane, ethane, propane, CO_2, and other fuel gases don't react or bind to hemoglobin. Getting the client to fresh air out of the source area of the gas, and supplemental oxygen is the treatment needed if the client is conscious and breathing. These gases have the common effect of crowding out oxygen and essentially suffocating the victim.
Nursing process step: Analysis

61. Which of the following is not a cause of noncardiac pulmonary edema?
[ ] **A.** Trauma
[ ] **B.** Aspiration
[ ] **C.** Sudden movement to a high altitude
[ ] **D.** Spontaneous pneumothorax

Correct answer—D. *Rationales:* A spontaneous pneumothorax wouldn't cause fluid accumulation in the pleural space. Trauma may cause rib fractures or thoracic compression, which can rupture alveoli. Aspiration may contribute to a collection of nonendogenous fluids in the alveoli. Sudden movement to a higher altitude may lead to high altitude pulmonary edema.
Nursing process step: Analysis

62. What's the treatment for high altitude pulmonary edema (HAPE)?
[ ] **A.** Diamox and acclimatization and Diamox
[ ] **B.** Antibiotics, because it's similar to pneumonia
[ ] **C.** Lasix and a decrease in altitude
[ ] **D.** No specific treatment exists

Correct answer—C. *Rationales:* A decrease in altitude allows the body to initiate "self-correction" of many altitude-related physiologic processes, but acclimatization will rarely be sufficient without adjunctive therapy. Diuretics such as Lasix have been shown to improve symptoms. Diamox is a treatment for high altitude cerebral edema. The mechanisms of HAPE aren't borne by bacteria and thus aren't treated as pneumonia.
Nursing process step: Intervention

63. Which of the following signs and symptoms may indicate that the client has aspirated fluid?
[ ] **A.** Crackles and altered mental status
[ ] **B.** Wheezing and poor skin turgor
[ ] **C.** Decreased urinary output and decreased mental status
[ ] **D.** Crackles and poor skin turgor

Correct answer—A. *Rationales:* Aspirated fluid will enter the alveoli, causing crackles and decreased oxygenation, which in turn may cause altered sensorium. Wheezing is adventitious lung sounds caused by airway constriction, not aspiration. Aspiration doesn't affect urinary output. Skin turgor is a sign of dehydration and is not caused by aspiration.
Nursing process step: Assessment

64. A client with a previous medical history of stroke is brought to the emergency department with altered mental status. The client's baseline mental status is alert and oriented to person, place, time, and event; however, at this time, he's responsive to painful stimuli only. His examination reveals hot, moist skin with a tympanic temperature of 102.2° F (39° C), adventitious lung sounds, and tachycardia. The nurse assesses that a possible reason for these signs is:
[ ] **A.** stroke.
[ ] **B.** myocardial infarction (MI).
[ ] **C.** aspiration pneumonia.
[ ] **D.** meningitis.

Correct answer—C. *Rationales:* A client who has had a stroke may be at high risk for aspiration, and although an acute onset of altered mental status may indicate a new stroke, the combination of warm, moist skin and adventitious lung sounds most likely results from aspiration. The assessment findings don't correlate to MI or meningitis.
Nursing process step: Assessment

65. A client is brought to the emergency department with mild respiratory distress. His oxygen saturation is 95% on 3 L of oxygen via nasal cannula, his respiratory rate is 28 breaths/minute, and his temperature is 101° F (38.3°C). He has decreased breath sounds over the base of the right lung, and he complains of a nonproductive cough. He has a history of tuberculosis. Based on these assessment findings, what should the nurse suspect this client has?
[ ] **A.** Empyema
[ ] **B.** Transudative effusion
[ ] **C.** Bronchiolitic effusion
[ ] **D.** Exudative effusion

Correct answer—A. *Rationales:* An empyema contains pus and can be caused by tuberculosis. Transudative effusion is common with heart failure, renal and liver disease, and exudative effusions are secondary to pulmonary malignancies, pulmonary embolus, and GI disease.
Nursing process step: Analysis

66. An unrestrained client who was involved in a high-speed motor vehicle collision is brought to the emergency department. He's complaining of chest pain. The paramedic states that there was extensive damage to the steering column. Assessment of the client's chest reveals a possible flail chest on the right side. The nurse's knowledge of flail chest helps her understand that the client is at risk for which of the following?
[ ] **A.** Myocardial contusion
[ ] **B.** Pneumonia
[ ] **C.** Rupture of the great vessels
[ ] **D.** Pulmonary contusions

Correct answer—D. *Rationales:* A pulmonary contusion is a common result of nonpenetrating chest trauma, especially flail chest. A myocardial contusion as well as rupture of the great vessels would be considered had the injury been on the left side. Also, rupture of the great vessels would lead to rapid cardiovascular instability and decline. Pneumonia wouldn't be a direct result of chest trauma.
Nursing process step: Analysis

67. A 24-year-old woman is in the early stage of an acute asthma attack. Knowing the pathology of asthma and the progression of an asthma attack and its correlation with arterial blood gases (ABGs), the nurse anticipates which of the following ABG results on this client?

[ ] **A.** Normal pH, normal $PaCO_2$, normal PaO_2
[ ] **B.** Elevated pH, decreased $PaCO_2$, decreased PaO_2
[ ] **C.** Decreased pH, increased $PaCO_2$, decreased PaO_2
[ ] **D.** Normal pH, normal $PaCO_2$, decreased PaO_2

Correct answer—B. *Rationales:* Early in an acute asthma attack, alveolar hyperventilation leads to hypocarbia, there's hypoxemia secondary to ventilation-perfusion mismatch, there's adequate alveolar ventilation, and carbon dioxide isn't being eliminated well. The other options are incorrect.

Nursing process step: Assessment

68. Which common laboratory test is used to assess for heart failure?

[ ] **A.** Brain natriuretic peptide (BNP)
[ ] **B.** D-dimer
[ ] **C.** Basic metabolic panel
[ ] **D.** Troponin T

Correct answer—A. *Rationales:* The BNP is secreted in the ventricles in response to changes in pressure that occur when heart failure occurs and worsens. A D-dimer is a nonspecific lab test to assess for the possibility of an embolus. A basic metabolic panel won't assess for heart failure. The troponin T is a cardiac enzyme that assesses heart damage during a myocardial infarction.

Nursing process step: Assessment

15 Shock

1. What's the initial rate at which a client in hemorrhagic hypovolemic shock should have I.V. crystalloid fluid replaced?

[ ] **A.** 5 to 10 mL/kg
[ ] **B.** 20 to 40 mL/kg
[ ] **C.** 80 to 90 mL/kg
[ ] **D.** 200 to 300 mL/kg

Correct answer–B. *Rationales:* The standard therapy for a hemodynamically unstable client in hemorrhagic hypovolemic shock is rapid infusion of crystalloid fluid at 20 to 40 mL/kg. The minimal rate of fluid replacement, 5 to 10 mL/kg, may not be sufficient to raise the circulating volume. A rate of 80 to 300 mL/kg may result in dilution of the remaining red blood cell mass, platelets, and coagulation factor. Clot formation in the injured vessels may be disrupted, and homeostasis of the injured site won't be maintained.
Nursing process step: Intervention

2. What's the priority intervention when assessing a client with multisystem trauma?

[ ] **A.** Airway management with cervical spine stabilization, breathing, level of consciousness and pupillary response, and circulation
[ ] **B.** Level of consciousness and pupillary response, airway management with cervical spine stabilization, breathing, and circulation
[ ] **C.** Breathing, airway management with cervical spine stabilization, circulation, and level of consciousness and pupillary response
[ ] **D.** Airway management with cervical spine stabilization, breathing, circulation, and level of consciousness and pupillary response

Correct answer–D. *Rationales:* The initial assessment of a client in shock must be rapid and begins with the primary survey. The airway, if not patent, must be opened while maintaining cervical spine stabilization. Breathing effectiveness needs to be assessed, and supplemental oxygen should be administered in the most appropriate route based on the client's condition. Assessment of circulation should be done by noting the client's skin temperature, moisture, and color. Capillary refill time in an adult (normal, 2 to 3 seconds; delayed, more than 3 seconds) is of questionable value but may still be included during the assessment as a baseline parameter. The client's level of consciousness must be evaluated next because cerebral perfusion may be affected by low-perfusion blood flow. If circulation is compromised, two I.V. lines with 14G to 16G catheters should be started with warmed normal saline or lactated Ringer's solution. Pupillary response assessment is performed to determine the equality of pupil size and response to light stimulation. The assessment is organized to identify and correct the most life-threatening conditions first.
Nursing process step: Assessment

3. A client was the driver of a compact automobile that had an impact on the driver's side; he wasn't wearing a seat belt at the time of the accident. He sustained severe abdominal injuries, bilateral fractured femurs, and a 4-cm laceration to the right arm. On arrival to the emergency department, the client was pale, diaphoretic, and talking incoherently. Vital signs on arrival were blood pressure, 50/40 mm Hg; heart rate, 130 beats/minute; respiratory rate, 36 breaths/minute; and tympanic temperature, 98.2° F (36.8° C). This client has which type of shock?

[ ] **A.** Cardiogenic
[ ] **B.** Septic
[ ] **C.** Hypovolemic
[ ] **D.** Neurogenic

Correct answer—C. *Rationales:* The client is hypotensive with a narrow pulse pressure, tachycardia, and altered level of consciousness. These signs and symptoms indicate that the client is in a compensatory phase of a hypovolemic shock condition. The mechanism of injury (unrestrained driver in a motor vehicle accident) suggests blunt trauma to the abdomen. The most common form of shock in trauma clients is hypovolemic shock. Cardiogenic shock is typically caused by myocardial infarction. Septic shock is most commonly caused by gram-negative and gram-positive bacteria. Neurogenic shock results from a severe brain stem injury at the level of the medulla, an injury to the spinal cord, or spinal anesthesia. A client with neurogenic shock has a different presentation than one with hypovolemic shock. Signs and symptoms of neurogenic shock include peripheral vasodilation and severe hypotension from loss of sympathetic tone. On assessment, the client is hypotensive with warm, flushed skin.

Nursing process step: Assessment

4. Which of the following values is an indication of poor prognosis in a client with septic shock?

[ ] **A.** Blood pressure, 90/56 mm Hg
[ ] **B.** Serum lactate, 6 mmol/L
[ ] **C.** Arterial blood gas (ABG), pH 7.35
[ ] **D.** Central venous pressure (CVP), 4 cm H_20 pressure

Correct answer—B. *Rationales:* An initial serum lactate value greater than 4 mmol/L is associated with increased client mortality. Serum lactate levels have been used for decades to identify and manage clients with progressive circulatory dysfunction secondary to sepsis. Successful hemodynamic resuscitation and continued monitoring are key components of the management of sepsis in the emergency department. An ABG pH of 7.35 is within normal limits. A CVP of 4 cm H_2O pressure is within normal limits; however, current research demonstrates that CVP isn't an accurate measure of fluid resuscitation. Hypotension is a symptom of septic shock and isn't the best indicator of the prognosis.

Nursing process step: Analysis

5. A client in the emergency department has a central venous pressure (CVP) reading of 3 cm H_2O and a blood pressure of 106/68 mm Hg. What is the most appropriate intervention for this client?

[ ] **A.** Fluid bolus
[ ] **B.** Reduce I.V. fluid rate
[ ] **C.** Administer dopamine at 6 mcg/kg per minute
[ ] **D.** Do nothing; these are appropriate values

Correct answer—A. *Rationales:* Normal CVP readings range from 4 to 10 cm H_2O. A reading above 10 cm H_2O indicate volume overload; readings below 4 cm H_2O identify a deficient fluid volume. Because the client is fluid deficient, a fluid bolus is appropriate and reducing the fluids is inappropriate. Dopamine should be administered after preexisting hypovolemia has been corrected. CVP is an unreliable estimate of what's happening to intravascular volume even in the healthiest client and the most stable situations.

Nursing process step: Analysis

6. What's the most common form of shock in trauma clients?

[ ] **A.** Hypovolemic
[ ] **B.** Cardiogenic
[ ] **C.** Neurogenic
[ ] **D.** Anaphylactic

Correct answer—A. *Rationales:* Hypovolemic shock is the most common form of shock in trauma clients. It occurs as a result of inadequate intravascular volume from the loss or redistribution of whole blood, plasma, or other body fluids. Hypovolemic shock is commonly caused by the loss of whole blood (hemorrhage). Additional causes are dehydration from body fluid loss and displaced fluid, as seen in thermal injuries. Cardiogenic shock is caused by myocardial infarction. Neurogenic shock is caused by loss of sympathetic tone brought on by spinal anesthesia or injury to the spinal cord. Anaphylactic shock is most commonly caused by an acute allergic reaction.
Nursing process step: Assessment

7. What's the recommended initial bolus of crystalloid fluid replacement for a pediatric client in shock?

[ ] **A.** 10 mL/kg
[ ] **B.** 15 mL/kg
[ ] **C.** 20 mL/kg
[ ] **D.** 30 mL/kg

Correct answer—C. *Rationales:* Fluid volume replacement must be calculated to the child's weight to avoid overhydration. Initial fluid bolus is administered at 20 mL/kg, followed by another 20 mL/kg bolus if there's no improvement in volume status. All other options are incorrect.
Nursing process step: Intervention

8. In which condition is use of a pneumatic antishock garment (PASG) contraindicated?

[ ] **A.** Bilateral femur fractures
[ ] **B.** Anaphylactic shock
[ ] **C.** Pelvic fracture
[ ] **D.** Right-sided tension pneumothorax

Correct answer—D. *Rationales:* Prehospital providers rarely use the PASG to control hemorrhage and support blood pressure; however, when it is used, inflation of the device causes tamponade of soft-tissue hemorrhage and raises blood pressure by increasing systemic vascular resistance. The PASG is contraindicated with a right-sided tension pneumothorax because it further elevates venous pressure associated with the tension pneumothorax. The PASG is also useful for unstable pelvic and femur fractures. In these cases, the garment stabilizes the fractures and tamponades retroperitoneal hemorrhage. Clients in anaphylactic shock may benefit from the PASG because it increases preload and enhances cardiac output.
Nursing process step: Intervention

9. What effect does alpha-adrenergic receptor stimulation have on the peripheral and central circulation vessels?

[ ] **A.** Vasodilation
[ ] **B.** No effect, vascular circulation
[ ] **C.** Vasoconstriction
[ ] **D.** Vasodilation, then vasoconstriction

Correct answer—C. *Rationales:* Alpha-adrenergic receptor stimulation results in vasoconstriction of the vascular beds. This occurs as a compensatory mechanism to enhance the central circulation by increasing diastolic blood pressure and maintaining systolic blood pressure. Beta-adrenergic receptor stimulation results in bronchodilation and postcapillary vasodilation. Options B and D are incorrect.
Nursing process step: Assessment

10. Which client has the lowest probability of developing septic shock?

[ ] **A.** A geriatric client with pneumonia

[ ] **B.** A client who has sustained second-degree burns to 30% of body surface area

[ ] **C.** A client with cancer who's receiving chemotherapy

[ ] **D.** A client with a 3-cm laceration to the hand sustained while washing dishes

Correct answer—D. *Rationales:* The most common organism responsible for septic shock is gram-negative bacteria, which releases endotoxins that activate various hormone and chemical mediators. Other causative organisms of septic shock are gram-positive bacteria, fungi, viruses, and rickettsiae. The client who received a 3-cm laceration on the hand while washing dishes has the lowest probability of developing septic shock because the injury occurred in a clean environment. Populations at risk for developing septic shock are the very young, the very old, multiple-injury clients, debilitated individuals, and immunosuppressed clients.
Nursing process step: Assessment

11. In addition to whole blood or packed red blood cells (RBCs), which clotting component should be replaced in a client with hemorrhagic shock?

[ ] **A.** Albumin

[ ] **B.** Dextran

[ ] **C.** Fresh frozen plasma or platelets

[ ] **D.** Washed red blood cells

Correct answer—C. *Rationales:* In addition to whole blood or packed RBCs, fresh frozen plasma or platelets should be replaced in a client with hemorrhagic shock. RBCs have minimal clotting factors and platelets available. To decrease the probability of the client developing coagulopathy deficits, 1 to 2 units of fresh frozen plasma or platelets are commonly administered after the infusion of 5 units of blood. Albumin is administered to expand the plasma volume rapidly and may not be necessary as long as blood has been replaced. Dextran and washed RBCs aren't clotting components.
Nursing process step: Intervention

12. A client with a 7.5-cm laceration on his right arm is admitted to the emergency department. The wound is bleeding profusely. Which nursing intervention should be performed immediately to control the bleeding?

[ ] **A.** Inject epinephrine into the wound.

[ ] **B.** Apply a tourniquet above the injury site.

[ ] **C.** Apply direct pressure to the wound.

[ ] **D.** Suture the wound.

Correct answer—C. *Rationales:* Direct pressure applied to the laceration is the most immediate nursing intervention to control bleeding. Applying a tourniquet above the injury may result in permanent damage to the circulatory and nervous pathways in the arm. Injecting epinephrine into the arm and suturing the wound are usually done by the medical staff.
Nursing process step: Implementation

13. What is the most common cause of cardiogenic shock?

[ ] **A.** Myocardial infarction (MI)

[ ] **B.** Myocardial contusion

[ ] **C.** Cardiac failure

[ ] **D.** Cardiac tamponade

Correct answer—A. *Rationales:* Cardiogenic shock occurs when the heart fails as a pump and results in reduced cardiac output. MI is the most common cause of cardiogenic shock. Myocardial contusion, cardiac temponade, and cardiac failure can also cause cardiogenic shock but they aren't the most common cause.
Nursing process step: Assessment

14. Distributive shock is caused by which condition?
[ ] **A.** Spinal shock
[ ] **B.** Cardiogenic shock
[ ] **C.** Septic shock
[ ] **D.** Hypovolemic shock

Correct answer—C. *Rationales*: Distributive shock results from a disruption in the tone of blood vessels that leads to vasodilation and maldistribution of blood volume. Examples of distributive shock include neurogenic shock, septic shock, and anaphylactic shock. "Spinal shock" term used to describe the flexia and flaccidity associated with complete cord injuries. Cardiogenic shock occurs when the heart fails as a pump. Hypovolemic shock results from inadequate circulating volume.
Nursing process step: Analysis

15. A client in septic shock has received a rapid infusion of 3 L of normal saline solution and now has a urine output of 35 mL/hour. Based on this finding, which action should be performed next?
[ ] **A.** Infuse another 2 L of normal saline solution.
[ ] **B.** Change I.V. fluid to dextrose 5% in water (D_5W).
[ ] **C.** Infuse normal saline solution at 125 mL/hour and continue to monitor urine output.
[ ] **D.** Rapidly infuse 1 L of normal saline solution.

Correct answer—C. *Rationales:* The client's urine output is within the normal range (equal to or greater than 30 mL/hour). The client is therefore experiencing adequate renal perfusion and the I.V. fluids should be decreased. The nurse should continue to monitor the urine output to determine whether the client is perfusing the viscera. It isn't necessary to infuse another 2 L of normal saline solution because the client has adequate urine output. It's inappropriate to switch to D_5W.
Nursing process step: Evaluation

16. A 16-year-old high school football player is brought into the emergency department with a suspected spinal injury. Which of the following signs most points to neurogenic shock?
[ ] **A.** Cool, diaphoretic skin
[ ] **B.** Distended jugular veins
[ ] **C.** Bradycardia
[ ] **D.** Hyperthermia

Correct answer—C. *Rationales*: The major clinical signs of neurogenic shock are hypotension and bradycardia. Clients are generally hypotensive with warm, dry skin. Cool, diaphoretic skin is more likely to be associated with shock from fluid loss. The loss of sympathetic tone may impair the ability to redirect blood flow from the periphery to the core circulation, leading to excessive heat loss and hypothermia. Bradycardia is a characteristic finding of neurogenic shock; however, it isn't universally present.
Nursing process step: Assessment

17. Which diagnosis best fits a client with a cervical spinal cord injury?
[ ] **A.** Hypovolemic shock
[ ] **B.** Neurogenic shock
[ ] **C.** Cardiogenic shock
[ ] **D.** Septic shock

Correct answer—B. *Rationales:* Injury to the cervical spinal cord affects the autonomic nervous system. Below the injury, the client will demonstrate blocking of sympathetic vasomotor regulation, resulting in extreme vasodilation and maldistribution of the circulating volume. Neurogenic shock occurs as a result of peripheral vasodilation with decreased venous return. The client's skin is warm, dry, and flushed. The client is hypotensive and bradycardic. The other options don't represent the client's assessment findings.
Nursing process step: Assessment

18. What significant fact is important to remember about distributive shock?
[ ] **A.** The heart is significantly less able to pump effectively.
[ ] **B.** The client has lost a significant amount of blood and fluids.
[ ] **C.** The circulating volume has stayed the same, but the systemic vascular resistance is decreased.
[ ] **D.** The circulating blood volume is reduced because of compression of the great vessels or the heart itself.

Correct answer—C. *Rationales*: Distributive shock results when the blood volume remains the same but vasodilatation causes decreased systemic vascular resistance. The heart is able to pump less effectively in cardiogenic shock. Hypovolemic shock results from a significant loss of blood and fluids. Obstructive shock results from compression of great veins, aorta, pulmonary arteries, or the heart.
Nursing process step: Assessment

19. A client with blunt trauma to the chest is admitted to the emergency department. The client has no breath sounds on the right side of the chest, jugular veins are distended, and the trachea is shifted to the left. Admission vital signs are blood pressure, 88/56 mm Hg; pulse rate, 128 beats/minute; respiratory rate, 32 breaths/minute; and a tympanic temperature of 98.4 F (36.9° C). The client's skin is pale, cool, and clammy. Which type of shock does this client have?
[ ] **A.** Hypovolemic
[ ] **B.** Obstructive
[ ] **C.** Septic
[ ] **D.** Neurogenic

Correct answer—B. *Rationales:* The client has a right-sided tension pneumothorax, creating an obstruction due to increased intrathoracic pressure displacing the inferior vena cava and obstructing venous return to the right atrium. Preload is decreased, and the client's vital signs exhibit a sympathetic response. Hypovolemic shock results in flat jugular veins from the low-volume state, and the trachea isn't affected. Clients with septic shock don't typically have alterations in the trachea, and jugular veins aren't generally distended. Neurogenic shock results in bradycardia from the depressed sympathetic nervous system innervation.
Nursing process step: Assessment

20. Early shock class I is characterized by which condition?
[ ] **A.** Falling systolic pressure and rising diastolic pressure
[ ] **B.** Normal to rising pulse pressure
[ ] **C.** Falling systolic and diastolic pressures
[ ] **D.** Increased systolic and diastolic pressures

Correct answer—B. *Rationales:* Early shock (class I) is characterized by normal or slightly increased pulse pressure and normal blood pressure. Narrowing pulse pressure is seen in class II shock when falling systolic pressure and rising diastolic pressure are seen. Sympathetic stimulation occurs as specialized cells in the carotid and aorta sense a decrease in oxygen and an increase in carbon dioxide in the circulating blood. Catecholamines are released to produce peripheral vasoconstriction and an increase in total peripheral resistance. This action results in an increase in diastolic pressure as a means of increasing preload and cardiac output. All other options are incorrect.
Nursing process step: Assessment

21. Rapid I.V. infusion of lactated Ringer's solution to a client in shock can best be accomplished by using a:
[ ] **A.** large-bore long catheter.
[ ] **B.** long I.V. tubing.
[ ] **C.** short I.V. pole.
[ ] **D.** large-bore short catheter.

Correct answer—D. *Rationales:* Rapid I.V. infusion of a crystalloid can best be accomplished by using a large-bore short catheter. A large-bore long catheter and long I.V. tubing or extension sets increase the infusion time. A short I.V. pole doesn't allow I.V. fluids to flow rapidly because of the decreased gravitational pull.
Nursing process step: Intervention

22. Blood products should be infused only through an I.V. line containing which crystalloid solution?

[ ] **A.** Lactated Ringer's solution
[ ] **B.** Dextrose 5% in water (D_5W)
[ ] **C.** Normal saline
[ ] **D.** Dextran

Correct answer—C. *Rationales:* Blood should be infused through an I.V. line with normal saline. Lactated Ringer's solution contains enough ionized calcium (3 mEq/L) to overcome the anticoagulant effect of CPDA-1 and allow the development of small clots, which may precipitate in the I.V. line. Dextran and D_5W contain glucose, which causes clumping of the red cells in the tubing and results in swelling and hemolysis of the red blood cells. The blood should be administered through a filter. Although filters come in mesh and microaggregate types, the latter is preferred, especially when transfusing multiple units of blood.
Nursing process step: Intervention

23. Which clinical manifestation indicates the late stage of shock in a pediatric client?

[ ] **A.** Cyanosis
[ ] **B.** Delayed capillary refill
[ ] **C.** Cool, clammy skin
[ ] **D.** Hypotension

Correct answer—D. *Rationales:* Hypotension is a late sign of shock in a pediatric client. A child's cardiovascular system is relatively healthy and may be capable of sustaining cardiac output for a period of time. During the early phase of shock, compensatory mechanisms are implemented to augment circulating volume and venous return. Cyanosis, delayed capillary refill, and cool, cold skin result from sympathetic nervous system innervation, which occurs in the early phase of shock.
Nursing process step: Evaluation

24. The abdominal section of the pneumatic antishock garment (PASG) shouldn't be inflated in the client with which condition?

[ ] **A.** Pelvic fractures
[ ] **B.** Pregnancy
[ ] **C.** Bilateral femur fractures
[ ] **D.** Blunt trauma to the abdomen

Correct answer—B. *Rationales:* The abdominal section of the PASG shouldn't be inflated in pregnant trauma clients because of potential injury to the fetus. Use of the PASG to augment circulating volume is controversial, but it can assist circulation by decreasing the volume loss from abdominal and extremity injuries.
Nursing process step: Intervention

25. A pediatric client with a history of vomiting and diarrhea for 2 days is admitted to the emergency department. Which assessment finding indicates that the child is in the late stages of shock?

[ ] **A.** Tachycardia
[ ] **B.** Bradycardia
[ ] **C.** Irritability
[ ] **D.** Urine output, 1 to 2 mL/kg/hour

Correct answer—B. *Rationales:* Bradycardia is a sign of late shock in a pediatric client. Cardiovascular dysfunction and impairment of cellular function lead to lowered perfusion pressures, increased precapillary arteriolar resistance, and venous capacitance. Decreased cardiac output occurs in late shock if the lost circulating volume isn't replaced. Sympathetic nervous innervation has limited compensatory mechanisms if the volume isn't replaced. Tachycardia and irritability occur during the early phase of shock as compensatory mechanisms are implemented to increase cardiac output. Normal urine output for a pediatric client is 1 to 2 mL/kg/hour; volumes less than this would indicate a decrease in renal perfusion and activation of the renin-angiotensin-aldosterone system to decrease water and sodium excretion.
Nursing process step: Evaluation

26. Which procedure should be completed before initiating antibiotic therapy on a client diagnosed with septic shock?
[ ] **A.** Urine culture, complete blood count (CBC), and one set of blood cultures
[ ] **B.** Lumbar puncture, urine culture, urinalysis, and CBC
[ ] **C.** CBC, urinalysis, serum electrolyte levels, prothrombin time, and partial thromboplastin time
[ ] **D.** Two separate sets of blood cultures from different venipuncture sites and a urine culture

Correct answer—D. *Rationales:* Before administering antibiotic therapy, the nurse should obtain cultures of blood and urine to identify the bacteria responsible for the septic condition. Blood cultures should be obtained from two separate venipuncture sites to avoid false results from skin contamination. Lumbar puncture should be done if a client has a clinical sign such as nuchal rigidity that indicates central nervous system infection. CBC, urinalysis, serum electrolyte levels, prothrombin time, and partial thromboplastin time are laboratory tests that should be done as part of the basic examination and don't need to be completed before initiating antibiotic therapy.
Nursing process step: Intervention

27. What's the major pulmonary cause of septic shock?
[ ] **A.** Tuberculosis
[ ] **B.** Bronchitis
[ ] **C.** Pulmonary embolus
[ ] **D.** Acute bacterial pneumonia

Correct answer—D. *Rationales:* The major pulmonary cause of septic shock is acute bacterial pneumonia. The most common causative organisms are *Streptococcus pneumoniae* and *Staphylococcus aureus.* Tuberculosis differs from other bacterial pulmonary diseases in that it's a chronic condition. After the organism has spread to the regional lymph nodes and disseminated hepatogenously, cell-mediated immunity occurs and halts further bacterial growth. Bronchitis is an inflammatory response of the bronchi caused by pollen, smoking, pollution, or inhalation of irritating substances. It's characterized by increased mucus production. Pulmonary embolus is caused by a clot lodging in the pulmonary artery (or one of the smaller branches) and obstructing blood flow distally.
Nursing process step: Assessment

28. Class III hemorrhagic shock is described as the loss of 30% to 40% of blood volume, or approximately 1,500 to 2,000 mL. What are the symptoms of class III shock?
[ ] **A.** Heart rate, 100 beats/minute; blood pressure, 110/70 mm Hg; urinary output, 30 mL/hour; respiratory rate, 20 breaths/minute
[ ] **B.** Heart rate, 90 beats/minute; blood pressure, 130/70 mm Hg; urinary output, 45 mL/hour; respiratory rate, 16 breaths/minute
[ ] **C.** Heart rate, 130 beats/minute; blood pressure 80/50 mm Hg; urinary output, 10 mL/hour; respiratory rate, 35 breaths/minute
[ ] **D.** Heart rate, 150 beats/minute; blood pressure, 70/40 mm Hg; oliguria; respiratory rate greater than 35 breaths/minute

Correct answer—C. *Rationales*: According to the American College of Surgeons Committee on Trauma, class III shock is characterized by a heart rate greater than 120 beats/minute, a decreased blood pressure, a decreased pulse pressure, a urinary output of 5 to 15 mL/hour, and a respiratory rate of 30 to 40 beats/minute. The other options are incorrect.
Nursing process step: Assessment

29. Which represents the estimated blood loss in a trauma client with bilateral femur fractures and a fractured pelvis?
[ ] **A.** 250 mL
[ ] **B.** 500 mL
[ ] **C.** 1,000 mL
[ ] **D.** 1,500 mL

Correct answer—D. *Rationales:* This client's blood loss is estimated to be more than 1,500 mL. A closed femur fracture can result in more than 1,000 mL of blood loss, and fractures of the pelvis can result in a blood loss of 1,500 to 3,000 mL. Pelvic fractures frequently disrupt adjacent blood vessels. The blood loss for pelvic fractures is gauged as 1 unit for each fracture of the pelvis. All other options are incorrect.
Nursing process step: Assessment

30. A client presents to the emergency department with complaints of cough, dyspnea, tachypnea, and fever for the past couple of days. Upon examination, the nurse notes small petechial hemorrhages on the face and chest. Based on these findings, what should the nurse suspect?
[ ] **A.** Disseminated intravascular coagulation (DIC)
[ ] **B.** Hemophilia
[ ] **C.** Anemia
[ ] **D.** Leukemia

Correct answer—A. *Rationales:* Clients with DIC present with cough, fever, dyspnea, tachypnea, and petechial hemorrhages due to thrombus formation in microcirculation. Hemophilia results in bleeding and bruising but doesn't produce any of the above respiratory symptoms. Anemia is a result of decreased red blood cells that leads to a decrease in the oxygen-carrying capacity of the blood. Leukemia is a malignant blood disorder.
Nursing process step: Analysis

31. The administration of dopamine would be the *most* beneficial in which shock state?
[ ] **A.** Hypovolemic
[ ] **B.** Septic
[ ] **C.** Cardiogenic
[ ] **D.** Neurogenic

Correct answer—A. *Rationales:* The administration of dopamine is most beneficial for a client in hypovolemic shock because raising the blood pressure with vasopressors increases the risk for mortality. Blood pressure in clients in hypovolemic shock should be raised by replacing red blood cells and circulating volume. Vasopressors are effective in raising blood pressure in all forms of shock in which peripheral vasodilation has occurred.
Nursing process step: Intervention

32. A client with increased urination and hunger and an elevated temperature for the past 3 days presents to the emergency department. His vital signs are as follows: blood pressure, 80/50 mm Hg; pulse rate, 132 beats/minute; respirations, 28 breaths/minute and shallow; temperature, 102° F (38.8° C). Laboratory studies reveal a blood glucose of 800 mg/dL and a serum potassium of 2.8 mEq/L with a serum osmolality of 370 mOsm/kg. Based on these findings, what is the client's diagnosis?
[ ] **A.** Hypoglycemia
[ ] **B.** Hyperglycemia
[ ] **C.** Diabetic ketoacidosis
[ ] **D.** Hyperosmolar hyperglycemic nonketotic syndrome (HHNS)

Correct answer—D. *Rationales:* HHNS is characterized by a serum osmolality greater than 350 mOsm/kg and a blood glucose greater than 600 mg/dL. Hypoglycemia is a serum glucose lower than 60 mg/dL. Hyperglycemia is a fasting blood sugar greater than 140 mg/dL. Diabetic ketoacidosis results in a serum glucose greater than 300 mg/dL.
Nursing process step: Analysis

33. Which intervention is most important for a client with hyperosmolar hyperglycemic nonketotic syndrome?

[ ] **A.** Insertion of an orogastric tube
[ ] **B.** Insertion of an indwelling urinary catheter
[ ] **C.** Initiation of an I.V. line
[ ] **D.** Collection of blood sample for culturing

Correct answer—C. *Rationales:* The most important intervention for this client is the initiation of an I.V. line for fluid replacement. Clients can lose up to 25% of total body water with HHNS; elderly clients can lose up to 50%. One-half of the estimated water deficit should be replaced during the first 12 hours and the remainder during the next 24 hours. Insertion of an orogastric tube isn't necessary at this time. Insertion of an indwelling urinary catheter can be completed to monitor urine output but isn't a priority before the replacement of circulating volume. The client's elevated temperature is probably caused by dehydration and doesn't require the collection of blood samples.

Nursing process step: Intervention

34. During the initial phase of fluid resuscitation, which I.V. solution should be infused?

[ ] **A.** Normal saline solution
[ ] **B.** 5% dextrose in water
[ ] **C.** Dextran 40
[ ] **D.** Plasma-Lyte A

Correct answer—A. *Rationales:* Initial fluid resuscitation should consist of normal saline solution. In clients who are hypertensive and have significant hypernatremia, a hypotonic saline solution (0.45% sodium chloride) should be used. Normal saline corrects the extracellular volume deficit, increases blood pressure, and maintains adequate urine output. After these physiologic conditions have been corrected, hypotonic saline can be administered to provide free water for correction of intracellular volume deficits. Dextran 40 is a glucose polysaccharide and worsens dehydration. Plasma-Lyte A contains glucagon and increases blood glucose levels. The use of 5% dextrose in water also increases blood glucose.

Nursing process step: Intervention

35. A pregnant trauma client in hemorrhagic shock can lose up to what percentage of her circulating volume before exhibiting hypotension?

[ ] **A.** 15%
[ ] **B.** 20%
[ ] **C.** 30%
[ ] **D.** 50%

Correct answer—C. *Rationales:* A pregnant client becomes hypervolemic during pregnancy, and blood volume increases 45% to 50% above normal by term. Because the increase in plasma is more than that of red blood cells, the client manifests a relative anemia. The increase in plasma volume allows the client to lose up to 30% of the circulating volume before vital signs change to reflect a hypovolemic state. All other options are incorrect.

Nursing process step: Assessment

36. Which statement best describes neurogenic shock?

[ ] **A.** Decrease in respiratory function
[ ] **B.** Loss of sympathetic vasomotor regulation
[ ] **C.** Inadequate cellular perfusion
[ ] **D.** Loss of parasympathetic vasomotor regulation

Correct answer—B. *Rationales:* Neurogenic shock follows compression or transection of the spinal cord above the 6th thoracic vertebrae and affects the autonomic nervous system. Other causes of neurogenic shock are the administration of anesthetic agents and the ingestion of drugs (barbiturates or tranquilizers). All causes block the sympathetic vasomotor regulation below the level of the injury. Parasympathetic stimulation is unopposed, resulting in venous dilation, decreased venous return, decreased cardiac output, and decreased tissue perfusion. A decrease in respiratory function may occur, depending on the level of injury. Venous vasodilation affects inadequate tissue perfusion because of decreases in cardiac output.

Nursing process step: Assessment

37. What's the best early clinical indicator of hypovolemic shock in a pediatric client?
[ ] **A.** Blood pressure
[ ] **B.** Respiratory rate
[ ] **C.** Pulse rate and skin temperature and color
[ ] **D.** Urine output

Correct answer—C. *Rationales:* The best early indicators of hypovolemic shock in a pediatric client are pulse rate and skin temperature and color. Low-volume receptors (baroreceptors) located in the aortic arch and carotid bodies sense a decrease in circulating volume and increase sympathetic nervous system stimulation. The sympathetic nervous system increases catecholamine release, which increases the heart rate. Peripheral vaso-constriction occurs in an effort to increase cardiac output. The peripheral vasoconstriction causes the skin temperature to become cool. If the low flow isn't corrected, the skin color will become cyanotic. Capillary refill may be longer than 3 seconds. During low-flow states, initial compensatory mechanisms maintain near normal blood pressure because the child has a relatively healthy cardiovascular system. Hypotension occurs late in a shock state. Respiratory rate may be unaffected in the initial low-flow state. Normal urine output may be affected in the initial low-flow state as a result of decreased perfusion to the kidneys. Urinary output must be monitored to identify alterations in renal perfusion.
Nursing process step: Assessment

38. An infant with an upper respiratory tract infection and irritability for 4 days is admitted to the emergency department. On admission, vital signs are blood pressure, 48/30 mm Hg; pulse rate, 160 beats/minute; respiratory rate, 60 breaths/minute; and tympanic temperature, 96.5° F (35.8° C). The infant is lethargic, extremities are cool and cyanotic, and capillary refill is delayed (longer than 3 seconds). There's a petechial rash on the abdomen. The clinical manifestations described indicate which type of shock condition?
[ ] **A.** Hypovolemia
[ ] **B.** Anaphylactic
[ ] **C.** Septic
[ ] **D.** Cardiogenic

Correct answer—C. *Rationales:* The clinical manifestations describe septic shock probably caused by a gram-negative organism. Endotoxin causes a decrease in intravascular volume from increased venous capacitance. Cardiac output falls as the compensatory mechanisms fail to support circulation with the initial increased sympathetic stimulation. Endotoxins injure the endothelium and alter platelet function, causing the activation of intrinsic clotting factors, which leads to the development of disseminated intravascular coagulation. This is evidenced by the petechial rash on the abdomen. Petechiae on the abdomen may be a sign of meningococcemia, and the client should be immediately isolated.
Nursing process step: Assessment

39. What's the priority intervention for a pediatric client with septic shock?

[ ] **A.** Initiate an I.V. line.

[ ] **B.** Obtain blood cultures.

[ ] **C.** Give oxygen therapy with the device best tolerated by the client.

[ ] **D.** Insert an indwelling urinary catheter to determine urine output.

Correct answer—C. *Rationales:* The priority intervention for this client is to support respirations with supplemental oxygen therapy. The nurse should use the device best tolerated by the child; fighting an oxygen device may use up the child's oxygen reserves. In septic shock, the child's respiratory efforts may quickly lead to fatigue, so the child requires close monitoring for signs of respiratory failure. Oxygen saturation can be monitored with pulse oximetry. Intubation and mechanical ventilation equipment should be readily accessible. Septic shock creates a hypovolemic state; therefore, fluid replacement should be started as soon as possible after the airway is secure. To isolate the causative organism, blood cultures and urine cultures should be done before antibiotics are administered. The nurse should insert an indwelling urinary catheter after stabilizing airway, breathing, and circulation.

Nursing process step: Intervention

40. Medication therapy for a child in septic shock should include which of the following?

[ ] **A.** Cefotaxime (Claforan)

[ ] **B.** Dobutamine

[ ] **C.** Diphenhydramine

[ ] **D.** Atropine sulfate

Correct answer—A. *Rationales:* Antibiotics are recommended after obtaining at least one blood culture. Cefotaxime is a third-generation cephalosporin used in the treatment of lower respiratory infections. Dobutamine isn't routinely used in septic shock because it can lower systemic vascular resistance, thus leading to a risk of hypotension. Diphenhydramine may be used in anaphylactic shock, which may be confused with septic shock. Atropine isn't indicated at this time. It is an anticholinergic drug that blocks parasympathetic action on the sinoatrial node. It thereby improves conduction through the atrioventricular node and results in an increased heart rate.

Nursing process step: Intervention

41. Which statement best describes anaphylactic shock?

[ ] **A.** Loss of sympathetic vasomotor function

[ ] **B.** Systemic antigen-antibody response

[ ] **C.** Endothelial surface damage from endotoxin

[ ] **D.** Decreased catecholamine release

Correct answer—B. *Rationales:* Anaphylactic shock occurs from a systemic antigen-antibody response in which massive quantities of chemical mediators are released from the mast cells and basophils throughout the body. For anaphylaxis to occur, there must be previous sensitization to a foreign substance. On reexposure to the substance, the foreign antigen binds to immunoglobulin E (IgE), which was made during the initial exposure. After the IgE bonds to the mast cells and basophils, chemical mediators (histamine, kallikrein, leukotrienes, heparin, prostaglandins, protease, and platelet-activating factor) are released. Loss of sympathetic vasomotor function occurs in neurogenic shock. Endothelial surface damage from endotoxin occurs in septic shock. Catecholamines are released during the stress response and result in tachycardia. Histamine, prostaglandins, and kallikrein lead to peripheral vasodilation regardless of the vasoconstrictive efforts of the catecholamines.

Nursing process step: Assessment

42. Adequate fluid resuscitation in pediatric clients is best characterized by which urine output?

[ ] **A.** 0.5 mL/kg/hour
[ ] **B.** 1 to 2 mL/kg/hour
[ ] **C.** 3 to 4 mL/kg/hour
[ ] **D.** 10 to 15 mL/kg/hour

Correct answer—B. *Rationales:* Adequate renal perfusion in pediatric clients is best characterized by a urine output of 1 to 2 mL/kg/hour. During fluid resuscitation, urine output must be monitored to assess the effectiveness of renal function. All other options are incorrect.
Nursing process step: Evaluation

43. What's the priority when implementing initial treatment of clients in anaphylactic shock?

[ ] **A.** Administering antihistamines
[ ] **B.** Maintaining airway patency
[ ] **C.** Establishing I.V. access
[ ] **D.** Infusing a bolus of 200 mL of lactated Ringer's solution

Correct answer—B. *Rationales:* The priority in the initial treatment of clients in anaphylactic shock is maintaining airway patency. Anaphylactic shock is associated with the sudden onset of severe respiratory distress. Bronchospasm and laryngeal edema may lead to airway obstruction. I.V. access should be initiated to administer antihistamines and other drugs. Infusing a bolus of crystalloids isn't necessary because the hypotension in this type of shock is caused by vasodilation, not hypovolemia. Therefore, the client's blood pressure would remain low even after the fluid bolus.
Nursing process step: Intervention

44. In the treatment of shock, when peripheral cannulation is unsuccessful, intraosseous cannulation is usually recommended in which age-group?

[ ] **A.** No age limit
[ ] **B.** Younger than age 2
[ ] **C.** Younger than age 6
[ ] **D.** Younger than age 13

Correct answer—A. *Rationales:* In the past, the use of intraosseous cannulation was limited to use in children; however, intraosseous infusion in adults (as has been shown in children) is an effective modality in both the prehospital and hospital settings. The newer devices, such as the drill insertion devices and sternal devices have been tested in both adults and the pediatric population. Rapid vascular access is required when the client is in hemodynamic or cardiac compromise. Intraosseous cannulation allows rapid access for fluid or drug resuscitation. An intraosseous infusion is started by inserting a rigid needle into the medullary cavity of a long bone or sternum. When initiating intraosseous access, only one attempt should be made in each bone. Drugs, fluids, and blood may be infused by this access.
Nursing process step: Intervention

45. A client who was stung by 30 hornets is brought to the emergency department in acute respiratory distress. What should be the initial intervention for this client?

[ ] **A.** Administer I.M. epinephrine.
[ ] **B.** Secure the airway.
[ ] **C.** Initiate a large-bore I.V. with isotonic crystalloid solution.
[ ] **D.** Administer I.V. diphenhydramine.

Correct answer—B. *Rationales:* Respiratory distress may occur from angioedema of the upper airways, and laryngeal and bronchial spasms may create an airway obstruction. Management of the airway is the first priority of care. After the airway is secure, all other options are appropriate.
Nursing process step: Intervention

46. During a shock state, the renin-angiotensin-aldosterone system has which expected outcome on renal function?

[ ] **A.** Decreased urine output, increased reabsorption of sodium and water

[ ] **B.** Decreased urine output, decreased reabsorption of sodium and water

[ ] **C.** Increased urine output, increased reabsorption of sodium and water

[ ] **D.** Increased urine output, decreased reabsorption of sodium and water

Correct answer—A. *Rationales:* The reninangiotensin-aldosterone system alters renal function by decreasing urine output and increasing reabsorption of sodium and water. Reduced renal perfusion stimulates the renin-angiotensin-aldosterone system in an effort to conserve circulating volume.

Nursing process step: Evaluation

47. A trauma client with a fractured femur and a fractured pelvis has been transfused with 2 units of packed red blood cells. Which measurements indicate that this client has received adequate replacement of circulating volume?

[ ] **A.** pH, 7.22; $PaCO_2$, 45; PaO_2, 88; HCO_3^-, 15

[ ] **B.** SaO_2, 76%

[ ] **C.** Blood pressure, 88/76 mm Hg; pulse, 120 beats/minute

[ ] **D.** pH, 7.35, $PaCO_2$, 40, PaO_2, 95; HCO_3^-, 22

Correct answer—D. *Rationales:* These blood gas values reflect a normal acid-base state, indicating that the client has received adequate blood replacement. All other assessments indicate a hypovolemic state that hasn't been corrected.

Nursing process step: Evaluation

48. An indwelling urinary catheter has been inserted in an adult client who was dehydrated from vomiting. Which urine output indicates that the client has received adequate fluid replacement?

[ ] **A.** 5 mL/hour

[ ] **B.** 15 mL/hour

[ ] **C.** 25 mL/hour

[ ] **D.** 30 mL/hour

Correct answer—D. *Rationales:* A urine output of 30 mL/hour or more indicates that the client has received adequate volume replacement and that renal perfusion is normal. All other options indicate the need for more fluids.

Nursing process step: Evaluation

49. What's the expected outcome of administering pharmacologic agents in the treatment of cardiogenic shock?

[ ] **A.** Decreased preload, increased contractility, increased peripheral resistance

[ ] **B.** Increased contractility, decreased peripheral resistance and afterload, increased cardiac output

[ ] **C.** Increased preload, increased peripheral resistance, increased afterload

[ ] **D.** Decreased cardiac output, decreased cardiac contractility, decreased peripheral resistance

Correct answer—B. *Rationales:* Administering dopamine (Intropin), dobutamine (Dobutrex), nitroprusside (Nipride), and nitroglycerine (Nitro-Bid) to treat cardiogenic shock should result in decreased peripheral resistance and afterload, increased contractility, and increased cardiac output. All other options are incorrect.

Nursing process step: Evaluation

50. Administering dopamine (Intropin) at 2 mcg/kg/minute results in:
[ ] **A.** decreased renal perfusion.
[ ] **B.** decreased reabsorption of sodium and water.
[ ] **C.** increased renal perfusion.
[ ] **D.** increased reabsorption of sodium and water.

Correct answer—C. *Rationales:* Dopamine, when administered at low doses of 0.5 to 3 mcg/kg/minute, produces primarily alpha-adrenergic effects and increases renal perfusion. Doses over 10 mcg/kg/minute result in renal vasoconstriction. Dopamine doesn't directly affect the reabsorption of sodium and water other than to dilate renal arterioles.
Nursing process step: Evaluation

51. A client with a fractured pelvis and retroperitoneal hemorrhage has received 10 units of packed red blood cells (RBCs). The nurse notices that blood is oozing from abrasions and puncture sites. What's the most appropriate intervention for this client?
[ ] **A.** Administer blood without warming it.
[ ] **B.** Administer fresh frozen plasma and platelets.
[ ] **C.** Discontinue further transfusion.
[ ] **D.** Administer cryoprecipitate.

Correct answer—B. *Rationales:* Packed RBCs and stored whole blood don't contain coagulation factors. One unit of fresh frozen plasma and six platelet packs are recommended for every 5 to 10 units of blood transfused. Hypothermia may also alter the coagulation cascade, so blood should be warmed to 98.6° F (37° C). There's no need to discontinue further blood transfusions; pelvic fractures and retroperitoneal hemorrhages may deplete all the circulating volume if they don't tamponade. Cryoprecipitate could be infused if more than 20 units of blood are administered. Cryoprecipitate contains clotting factors that may be lacking in a client requiring multiple transfusions.
Nursing process step: Intervention

52. A 71-year-old female client presents with increased shortness of breath over a 6-day period, followed by acute onset of severe back and interscapular pain. She is obese, has a history of hypertension, and has type 2 diabetes. Presenting vital signs are blood pressure, 80/40 mm Hg; pulse rate, 110 beats/minute; and respiratory rate, 36 breaths/minute. This client is diagnosed with pulmonary embolus causing obstructive shock. What is the priority of treatment for this client?
[ ] **A.** Administration of a thrombolytic
[ ] **B.** Fluid resuscitation
[ ] **C.** Intubation
[ ] **D.** Surgical embolectomy

Correct answer—C. *Rationales:* Pulmonary embolism severe enough to cause obstructive shock requires respiratory support prior to other interventions. Fluid resuscitation must be managed carefully so as to not cause fluid overload. After the airway is stabilized, either a thrombolytic or a surgical embolectomy may be used to manage the clot. Acute major pulmonary embolism is associated with right ventricular dysfunction and shock. This condition is frequently lethal despite thrombolysis. Survival depends on rapid recanalization of the pulmonary arterial occlusion and reduction of the right ventricular afterload. Pulmonary embolism can also result in cardiogenic shock; the important point is the rapid identification and treatment of the clot.
Nursing process step: Intervention

53. A trauma client is transferred from another hospital where his initial hematocrit was 40%. After receiving 4 L of normal saline solution, the hematocrit is 32%. This decrease is probably related to which condition?
[ ] **A.** Additional blood was lost.
[ ] **B.** Hemodilution occurred from the infusion of crystalloids.
[ ] **C.** The specimen was drawn above the I.V. site.
[ ] **D.** A hemolyzed blood specimen was spun.

Correct answer—B. *Rationales:* Hemodilution from an infusion of crystalloid solution has caused the hematocrit decrease from 40% to 32% and occurs when the ratio of plasma to red cells increases. Additional blood loss may decrease the hematocrit level, but this decrease is probably caused by hemodilution. Specimens drawn above the I.V. site would increase the hematocrit. Hematocrit can be obtained even when a specimen is hemolyzed.
Nursing process step: Evaluation

54. Children may lose up to which percentage of their circulating volume before clinical manifestations of shock occur?
[ ] **A.** 5%
[ ] **B.** 15%
[ ] **C.** 25%
[ ] **D.** 35%

Correct answer—C. *Rationales:* Children may lose up to 25% of their circulating volume before they manifest signs of shock. The normal blood volume for children is 80 to 85 mL/kg. When fluid losses occur, intrinsic compensatory mechanisms initiate changes to augment circulation: venous capacitance decreases, fluid shifts from the interstitial to the intravascular compartments, and arteriolar constriction increases.
Nursing process step: Assessment

55. Which compensatory mechanisms are responses to shock?
[ ] **A.** Increased renal perfusion and retention of sodium and water
[ ] **B.** Decreased renal perfusion and excretion of sodium and water
[ ] **C.** Increased renal perfusion and excretion of sodium and water
[ ] **D.** Decreased renal perfusion and retention of sodium and water

Correct answer—D. *Rationales:* Vasoconstriction in response to a low-flow state decreases renal perfusion. Reduction of renal blood flow and stimulation of the renin-angiotensin-aldosterone system increase reabsorption of sodium and water, thus decreasing urine output. None of the other options reflects the compensatory state of shock.
Nursing process step: Evaluation

56. What's the normal range for serum lactate levels?
[ ] **A.** 0.5 to 2.2 mmol/L
[ ] **B.** 1.5 to 0.5 mmol/L
[ ] **C.** 2.5 to 5.5 mmol/L
[ ] **D.** 5.5 to 7.2 mmol/L

Correct answer—A. *Rationales:* The normal range for serum lactate levels is 0.5 to 2.2 mmol/L for venous blood and 0.5 to 1.6 mmol/L for arterial blood. If oxygen isn't readily available to body cells, anaerobic metabolism occurs, with lactic acid as a by-product. A serum lactate level measures the amount of lactic acid in the blood and is a fairly sensitive and reliable indicator of tissue hypoperfusion and hypoxia.
Nursing process step: Assessment

57. Treatment for a client in anaphylactic shock includes administering antihistamines, bronchodilators, and epinephrine. Which other histamine$_2$ (H_2) blocker could be administered?
[ ] **A.** Atenolol (Tenormin)
[ ] **B.** Methylprednisolone (Solu-Medrol)
[ ] **C.** Diphenhydramine (Benadryl)
[ ] **D.** Cimetidine (Tagamet)

Correct answer—D. *Rationales:* Initial treatment of anaphylactic shock includes administering antihistamines, bronchodilators, and epinephrine. It also includes administering H_2 blockers and cimetidine 300 mg I.V. Administration of H_2 blockers and cimetidine is repeated every 6 to 8 hours. Atenolol is a beta-adrenergic blocker, so these clients may require higher doses of epinephrine to counteract the effects of the mediators released from the mast cells and basophils. Diphenhydramine is an antihistamine. An initial dose of 50 mg is administered I.V. and may be repeated every 6 to 8 hours. Methylprednisolone is a glucocorticoid and may prevent or lessen the delayed reactions from the antigen-antibody reaction.
Nursing process step: Intervention

58. The client's urine specific gravity is 1.050. What does this indicate?
[ ] **A.** Dehydration with altered renal tissue perfusion
[ ] **B.** Adequate fluid resuscitation
[ ] **C.** Overhydration
[ ] **D.** Urinary tract infection

Correct answer–A. *Rationales:* Normal urine specific gravity ranges from 1.003 to 1.040. A urine specific gravity greater than 1.050 indicates dehydration with altered renal tissue perfusion. The compensatory mechanism during a low-flow state is to shunt blood from the skin and the GI and renal systems to maintain heart and brain functions. Decreased renal perfusion results in decreased water excretion and reabsorption and decreased sodium. Hypervolemia is usually evidenced by a decrease in urine specific gravity.
Nursing process step: Assessment

59. A client with blunt trauma to the abdomen has received 2 L of lactated Ringer's solution. What's the most appropriate intervention in response to the following arterial blood gas (ABG) values: pH, 7.21; $PaCO_2$, 45; PaO_2, 84; HCO_3^-, 15?
[ ] **A.** Infuse lactated Ringer's solution at a keep-vein-open rate.
[ ] **B.** Infuse a bolus with lactated Ringer's solution at 40 mL/kg.
[ ] **C.** Infuse whole blood or packed red cells.
[ ] **D.** Administer sodium bicarbonate.

Correct answer–C. *Rationales:* The ABG values reveal that the client is in metabolic acidosis because of decreased tissue perfusion from hemorrhage. Blunt trauma to the abdomen may result in injury to the solid viscera (spleen and liver) and produce severe loss of circulating volume and oxygen. When tissues don't have adequate oxygenation, an anaerobic environment occurs and produces a buildup of lactic acid. The replacement of red blood cells (RBCs) decreases the anaerobic environment. Replacement may be with whole blood or packed RBCs. The infusion of crystalloids, such as lactated Ringer's solution or normal saline, will replace circulating volume; however, hemodilution of existing RBCs will occur. During the initial shock phase, metabolic acidosis is treated with blood and fluid replacement. If acidosis continues, sodium bicarbonate may be administered.
Nursing process step: Intervention

60. A listless 3-year-old child is brought into the emergency department. The father relates that the child had been eating a peanut butter sandwich when she began crying and rubbing her mouth. Immediately, her lips and eyes became swollen and she developed a raised rash on her trunk and extremities. Her breathing is labored, and audible wheezing can be heard. Vital signs are as follows: blood pressure, 86/33 mm Hg; pulse, 185 beats/minute; respiratory rate, 48 breaths/minute; oxygen saturation, 90% on room air. The doctor decides to treat for anaphylaxis. Which of the following medications would be contraindicated?
[ ] **A.** Racemic epinephrine
[ ] **B.** Ipratropium inhaler
[ ] **C.** Albuterol nebulizer
[ ] **D.** Diphenhydramine

Correct answer–B. *Rationales*: Ipratropium inhaler should be avoided in clients with soya lecithin allergies (soybean and peanut) because of a preservative the inhaler contains. Clients have been known to adversely react to this medication when in this form. Albuterol nebulizers are safe in this client population because they don't contain the preservative. The other treatments listed are appropriate for anaphylaxis.
Nursing process step: Intervention

61. What's the best unit of measure for identifying early shock in a trauma client?
[ ] **A.** Hemoglobin and hematocrit
[ ] **B.** Central venous pressure (CVP)
[ ] **C.** Blood pressure
[ ] **D.** Heart rate

Correct answer—B. *Rationales:* Central venous pressure (CVP) is the best unit of measure for identifying shock in a trauma client. CVP measures the right-sided heart pressure, which reflects blood and fluid status. A normal CVP measurement is 4 to 10 cm H_2O pressure. A value less than 4 cm may indicate hypovolemia or vasodilation. Hemoglobin and hematocrit aren't the best indicators of early shock in a trauma client because they may be normal in early shock unless there has been massive blood loss. It normally takes 4 to 6 hours for blood loss to be reflected in hemoglobin and hematocrit levels.
Nursing process step: Assessment

62. Which of the following values best identifies tissue hypoperfusion and shock in the presence of normal vital signs?
[ ] **A.** Serum lactate, 6 mmol/L
[ ] **B.** Arterial blood gas (ABG), pH 7.5
[ ] **C.** Hematocrit of 18
[ ] **D.** Base excess–1

Correct answer—A. *Rationales*: A serum lactate of 6 mmol/L reflects cellular hypoxia. An ABG pH of 7.5 is within normal limits. Although a hematocrit of 18 may be considered low, there are many causes for it; it's a poor indicator of shock or blood loss and it doesn't correlate well with hypoperfusion. Base excess also can reflect hypoxia; however, a level of –1 is within normal limits. Greater than –4 may indicate acidosis.
Nursing process step: Analysis

63. A client who's receiving beta-adrenergic blockers shows which response to a shock state?
[ ] **A.** Increased pulse rate and hypotension
[ ] **B.** Bradycardia, hypotension, and decreased renin secretion
[ ] **C.** Increased pulse rate and hypertension
[ ] **D.** Bradycardia and hypertension

Correct answer—B. *Rationales:* Beta-adrenergic blockers may mask the signs of shock. The sympathetic stimulation causing an increase in heart rate is blocked by beta-adrenergic blockers. The client may show bradycardia and hypotension with a decrease in renin secretion.
Nursing process step: Evaluation

64. A young mother brings her 6-month-old baby to the emergency department. The baby is pale and responsive, has cool extremities, and has a capillary refill time of 3 seconds. The heart rate is 200 beats/minute apically, the respiratory rate is 28 breaths/minute, and the temperature can't be obtained. The baby's diaper is soaked with yellow-green liquid. A bedside serum glucose is 40 mg/dL. The nurse is unable to obtain a tympanic temperature measurement. The baby had a day and a half of vomiting and diarrhea, which seemed to get better. What intervention should the nurse perform?
[ ] **A.** Provide education to the mother on dehydration and recommend she make an appointment at the clinic the next day.
[ ] **B.** Have the child taken immediately to a resuscitation area for immediate intervention.
[ ] **C.** Return the mother and child to the waiting room to await their turn to see a provider, recommending to the mother that she encourage fluids while she waits.
[ ] **D.** Place the child in an exam room and place the chart in the rack for the physician.

Correct answer—B. *Rationales:* This child is in compensated shock and requires immediate oxygenation and fluid. The symptoms in compensated shock can be subtle and must be identified. The critical findings of cool extremities, poor capillary refill, and the baby's relative tachycardia signals his heart's limited compensatory effort to improve cardiac output. The young heart has limited ability to increase stroke volume when stressed, so the primary cardiac compensatory mechanism of the pediatric heart is increased rate. Infants have limited stores of glycogen, and hypoglycemia may both mimic and contribute to the clinical state of shock. If compensated shock isn't immediately corrected, it will quickly deteriorate into an uncompensated state.
Nursing process step: Analysis

65. Which of the following medications can make anaphylaxis worse?
[ ] **A.** Corticosteroids
[ ] **B.** Antihistamines
[ ] **C.** Beta-adrenergic blockers
[ ] **D.** Epinephrine

Correct answer—C. *Rationales:* Beta-adrenergic blockers are medicines that can worsen anaphylaxis and make treatment with drugs like epinephrine less effective. Beta-adrenergic blockers can turn a bearable skin reaction to anaphylaxis into a dangerous reaction with shock. All other drugs listed are treatment modalities for anaphylaxis.
Nursing process step: Intervention

16 Substance abuse and toxicologic emergencies

1. A client with a history of alcohol abuse comes to the emergency department 12 hours after his last drink complaining of nausea, palpitations, and feeling anxious. The client is tremulous. Which medication can the nurse anticipate to be the first ordered for this client?

[ ] **A.** Thiamine
[ ] **B.** Lorazepam (Ativan)
[ ] **C.** Phenytoin
[ ] **D.** Haloperidol (Haldol)

Correct answer—B. *Rationales:* Benzodiazepines such as lorazepam are considered to be first-line therapy for the treatment of acute withdrawal syndrome and the prevention and treatment of seizure activity and delirium tremens. Antiepileptic therapy has long been studied for the prevention of seizures in acute withdrawal syndrome for lessening the overall syndrome. Placebo-controlled trials have demonstrated that phenytoin is ineffective for the secondary prevention of alcohol withdrawal seizures. In addition, phenobarbital use has been attributed to respiratory depression in high doses or when combined with alcohol. For the treatment of Wernicke's encephalopathy and thiamine deficiency, the administration of thiamine is recommended; however, this would not be a first-line therapy. Haloperidol has also been used to control the psychiatric symptoms of alcohol withdrawal, including combativeness, delirium, and anxiousness. However, it has been shown to be significantly less effective than benzodiazepines in preventing delirium and can cause torsades de pointes by prolonging the QT interval.
Nursing process step: Analysis

2. A 20-year-old client complaining of substernal chest pain comes to the emergency department triage desk. Breath sounds are clear, and the client is negative for a history of medical problems. The nurse should ask specifically about the use of which of these drugs?

[ ] **A.** Tricyclic antidepressants
[ ] **B.** Benzodiazepines
[ ] **C.** Opioids
[ ] **D.** Cocaine

Correct answer—D. *Rationales:* Cocaine has direct effects on the heart that include increased myocardial oxygen consumption, coronary artery spasm, ischemia, and myocardial infarction. Tricyclic antidepressants cause arrhythmias in overdoses. Benzodiazepines cause drowsiness and confusion in overdoses. Opioids cause respiratory depression.
Nursing process step: Assessment

3. Appropriate nursing interventions for a client who's actively hallucinating and agitated after ingesting D-lysergic acid diethylamide (LSD) include all of these *except*:

[ ] **A.** instructing the client to keep his eyes open.
[ ] **B.** keeping the room well lit.
[ ] **C.** reassuring the patient.
[ ] **D.** restraining the client.

Correct answer—D. *Rationales:* Restraining the client will increase his agitation. Reassure him that he isn't losing his mind and that the effects of the drug will wear off. Instruct him to keep his eyes open to decrease the intensity of hallucinations. Keeping the room well lit reduces shadows that may be misinterpreted by the client, thereby adding to his agitation.
Nursing process step: Intervention

4. When planning care for a client who has ingested phencyclidine (PCP), what's the highest priority?
[ ] **A.** Client's physical needs
[ ] **B.** Client's safety needs
[ ] **C.** Client's psychosocial needs
[ ] **D.** Client's medical needs

Correct answer—B. *Rationales:* The highest priority for a client who has ingested PCP is meeting safety needs of the client—as well as those of the staff. PCP effects are unpredictable and prolonged, and the client may lose control easily. After safety needs have been met, the client's physical, psychosocial, and medical needs can be met.
Nursing process step: Intervention

5. Which drug should the nurse prepare to administer to a client with a toxic acetaminophen (Tylenol) level?
[ ] **A.** Deferoxamine (Desferal)
[ ] **B.** Succimer (Chemet)
[ ] **C.** Flumazenil (Romazicon)
[ ] **D.** Acetylcysteine (Acetadote)

Correct answer—D. *Rationales:* The antidote for acetaminophen toxicity is acetylcysteine, which enhances conversion of toxic metabolites to nontoxic metabolites. Deferoxamine mesylate is the antidote for iron intoxication. Succimer is an antidote for lead poisoning, and flumazenil reverses the sedative effects of benzodiazepines.
Nursing process step: Intervention

6. Interventions for hydrofluoric acid exposure may be deemed effective if:
[ ] **A.** glucose level returns to normal.
[ ] **B.** calcium level returns to normal.
[ ] **C.** magnesium level returns to normal.
[ ] **D.** potassium level returns to normal.

Correct answer—B. *Rationales:* Fluoride ions in hydrofluoric acid bind with calcium and cause severe hypocalcemia, which can lead to tetany and death. Chvostek's sign is elicited by tapping the side of the face over the facial nerve. If hypocalcemia is present, the client's facial muscles will contract. Fluoride ions don't directly affect glucose, magnesium, or potassium levels.
Nursing process step: Evaluation

7. An inebriated client is brought to the emergency department by the police. The nurse suspects that the client has ingested methanol after she notes which odor on the client's breath?
[ ] **A.** Bitter almond
[ ] **B.** Moth balls
[ ] **C.** Formalin
[ ] **D.** Garlic

Correct answer—C. *Rationales:* Formalin is a characteristic breath odor in methanol poisoning because formic acid is a metabolite of methanol. The client's urine may also have a formalin odor. A number of poisons may be indicated by the presence of associated breath odors. Bitter almond, for example, is characteristic of cyanide. The odor of moth balls is characteristic of camphor and naphthalene. Garlic is characteristic of arsenic, organophosphates, phosphorous, selenium, and thallium.
Nursing process step: Analysis

8. Nursing assessment of the client undergoing therapy for ethylene glycol ingestion includes monitoring for:
[ ] **A.** hypercalcemia.
[ ] **B.** hypokalemia.
[ ] **C.** hypertension.
[ ] **D.** ethanol levels.

Correct answer—D. *Rationales:* Medical therapy for ethylene glycol ingestion includes blocking the metabolism of the drug by saturating alcohol dehydrogenase sites with ethanol to prevent the production of toxic metabolites. The dehydrogenase sites are saturated when ethanol levels are 100 mg/dL. Hypercalcemia isn't present because ethylene glycol toxicity causes hypocalcemia from chelation of calcium by oxalates. Hypokalemia isn't present because metabolites cause severe acidosis and hyperkalemia. Ethylene glycol toxicity doesn't cause hypertension although the client may become hypotensive 4 to 12 hours after ingestion.
Nursing process step: Assessment

9. A 6-year-old child who is brought to the emergency department by his grandmother appears to be intoxicated. The grandmother reports that the child was helping her clean out the garage. She reports that the child may have opened the antifreeze bottle. Which nursing action takes highest priority?

[ ] **A.** Sending labwork to determine methanol level
[ ] **B.** Administering I.V. fluids
[ ] **C.** Providing airway support
[ ] **D.** Educating the grandmother on the risks of hazardous household materials

Correct answer–C. *Rationales:* Although all of the options can be anticipated during the care of this client, supporting the child's airway take priority. Clients with methanol intoxication are at risk for sudden respiratory arrest because methanol and its metabolites depress the brain stem.
Nursing process step: Analysis

10. Which would the nurse expect to find in a client with a known amphetamine overdose?

[ ] **A.** Hypotension
[ ] **B.** Tachycardia
[ ] **C.** Hot, dry skin
[ ] **D.** Constricted pupils

Correct answer–B. *Rationales:* Amphetamines are central nervous system stimulants that cause sympathetic stimulation, including hypertension, tachycardia, vasoconstriction, and hyperthermia. Hot, dry skin is seen with anticholinergic agents such as jimsonweed. Pupils are dilated, not constricted, with amphetamine overdose.
Nursing process step: Assessment

11. A comatose client with a suspected barbiturate overdose is admitted to the emergency department. Gastric lavage is ordered. How does the nurse perform this procedure correctly in an adult client?

[ ] **A.** By instilling 300 mL of fluid
[ ] **B.** By placing the client in the right lateral Trendelenburg position
[ ] **C.** By inserting an 18 French gastric tube
[ ] **D.** By instilling activated charcoal before lavage

Correct answer–A. *Rationales:* A client receiving gastric lavage should have 100 to 300 mL of fluid instilled. The fluid should then be removed by gravity or gentle suction. Larger amounts may cause the pyloric sphincter to open and force the toxins into the intestine. The client should be placed in the left lateral Trendelenburg position. A large-bore gastric tube (22 to 36 French) should be used. The average size for an adult is 32 to 36 French. Activated charcoal is usually instilled after lavage has been completed.
Nursing process step: Intervention

12. While caring for a client with carbon monoxide poisoning, which of the following is the most likely cause of the client's confusion?

[ ] **A.** Impaired gas exchange
[ ] **B.** Airway compromise
[ ] **C.** Ingestion of other substances
[ ] **D.** Underlying dementia

Correct answer–A. *Rationales:* The primary problem is impaired gas exchange at the cellular level. Carbon monoxide displaces oxygen on the hemoglobin, which leads to hypoxia, thereby causing confusion. Carbon monoxide poisoning won't cause a primary airway compromise. The other two options are incorrect.
Nursing process step: Analysis

13. After swallowing evidence during an arrest, a client with a possible cocaine overdose is brought to the emergency department. Which sign should the nurse assess for cocaine overdose?

[ ] **A.** Hypotension
[ ] **B.** Hypothermia
[ ] **C.** Constricted pupils
[ ] **D.** Tachycardia

Correct answer–D. *Rationales:* Cocaine is a stimulant drug. It causes hypertension, hyperthermia, dilated pupils, seizures, and tachycardia.
Nursing process step: Assessment

14. A client with known acute cyanide ingestion is admitted to the emergency department. Which intervention takes highest priority?

[ ] **A.** Administer cyanide antidote.
[ ] **B.** Perform gastric lavage.
[ ] **C.** Administer activated charcoal.
[ ] **D.** Manage seizures.

Correct answer—A. *Rationales:* The cyanide antidote should be administered before decontaminating the GI tract. Because cyanide is rapidly absorbed and causes cellular hypoxia, reversing the hypoxia takes priority. The Lilly Cyanide Kit, used to treat cyanide poisoning, contains an amyl nitrite inhaler and sodium nitrite, which create methemoglobin and attract cyanide away from the respiratory enzyme cytochrome oxidase. Sodium thiosulfate is also used; it forms nontoxic thiocyanate. Performing gastric lavage, administering activated charcoal, and managing seizures are correct, but not immediate, interventions.
Nursing process step: Intervention

15. A client is admitted to the emergency department with arsenic poisoning. Which medication should the nurse prepare to administer?

[ ] **A.** Deferoxamine (Desferal)
[ ] **B.** Dimercaprol (BAL in Oil)
[ ] **C.** Calcium EDTA (calcium disodium versenate)
[ ] **D.** Succimer (Chemet)

Correct answer—B. *Rationales:* Arsenic is a heavy metal. Effective chelating agents for it include dimercaprol and D-penicillamine. Other measures include alkalinization of the urine and hemodialysis. Deferoxamine mesylate is used for iron intoxication. Calcium EDTA and succimer are indicated for lead poisoning.
Nursing process step: Intervention

16. A pediatric client is admitted to the emergency department after swallowing his mother's prenatal vitamins. The client has abdominal pain and diarrhea. After determining that he has ingested more than 20 mg/kg of elemental iron, chelation therapy is started. Which of the following indicates a positive response to deferoxamine (Desferal)?

[ ] **A.** Urine color turns orange-red.
[ ] **B.** Diarrhea stops.
[ ] **C.** Acid-base balance returns to normal.
[ ] **D.** Vital signs return to normal.

Correct answer—A. *Rationales:* After deferoxamine chelates iron, it's excreted as pink to orange-red urine. This is the earliest indication of a positive response to chelation therapy. The symptoms displayed by a pediatric client with iron poisoning depend on how quickly medical attention is received. Early symptoms are GI irritation, hematemesis, abdominal pain, and lethargy. This is followed by a latent period in which the client appears to improve. The third phase includes shock, acidosis, and fever.
Nursing process step: Evaluation

17. A client with depressed mental status and slowed respirations is brought to the emergency department by emergency medical personnel. They state that no pill bottles or needles were found at the scene, but they did find a white powder substance and a pipe that the client appeared to have been inhaling. What should the nurse assess for next?

[ ] **A.** Hypertension
[ ] **B.** Tachycardia
[ ] **C.** Pinpoint pupils
[ ] **D.** Hot, dry skin

Correct answer—C. *Rationales:* This client shows signs of a possible opioid overdose. Opioids, except for meperidine, cause pinpoint pupils. The nurse should rapidly assess the client's pupils before taking the client's blood pressure and pulse. Hypertension and tachycardia aren't present because opioids cause bradycardia and hypotension. Hot, dry skin is seen with an anticholinergic overdose.
Nursing process step: Assessment

18. The nurse should prepare to administer which drug to the client with symptoms of organophosphate overdose?

[ ] **A.** Physostigmine
[ ] **B.** Flumazenil (Romazicon)
[ ] **C.** Glucagon
[ ] **D.** Atropine

Correct answer—D. *Rationales:* The symptoms of organophosphate poisoning result from cholinergic overactivity; the antidote is the anticholinergic agent atropine. Physostigmine is a cholinergic agent and will worsen symptoms. Flumazenil reverses the sedative effects of benzodiazepines. Glucagon is the antidote for beta-adrenergic blockers.
Nursing process step: Intervention

19. When evaluating the effectiveness of antidote therapy for organophosphate poisoning, the nurse should prepare to administer additional antidote if the client continues to display which sign or symptom?

[ ] **A.** Hot, dry skin
[ ] **B.** Pinpoint pupils
[ ] **C.** Tachycardia
[ ] **D.** Drying of mucous membranes

Correct answer—B. *Rationales:* Atropine, the antidote for organophosphate poisoning, is an anti-cholinergic agent. The nurse will find pupil dilation if the client has received an adequate dose of atropine. Hot, dry skin as well as tachycardia and dry mucous membranes are signs that the atropine has been effective.
Nursing process step: Evaluation

20. A teenager is brought to the hospital by friends after accidentally ingesting gasoline while siphoning it from a car. Based on the nurse's knowledge of petroleum distillates, which system should be the priority assessment?

[ ] **A.** GI system
[ ] **B.** Respiratory system
[ ] **C.** Neurologic system
[ ] **D.** Cardiovascular system

Correct answer—B. *Rationales:* The primary concern with petroleum distillate ingestion is its effect on the pulmonary system. Aspiration or absorption of petroleum distillates can cause severe chemical pneumonitis and impaired gas exchange. The GI, neurologic, and cardiovascular systems may also be affected if the petroleum contains additives such as pesticides, but the respiratory system is the first priority.
Nursing process step: Assessment

21. A client who's actively hallucinating is brought to the emergency department by friends. They say that the client used either D-lysergic acid diethylamide (LSD) or phencyclidine (PCP) at a concert. During triage, which assessment finding indicates that the client may have ingested PCP?

[ ] **A.** Dilated pupils
[ ] **B.** Nystagmus
[ ] **C.** Paranoia
[ ] **D.** Altered mood

Correct answer—B. *Rationales:* Phencyclidine is an anesthetic with severe psychological effects. It blocks the reuptake of dopamine and directly affects the midbrain and thalamus. Nystagmus and ataxia are common physical findings of PCP use. Dilated pupils are evidence of LSD ingestion. Paranoia and altered mood occur with both PCP and LSD ingestion.
Nursing process step: Assessment

22. After chewing rhubarb leaves, a 3-year-old is brought to the emergency department by her parents. The nurse should expect to find which condition?

[ ] **A.** Lethargy
[ ] **B.** Bradycardia
[ ] **C.** Hypertension
[ ] **D.** Dysphagia

Correct answer—D. *Rationales:* Rhubarb leaves contain oxalic acid, a toxin that irritates the mouth and throat. The acid may cause edema of the mouth and throat, dysphagia, and increased salivation. Systemic effects include hypocalcemia. Calcium oxalate crystals may be found in the urine. Lethargy may occur after ingestion of a number of plants, especially of the amygdalin-glycoside-cyanide category. Bradycardia is found after ingestion of plants that contain cardiac glycosides. Hypertension occurs after ingestion of plants that contain anticholinergic agents.
Nursing process step: Assessment

23. A 15-year-old presents to the emergency department with dry, flushed skin; confusion; and restlessness. He's tachycardic. His friends say that they were all at a party and ate some "stinkweed." Recognizing this as jimson weed, the nurse should anticipate all but which one of the following actions?
[ ] **A.** Providing a cooling blanket
[ ] **B.** Preparation for intubation
[ ] **C.** Administering physostigmine
[ ] **D.** Administration of I.V. crystalloid solution

Correct answer—B. *Rationales:* A client who has ingested jimson weed usually doesn't have airway problems. Cooling measures, such as cooling blankets or cool cloths and cooled I.V. fluids, may be used to treat hyperpyrexia. Physostigmine is an acetylcholinesterase inhibitor and can therefore reverse the peripheral and central manifestations of anticholinergic excess.
Nursing process step: Analysis

24. The physician orders physostigmine 1 mg slow I.V. push for a client who has ingested deadly nightshade. After administering the medication, the nurse should look for which change to determine if the medication has been effective?
[ ] **A.** Heart rate increases.
[ ] **B.** Blood pressure rises.
[ ] **C.** Hallucinations subside.
[ ] **D.** Pupils dilate.

Correct answer—C. *Rationales:* Physostigmine is given to reverse the effects of severe poisoning by deadly nightshade, which has anticholinergic properties. Increased heart rate and blood pressure and dilated pupils are all signs of an anticholinergic effect.
Nursing process step: Evaluation

25. An elderly client comes to the triage desk and complains of arthritis pain and tinnitus. The client has been taking nonprescription medications for pain relief. Based on the client's chief complaints, the nurse should ask him about the use of:
[ ] **A.** ibuprofen (Motrin).
[ ] **B.** acetaminophen (Tylenol).
[ ] **C.** naproxen (Aleve).
[ ] **D.** aspirin.

Correct answer—D. *Rationales:* Tinnitus is the most common central nervous system sign of mild salicylate toxicity. Clients taking medications that contain salicylates at doses prescribed for arthritis may develop mild toxicity (salicylism). Ibuprofen usually causes GI upset and blurred vision. Acetaminophen toxicity causes liver failure. Naproxen may cause GI bleeding without other GI symptoms. It may also mask infection.
Nursing process step: Assessment

26. Flumazenil (Romazicon) has been ordered for a client who has overdosed on oxazepam (Serax). Before administering the medication, the nurse should be prepared for which potential immediate outcome?
[ ] **A.** Seizures
[ ] **B.** Shivering
[ ] **C.** Anxiety
[ ] **D.** Chest pain

Correct answer—A. *Rationales:* The most common serious adverse effect of using flumazenil to reverse benzodiazepine overdose is seizures. The effect is magnified if the client has a combined tricyclic antidepressant and benzodiazepine overdose. Less common adverse effects include shivering, anxiety, and chest pain.
Nursing process step: Evaluation

27. An awake, alert client is brought to the emergency department by family members. Fifteen minutes earlier, he ingested the entire contents of a new prescription for the tricyclic antidepressant amitriptyline (Elavil). Which of the following isn't indicated for this client?
[ ] **A.** Activated charcoal
[ ] **B.** Ipecac
[ ] **C.** Gastric lavage
[ ] **D.** Electrocardiogram (ECG)

Correct answer—B. *Rationales:* Ipecac is contraindicated in tricyclic antidepressant overdose. Rapid deterioration with cardiovascular collapse and seizures can occur in a client who's initially awake and alert. Airway compromise may occur from aspiration. Gastric lavage should be ordered with endotracheal intubation with proper cuff inflation and mechanical ventilation. Administration of activated charcoal may be delayed. A baseline ECG may be ordered. The client should be placed on a cardiac monitor because arrhythmias and cardiac conduction delays are common.
Nursing process step: Intervention

28. A comatose client, who had ingested the tricyclic antidepressant doxepin (Sinequan), is brought to the emergency department. In addition to supportive measures, the nurse administers ordered sodium bicarbonate I.V. push. When evaluating the effectiveness of the medication, the nurse should monitor:
[ ] **A.** neurologic status.
[ ] **B.** respiratory status.
[ ] **C.** acid-base status.
[ ] **D.** cardiovascular status.

Correct answer—D. *Rationales:* Management of tricyclic antidepressant overdose is focused on reversing cardiotoxicity. The primary effect of administering sodium bicarbonate is to reverse QRS prolongation and hypotension. The actual mechanism of action is unclear. Sodium bicarbonate may inhibit binding of tricyclic antidepressants to the myocardial sodium channels. Seizures may occur, but administration of benzodiazepines will suppress them. The administration of sodium bicarbonate doesn't directly affect respiratory status. Acid-base status should also be monitored, but effectiveness is based on cardiac response.
Nursing process step: Evaluation

29. A mother brings her 3-year-old child to the emergency department. She has also brought a can of crystalline Drano, and she thinks the child may have ingested some of the crystals. What should the triage nurse do first?
[ ] **A.** Ask the mother how full the Drano container had been.
[ ] **B.** Note whether the child is drooling.
[ ] **C.** Contact the poison control center immediately.
[ ] **D.** Give the child milk to dilute the poison.

Correct answer—B. *Rationales:* Crystalline Drano is an alkaline substance and causes severe tissue necrosis. Signs of tissue necrosis include dysphagia and drooling from burns to the oral mucosa and esophagus. The priority is to assess the child for signs of poisoning and airway compromise. Even small amounts of alkali can cause severe burns. The poison control center should be contacted if the client care team is unfamiliar with the treatment of alkali poisoning. Milk or water may be used to dilute the poison if there are no signs of drooling and dysphagia. If such signs are present, the child may have a severe burn. In that case, more damage may occur if the child's esophagus has perforated and water or milk enters the mediastinum.
Nursing process step: Assessment

30. A 2-year-old has swallowed an alkaline button battery. The nurse is talking with the parents about the procedures and care that the child is about to receive. The parents ask about any long-term effects regarding the battery ingestion. What would be the nurse's best response to the parents?
[ ] **A.** "There are no long-term effects."
[ ] **B.** "Your child may experience swallowing difficulties due to esophageal strictures."
[ ] **C.** "Your child will experience painful swallowing for the rest of his life."
[ ] **D.** "Your child will require a feeding tube."

Correct answer—B. *Rationales*: Scarring of the esophagus, which occurs during the healing phase of esophageal burns caused by alkalis, leads to strictures and narrowing of the esophagus. Pain is generally more prevalent with acid battery ingestion; the preventive coating of alkaline batteries results in a slower release of the alkaline substance. Resting the esophagus and determining the extent of damage will dictate the need for adjunctive enteral nutrition. The other options are incorrect.
Nursing process step: Analysis

31. During the past 2 to 3 hours, several adult clients with similar GI symptoms have arrived at the emergency department. Symptoms include vomiting, severe diarrhea, and abdominal cramps. Each of these clients ate at the same restaurant the evening before. None has anything else in common. Based on this information, the triage nurse suspects that these clients are suffering from which type of food poisoning?
[ ] **A.** Staphylococcal
[ ] **B.** Listeriosis
[ ] **C.** Botulism
[ ] **D.** Salmonella

Correct answer—D. *Rationales:* Signs of Salmonella poisoning appear from 12 to 24 hours after the ingestion of contaminated food. Common foods contaminated with Salmonella include milk, custards and other egg dishes, salad dressings, sandwich fillings, polluted shellfish, and poultry. Staphylococcal symptoms appear suddenly 1 to 6 hours after exposure and also include headache and fever. Listeriosis occurs 3 to 21 days after exposure, and in addition to diarrhea, fever, and headache, it may result in pneumonia, meningitis, and endocarditis. Botulism doesn't usually cause diarrhea.
Nursing process step: Analysis

32. A child is brought to the emergency department after ingesting oleander. The nurse should monitor the client for:
[ ] **A.** dysarthria.
[ ] **B.** drooling.
[ ] **C.** bradycardia.
[ ] **D.** diarrhea.

Correct answer—C. *Rationales:* Oleander is a plant that can produce cardiac glycoside effects. Symptoms of toxicity are similar to those of digoxin toxicity, so bradycardia may be evident. Dysarthria, drooling, and diarrhea aren't associated with oleander toxicity.
Nursing process step: Assessment

33. Two hours after taking an overdose of acetaminophen (Tylenol), a client arrives at the emergency department. Based on the nomogram for acute ingestion, when can the nurse expect to draw a blood acetaminophen level?
[ ] **A.** Immediately
[ ] **B.** In 1 hour
[ ] **C.** In 2 hours
[ ] **D.** In 4 hours

Correct answer—D. *Rationales:* Based on the nomogram for acute ingestion, serum acetaminophen levels should be drawn 4 hours after ingestion. Levels drawn sooner or later wouldn't reflect the peak acetaminophen level. An acetaminophen level greater than 150 g/mL 4 hours after ingestion indicates toxicity.
Nursing process step: Intervention

34. After ingesting 10 mg of the antihypertensive drug clonidine (Catapres) in a suicide attempt, a client comes to the emergency department with a depressed level of consciousness. After the airway is secured and I.V. access has been obtained, the nurse should anticipate administering:
[ ] **A.** naloxone.
[ ] **B.** calcium chloride.
[ ] **C.** magnesium sulfate.
[ ] **D.** sodium bicarbonate.

Correct answer—A. *Rationales:* Clonidine is an imidazoline antihypertensive agent that stimulates alpha-adrenergic receptors in the central nervous system. Clonidine may also stimulate the production of an opioid-like substance. Investigational uses include detoxification of opioid dependence. Calcium chloride, magnesium sulfate, and sodium bicarbonate aren't indicated.
Nursing process step: Intervention

35. A client is brought to the emergency department after ingesting an overdose of the beta-adrenergic blocker propranolol (Inderal). The nurse should prepare to administer which medication to reverse the effects of propranolol?
[ ] **A.** Calcium chloride
[ ] **B.** Glucagon
[ ] **C.** Furosemide (Lasix)
[ ] **D.** Sodium bicarbonate

Correct answer—B. *Rationales:* Glucagon is a first-line therapy for beta blocker overdose. It reverses bradycardia as well as the cardiac depression that beta-adrenergic blockers cause. Adverse effects of glucagon therapy include nausea and vomiting. Calcium chloride may be given in calcium channel blocker overdose. Furosemide doesn't reverse the effects of propranolol. Sodium bicarbonate doesn't reverse the effects of beta-adrenergic blocker toxicity.
Nursing process step: Intervention

36. A client has been admitted to the emergency department after ingesting an overdose of sustained-release theophylline. Theophylline levels continue to rise after administration of activated charcoal, and the physician orders whole-bowel irrigation with isotonic polyethylene glycol and electrolyte solution (GoLYTELY). The client will no longer require administration of the solution when which occurs?
[ ] **A.** Serum levels return to normal.
[ ] **B.** The client has a bowel movement.
[ ] **C.** Pulse rate returns to normal.
[ ] **D.** The client has clear rectal effluent.

Correct answer—D. *Rationales:* Whole bowel irrigation is a safe technique for treatment of overdoses of sustained-release products that are absorbed in the intestine. The technique is also safe for lithium, lead, and iron overdose. To confirm that all the pills have been removed, treatment should continue until rectal effluent is clear. Stopping after the first bowel movement is too soon. This treatment doesn't directly affect serum levels or pulse rate.
Nursing process step: Evaluation

37. Which symptom of opiate overdose is the most life-threatening?
[ ] **A.** Respiratory depression
[ ] **B.** Coma
[ ] **C.** Hypothermia
[ ] **D.** Miosis

Correct answer—A. *Rationales:* Opiate overdose will cause respiratory depression. Miosis is a sign of the overdose, not a condition to treat. Hypothermia is more readily amenable to treatment. Level of consciousness isn't a good indicator of severity except as it relates to respiratory depression.
Nursing process step: Assessment

38. Which drug is most commonly used to treat anticholinergic delirium?
[ ] **A.** Naloxone
[ ] **B.** Lithium
[ ] **C.** Physostigmine
[ ] **D.** Atropine

Correct answer—C. *Rationales:* Physostigmine acts by interfering with the metabolism of acetylcholine. Naloxone is used in opiate overdose. Lithium isn't used as an antidote in any scenario. Atropine is used in beta-adrenergic blocker, calcium channel blocker, and organophosphate and physostigmine poisonings.
Nursing process step: Intervention

39. What's a common drug used to treat central nervous system stimulation due to amphetamine overdose?
[ ] **A.** Naloxone
[ ] **B.** Flumazenil (Romazicon)
[ ] **C.** Physostigmine
[ ] **D.** Haloperidol (Haldol)

Correct answer—D. *Rationales*: Haloperidol is used to treat agitation. Physostigmine is used in anticholinergic delirium. Flumazenil is used in benzodiazepine poisoning. Naloxone is used to treat opiate toxicity.
Nursing process step: Intervention

40. A client is brought to the emergency department after inhaling a large amount of cocaine at a party. The client is very anxious. Vital signs are as follows: pulse, 130 beats/minute; blood pressure, 180/100 mm Hg; respirations, 22 breaths/minute; temperature, 72° F (40° C). What's the nursing priority for this client?
[ ] **A.** Administer activated charcoal.
[ ] **B.** Administer I.V. propranolol.
[ ] **C.** Administer oral propranolol.
[ ] **D.** Administer I.V. diazepam.

Correct answer—D. *Rationales:* Diazepam is used to treat the tachycardia associated with cocaine toxicity. Activated charcoal works by binding to substances in the gut. Propranolol is indicated for treatment of tachydysrhythmia but not tachycardia associated with cocaine toxicity.
Nursing process step: Intervention

17 Wound management

1. Rabies is least likely to be transmitted to humans through bites from which animal?

[ ] **A.** Dogs
[ ] **B.** Bats
[ ] **C.** Rats
[ ] **D.** Skunks

Correct answer—C. *Rationales:* Rabies isn't generally transmitted through the bites of rodents. Members of the rodent family include rats, mice, hamsters, gerbils, squirrels, and chipmunks. Rabies is primarily transmitted through the saliva of carnivorous animals. All wild carnivorous animals should be considered rabid unless proven otherwise by laboratory analysis. Domestic animals that don't have veterinary documentation of immunization should be observed for 10 days for development of symptoms.
Nursing process step: Assessment

2. Pharmacologic interventions for a client who has been bitten by a wild animal should include all of the following *except*:

[ ] **A.** administration of corticosteroids.
[ ] **B.** administration of tetanus toxoid.
[ ] **C.** administration of rabies immune globulin.
[ ] **D.** administration of human diploid cell vaccine (HDCV).

Correct answer—A. *Rationales:* Corticosteroids shouldn't be given to a client who's receiving rabies immunization. The anti-inflammatory properties of corticosteroids interfere with active immunity. Administering tetanus toxoid is an appropriate choice for a break in skin integrity from a potentially contaminated source. Rabies immune globulin and the HDCV should be administered as soon as possible after the bite.
Nursing process step: Intervention

3. To which classification is coral snake venom assigned?

[ ] **A.** Neurotoxic
[ ] **B.** Hemotoxic
[ ] **C.** Proteolytic
[ ] **D.** Coagulopathic

Correct answer—A. *Rationales:* The coral snake is an elapid, and its venom is neurotoxic. The effects are primarily systemic; local wound signs or symptoms are few or absent. Hemotoxic and proteolytic venoms are associated with pit vipers. Coagulopathic venom isn't a category of snake venom.
Nursing process step: Analysis

4. A client who has been bitten by a copperhead snake is at risk for developing:

[ ] **A.** slurred speech.
[ ] **B.** compartment syndrome.
[ ] **C.** respiratory paralysis.
[ ] **D.** muscle weakness.

Correct answer—B. *Rationales:* Pit viper bites (copperheads, water moccasins, and rattlesnakes) are associated with proteolytic and hemotoxic reactions. Their bites are painful, and blood usually oozes from visible fang marks. Edema of the affected area can lead to compartment syndrome. Other signs and symptoms include erythema, ecchymosis, blisters, hypotension, shock, and coagulopathies. Slurred speech, respiratory paralysis, and muscle weakness are associated with the neurotoxic venom of elapids (coral snakes and cobras).
Nursing process step: Assessment

5. If the client won't receive antivenin for more than 2 hours, which intervention should be taken?
[ ] **A.** Immobilize the affected extremity.
[ ] **B.** Elevate the affected extremity above the level of the heart.
[ ] **C.** Apply a tightly constricting band above the site of envenomation.
[ ] **D.** Apply ice to the affected extremity.

Correct answer—A. *Rationales:* Because venom is spread through the lymphatic system, immobilization of the extremity reduces lymph production. The affected extremity should be placed slightly lower than the heart to decrease the spread of the venom. Applying tight or constricting bands isn't recommended. Instead, a moderately constricting band may be placed about 4″ (10 cm) proximal to the bite. The purpose of the band is to slow lymphatic flow. Care should be taken to avoid impeding arterial or venous flow. Applying ice to the affected extremity won't reduce the spread of the venom.
Nursing process step: Intervention

6. What's the initial intervention for a client with external bleeding?
[ ] **A.** Elevation of the extremity
[ ] **B.** Pressure point control
[ ] **C.** Direct pressure
[ ] **D.** Application of a tourniquet

Correct answer—C. *Rationales:* Applying direct pressure to an injury is the initial step in controlling bleeding. For severe or arterial bleeding, pressure point control can be used. Pressure points are those areas where large blood vessels can be compressed against bone: femoral, brachial, facial, carotid, and temporal artery sites. Elevation reduces the force of flow, but direct pressure is the first step. A tourniquet may further damage the injured extremity and should be avoided unless all other measures have failed.
Nursing process step: Intervention

7. After receiving treatment for multiple human bites, a client is discharged with a prescription for tetracycline (Achromycin). Which statement indicates that the client understands the antibiotic treatment?
[ ] **A.** "I should limit my exposure to the sun because I now have an increased risk of burning."
[ ] **B.** "I should take the medication with food so I don't irritate my stomach."
[ ] **C.** "Rash and itching are expected side effects. I can still continue my medications."
[ ] **D.** "I can take Mylanta to prevent nausea."

Correct answer—A. *Rationales:* Clients taking tetracycline are photosensitive and have exaggerated sunburn reaction. At the first sign of skin erythema, clients should stop taking the drug and notify their physicians; rash and itching are signs of a hypersensitivity reaction. Tetracycline should be taken with a full glass of water 1 hour before or 2 hours after meals because taking it with food or milk interferes with its absorption. Antacids that contain aluminum, calcium, or magnesium impair absorption of tetracycline.
Nursing process step: Evaluation

8. Which medication is used in the treatment of tetany?
[ ] **A.** Tetanus immune globulin
[ ] **B.** Anticonvulsants
[ ] **C.** Opioid analgesics
[ ] **D.** Cephalosporins

Correct answer—A. *Rationales:* Tetanus immune globulin should be administered I.M. (3,000 to 5,000 units) along with tetanus toxoid. Seizures aren't associated with tetany. Sedatives and muscle relaxants can be used to reduce pain. Because of their effect against *Clostridia,* penicillin and tetracycline are the antibiotics of choice.
Nursing process step: Intervention

9. Prophylaxis for exposure to rabies for clients not previously vaccinated includes administration of which medication?

[ ] **A.** 20 IU/kg of rabies immune globulin in one I.M. injection

[ ] **B.** Tetanus toxoid, regardless of date of last immunization

[ ] **C.** Human diploid cell vaccine, I.M. on days 0, 3, 6, and 14

[ ] **D.** Human diploid cell vaccine on days 0, 3, 7, 14, and 28

Correct answer—D. *Rationales:* Postexposure rabies prophylaxis includes administration of human diploid cell vaccine on days 0, 3, 7, 14, and 28. If human diploid cell vaccine is being administered as a preexposure immunization, only days 0 and 3 are necessary. Rabies immune globulin is administered in a dose of 20 IU/ kg. The full dose is administered locally, around the wound; any remaining volume should be administered I.M. Option C is an incorrect schedule for administering this immunization.

Nursing process step: Intervention

10. A hiker with complaints of fever, headache, abdominal pain, and generalized muscle discomfort comes to the emergency department. Symptoms began 1 week after returning from a summer camping trip in Virginia. Physical examination reveals a 3-day-old, deep-red rash on the ankles, soles, wrists, and palms. The rash now appears petechial and purpuric. Based on the information provided, the client is diagnosed with which condition?

[ ] **A.** Meningococcemia

[ ] **B.** Rocky Mountain spotted fever

[ ] **C.** Poison ivy

[ ] **D.** Measles

Correct answer—B. *Rationales:* Found in every state, Rocky Mountain spotted fever has the highest incidence in North Carolina, South Carolina, Oklahoma, and Virginia. The disease is primarily seen in the warmer months of late spring, summer, and early fall. Symptoms of the fever appear 2 to 14 days after contact with infected ticks, and a rash develops over the soles, palms, hands, feet, wrists, and ankles on the 2nd to 5th day. The rash becomes petechial and eventually spreads to the rest of the body. The client may develop edema, hypotension, and delirium. Meningococcemia typically follows a mild upper respiratory tract infection. A petechial rash appears on the trunk and lower portion of the body. Poison ivy erupts in linear streaks that correspond to the areas that have come in contact with the vines or stems of the ivy. Additional lesions can spread to new locations and may have accompanying blisters and edema. Measles begin as a red maculopapular rash on the face that rapidly spreads over the trunk and arms.

Nursing process step: Assessment

11. What's the best method for removing a tick?

[ ] **A.** Grasping the tick close to the skin with tweezers and then pulling the tick away from the skin

[ ] **B.** Applying nail polish to the tick's body

[ ] **C.** Applying isopropyl alcohol to the tick's body

[ ] **D.** Touching a hot match to the tick's body

Correct answer—A. *Rationales:* The best method for removing a tick is to grasp it gently with tweezers close to the skin. Slowly pull it away from the skin while applying gentle traction. Take care not to squeeze the tick because toxins or viruses could be injected into the client. The other options aren't recommended because they may cause the tick to regurgitate or salivate into the wound.

Nursing process step: Intervention

12. Early administration of which antimicrobial is the most effective treatment of Rocky Mountain spotted fever?

[ ] **A.** Amoxicillin

[ ] **B.** Doxycycline

[ ] **C.** Co-trimoxazole (Bactrim)

[ ] **D.** Erythromycin

Correct answer—B. *Rationales:* Doxycycline is the first-line treatment for adults and children and should be initiated immediately. Amoxicillin, co-trimoxazole, and erythromycin, although antimicrobials, aren't effective for treating *Rickettsia rickettsii* (Rocky Mountain spotted fever).

Nursing process step: Intervention

13. What is an early symptom of Rocky Mountain spotted fever?

[ ] **A.** Joint pain
[ ] **B.** Fever
[ ] **C.** Diarrhea
[ ] **D.** Rash

Correct answer—B. *Rationales:* The early symptoms of Rocky Mountain spotted fever are nonspecific, such as fever (usually greater than 102° F [38.9° C]), nausea, vomiting, headache, muscle aches, and fatigue. These symptoms are commonly ignored or attributed to other causes. The rash, abdominal pain, joint pain, and diarrhea usually develop about 2 to 14 days after a bite by an infected tick. The rash usually begins on the wrists and ankles and spreads, but some individuals (about 10% to 15%) don't develop it. Other symptoms that may occur are loss of appetite, hallucinations, photosensitivity, and excessive thirst.
Nursing process step: Evaluation

14. What is the recommended treatment for scabies in a pediatric client younger than age 1?

[ ] **A.** Lindane
[ ] **B.** Tolnaftate (Tinactin)
[ ] **C.** Thiabendazole
[ ] **D.** Permethrin (Elimite)

Correct answer—D. *Rationales:* Permethrin is supplied in a cream. It should be massaged into the skin from the head to the soles. Although permethrin is the treatment of choice for children younger than age 1, its safety hasn't been established for those younger than age 2 months. Lindane, a treatment for scabies, isn't recommended for children younger than age 1, and it shouldn't be used on children older than age 1 if they won't be supervised. The hands and feet of a child should be covered during treatment to prevent him from ingesting the cream or lotion. Young children may be more sensitive to central nervous system toxicity from the drug. Tolnaftate is used to treat ringworm. Thiabendazole is used to treat hookworm, roundworm, threadworm, and whipworm.
Nursing process step: Intervention

15. Which statement shows that a client diagnosed with scabies doesn't have an understanding of discharge instructions?

[ ] **A.** "My symptoms might not disappear for 1 to 2 weeks after I begin my treatment."
[ ] **B.** "It isn't necessary to treat my family members if they don't have symptoms."
[ ] **C.** "I should apply the prescribed lotion to all body areas below my neck."
[ ] **D.** "I should machine-wash all clothing and bed linen in very hot water."

Correct answer—B. *Rationales:* Because scabies is transmitted through prolonged contact, it commonly affects all family members. Most clients are infested before obvious symptoms appear. The other options represent information that should be included in discharge instructions.
Nursing process step: Evaluation

16. Which characteristic identifies the brown recluse spider?

[ ] **A.** Violin-shaped mark anterodorsally
[ ] **B.** Hourglass shape ventrally
[ ] **C.** Velvety black abdomen with brushes of red hair
[ ] **D.** Two circular black markings on a brown anterodorsal area

Correct answer—A. *Rationales:* The brown recluse spider has a light brown color with a darker brown violin shape on its back and is commonly found in southern portions of the United States. Circular black markings and a velvety black abdomen with brushes of red hair aren't found on the brown recluse spider. The black widow spider can be identified by its black body and a bright red hourglass on its abdomen.
Nursing process step: Analysis

17. Which skin reaction can be expected several hours after a bite by a brown recluse spider?
[ ] **A.** Slight erythema with tiny visible punctum
[ ] **B.** Eschar
[ ] **C.** Reddish blue halo surrounding the area
[ ] **D.** Petechiae on the affected extremity

Correct answer—C. *Rationales:* Initially, a mild stinging sensation occurs at the site of the brown recluse's bite. Next, a reddish blue halo and local edema appear. Erythema and necrosis of the tissue follow by the end of the fourth day. Eschar forms by day 14, and healing is completed by day 21. The client experiences joint pain, malaise, nausea, and vomiting. Treatment includes corticosteroids, antibiotics, and antihistamines. Slight erythema with tiny visible punctum is a sign of the black widow spider's bite. An eschar is a later symptom and forms on the 14th day after the bite. Petechiae on the same extremity as a bite injury indicate Rocky Mountain spotted fever.
Nursing process step: Assessment

18. What's the primary intervention for a client having a severe reaction to a black widow spider's bite?
[ ] **A.** Administration of black widow spider antivenin
[ ] **B.** Application of ice to the injury site
[ ] **C.** Administration of opioids for pain relief
[ ] **D.** Administration of oxygen

Correct answer—D. *Rationales:* Maintaining an airway should always be the primary focus in an emergency. The nurse should prepare to intubate if the client develops severe respiratory distress or signs and symptoms of anaphylaxis. Black widow spider antivenin (one ampule in 10 to 50 mL of saline in a slow I.V.) can be administered after skin testing. Applying ice slows the venom's absorption rate, but this action should be taken after airway, breathing, and circulation have been assessed and maintained. Opioids are helpful in pain management but should be used cautiously to prevent respiratory depression.
Nursing process step: Intervention

19. A client comes to the emergency department after being stung by a Portuguese man-of-war. The client is wheezing and tachycardic and has diffuse edema at the site of injury. Which indicates that interventions have decreased the potential for poisoning?
[ ] **A.** Minimal edema progression
[ ] **B.** Positive response to antivenin sensitivity testing
[ ] **C.** Quiet breath sounds
[ ] **D.** Stable vital signs

Correct answer—A. *Rationales:* Treatment is effective in a hazardous marine life poisoning if the client has stable vital signs, minimal edema, a negative response to antivenin sensitivity testing, and slowed symptom progression. A positive response to antivenin sensitivity testing indicates that this is an incompatible alternative for this client. Wheezing that progresses to quiet breath sounds is an ominous finding because it indicates that air exchange in the lungs is decreasing.
Nursing process step: Evaluation

20. A client comes to the emergency department after sustaining an injury while operating a table saw. The first and third digits have been amputated below the distal phalanx and another digit has a tip avulsion. Which intervention is appropriate?
[ ] **A.** Wrap the amputated parts in a sterile dressing and place them on dry ice.
[ ] **B.** Wrap the amputated parts in povidone-iodine-soaked dressings.
[ ] **C.** Wrap the amputated parts in gauze moistened with normal saline, place in a sealed plastic bag, and submerge the bag in ice water.
[ ] **D.** Wrap the amputated parts in sterile gauze and place in a bath of sterile saline.

Correct answer—C. *Rationales:* Sterile technique should be used whenever handling amputated parts. The part should be cleaned of debris by gently irrigating with sterile saline, water, or lactated Ringer's solution. It should then be wrapped in gauze (dry or moistened) and placed in a plastic bag. The bag should then be submerged in a container of ice water until reimplantation occurs. Placing the amputated part on dry ice increases tissue damage (necrosis) because of the excessively cold temperature. Wrapping the part in povidone-iodinesoaked dressings causes the subcutaneous tissue to dry out. Placing the amputated parts directly in a solution leads to tissue sloughing and maceration.
Nursing process step: Intervention

21. Which bites have the highest rate of infection?
[ ] **A.** Cats
[ ] **B.** Dogs
[ ] **C.** Humans
[ ] **D.** Scorpions

Correct answer—C. *Rationales:* Human bites have the highest infection rate. Human saliva contains *Staphylococcus aureus, Streptococcus, Proteus, Klebsiella,* and *Escherichia coli.* Typically there's an open wound that presents as a laceration, puncture, tear, crush injury, avulsion, or amputation. Cat bites are second in infection rate because of their frequent mouth contact with rodents. Dogs are more a source of disfigurement than of infection. There's no evidence that scorpion bites are an infection risk.
Nursing process step: Analysis

22. A client with a scorpion sting may initially exhibit:
[ ] **A.** bradycardia.
[ ] **B.** hypotension.
[ ] **C.** decreased respiratory drive.
[ ] **D.** wheezing.

Correct answer—D. *Rationales:* Signs and symptoms of scorpion stings include pain and swelling at the sting site, tachycardia, hypertension, tachypnea, wheezing, ataxia, visual disturbances, and anaphylaxis.
Nursing process step: Assessment

23. Treatment of stings caused by a Portuguese man-of-war should include:
[ ] **A.** immediate rinsing with fresh water.
[ ] **B.** soaking the wound in salt water.
[ ] **C.** applying ice to the sting sites.
[ ] **D.** soaking the wound in fresh water.

Correct answer—B. *Rationales:* Treatment of a Portuguese man-of-war sting consists of soaking the wound in salt water. To prevent discharge of additional venom into the client, any tentacles still clinging to the skin should be inactivated by rinsing with acetic acid. Tentacles can then be scraped off the skin. Ice shouldn't be applied because of vasoconstriction.
Nursing process step: Intervention

24. During trauma resuscitation, clothing saturated with blood is cut from the victim of a gunshot wound. The client is pronounced dead after efforts at resuscitation are unsuccessful. Proper handling of the client's belongings should include which procedure?
[ ] **A.** Disposal with other biohazardous materials
[ ] **B.** Release to family members at their request
[ ] **C.** Release of clothing to police
[ ] **D.** Clothing kept with the victim

Correct answer—C. *Rationales:* A gunshot wound should be reported to law enforcement agencies. The victim's clothing should be treated as evidence from the moment the victim arrives in the emergency department. Care should be taken not to cut clothing through bullet holes. While handling clothing, gloves should be worn for standard precautions as well as for preserving evidence. When a suspect dies, the coroner can claim the body. At that time, police are free to gather any evidence that won't mutilate the body. A dead body has no constitutional rights. Disposal of the clothing will destroy the evidence in this case. The family can't claim the victim's belongings until they are released from the coroner. Sending belongings to the morgue along with the victim doesn't guarantee safekeeping of the evidence. Suspects and victims of crime should remain secure in the emergency department until released to the morgue by the coroner or released to a law enforcement agency.
Nursing process step: Intervention

25. What's the classification of a degloving injury?
[ ] **A.** Burn
[ ] **B.** Laceration
[ ] **C.** Avulsion
[ ] **D.** Abrasion

Correct answer—C. *Rationales:* An avulsion is full-thickness skin loss that doesn't allow for reapproximation of the skin. In a degloving injury, the skin is pulled away from the remainder of the extremity, usually a hand or foot. Burns are tissue injuries that occur as a result of prolonged exposure to thermal, chemical, radioactive, or electrical agents. A laceration is a tear in the flesh. Abrasions are caused by friction that may remove the epithelial or epidermal layers of the skin.
Nursing process step: Analysis

26. Which intervention is appropriate for a client with a contusion to the lower leg following a fall?
[ ] **A.** Application of dry sterile dressing
[ ] **B.** Administration of tetanus toxoid if it has been more than 5 years since the last immunization
[ ] **C.** Application of a firm pressure bandage
[ ] **D.** Application of cold

Correct answer—D. *Rationales:* Applying cold to a contused area helps to decrease swelling and discomfort. Applying a dry sterile dressing and administering tetanus toxoid are unnecessary because the skin remains intact and the chance of the area becoming infected is minimal. Applying a pressure dressing should be avoided; prolonged pressure to an area with edema can lead to compartment syndrome.
Nursing process step: Intervention

27. In gunshot wounds, *yaw* refers to:
[ ] **A.** the mass of the bullet.
[ ] **B.** the length of the gun barrel.
[ ] **C.** the rotation of the missile.
[ ] **D.** the missile's angle of entry into the body.

Correct answer—D. *Rationales:* Yaw is the deviation of the bullet from a straight path. The degree of wound produced from a gunshot varies, depending on the bullet mass, gun barrel length, missile velocity, and angle of yaw. The longer the gun barrel, the higher the velocity of the bullet. This usually results in a small entrance wound and a large exit wound. When the bullet strikes a soft surface (a person), the degree of deformation is influenced by the size of the bullet, the yaw, and the rotation of the bullet (tumbling).
Nursing process step: Analysis

28. A client is being treated for a lower-leg laceration sustained from a metal bar. He states that he has never received tetanus immunization. Considering this information, the nurse should anticipate an order for which drug?
[ ] **A.** 0.5 mL of adsorbed tetanus toxoid
[ ] **B.** 250 units of tetanus immune globulin
[ ] **C.** 1 mL of adsorbed tetanus toxoid
[ ] **D.** 0.5 mL of adsorbed tetanus toxoid and 250 units of tetanus immune globulin

Correct answer—D. *Rationales:* A client who has never received tetanus immunization or has received only a partial series of injections (one or two) should receive 0.5 mL of adsorbed tetanus toxoid and 250 units of tetanus immune globulin. For a client who has received two or more tetanus injections or who received a dose 10 or more years ago, 0.5 mL of adsorbed tetanus toxoid is recommended. Tetanus immune globulin (250 units) is delivered as an adjunct to adsorbed tetanus toxoid. Option C, 1 mL, is an incorrect dose for adsorbed tetanus toxoid.
Nursing process step: Intervention

29. A client with a laceration to his upper arm is now unable to extend his thumb into a hitchhiker's sign. This indicates damage to which nerve?
[ ] **A.** Pilomotor nerve
[ ] **B.** Median nerve
[ ] **C.** Radial nerve
[ ] **D.** Ulnar nerve

Correct answer—C. *Rationales:* Damage to the radial nerve results in the client's inability to extend his thumb. The pilomotor nerve innervates the pilorum muscles of hair follicles. Damage to the median nerve results in an inability to sense pain in the tip of the index finger. Ulnar nerve damage results in the client's inability to sense pain in the tip of the little finger.
Nursing process step: Assessment

30. A pediatric client received multiple lacerations and puncture wounds to the face, arms, and legs after being attacked by a dog. Conscious sedation was used to assist in reducing pain and anxiety in the client during repair. When alert and oriented, the client is discharged with his parents. This level of consciousness is associated with which Ramsey score?

[ ] **A.** 1
[ ] **B.** 2
[ ] **C.** 6
[ ] **D.** 10

Correct answer—B. *Rationales:* The Ramsey score is an evaluation of the level of sedation. Scores are as follows: 1, irritable and anxious; 2, alert and oriented; 3, responds to verbal stimuli; 4, responds to tactile stimuli; 5, responds to noxious stimuli; and 6, doesn't respond to stimuli. After receiving conscious sedation, a client should be alert and oriented, have the ability to ambulate, and be able to tolerate fluids.
Nursing process step: Evaluation

31. A 5-year-old client is brought to the emergency department after being stung multiple times on the face by yellow jackets. Which symptom of anaphylaxis requires priority medical intervention?

[ ] **A.** Blood pressure of 90/52 mm Hg
[ ] **B.** Diffuse facial urticaria
[ ] **C.** Respiratory rate of 28 breaths/minute
[ ] **D.** Pulse rate of 60 beats/minute

Correct answer—D. *Rationales:* Bradycardia is an ominous sign in pediatric clients. Older children initially demonstrate tachycardia in response to hypoxemia. When tachycardia can no longer maintain tissue oxygenation, bradycardia follows. The development of bradycardia usually precedes cardiopulmonary arrest. The average systolic blood pressure of a client older than 1 year can be determined by this formula: 80 mm Hg + (2× the age). Thus, an average systolic blood pressure for a 5-year-old client is 80 mm Hg + (2 × 5) = 90 mm Hg. Urticaria should be treated after airway control has been established. The normal respiratory rate for a 5-year-old is 20 to 25 breaths/minute.
Nursing process step: Assessment

32. Verbal understanding of discharge instructions for a client who exhibits anaphylactic reactions to bee stings should include all of the following *except:*

[ ] **A.** "I don't want to use the Epi-Pen unless I have trouble breathing."
[ ] **B.** "I should avoid wearing bright colors when I go outside."
[ ] **C.** "I should avoid using perfumed soaps and shampoos."
[ ] **D.** "I should wear long pants and shirts when I'm around flowers."

Correct answer—A. *Rationales:* The client with severe anaphylactic reactions to bee stings should be advised to use the Epi-Pen immediately after being stung. The nurse should instruct the client that waiting until dyspnea develops may put the client at risk for respiratory arrest. The other options are correct responses.
Nursing process step: Evaluation

33. What's an early sign associated with Lyme disease?

[ ] **A.** Synovitis
[ ] **B.** Arthritic pain
[ ] **C.** Reddened lesion with central clearing
[ ] **D.** Myocarditis

Correct answer—C. *Rationales:* Lyme disease is a tick-borne disease that progresses through distinctly separate stages. In the first stage, the disease presents with red-ringed circular skin lesions, called erythema chronicum migrans. At the same time the lesions appear, the client commonly experiences headache, stiff neck, fever, and malaise. During stage two, cardiomegaly, neuritis, and myopericarditis may appear. The final stage includes arthritic pain, chronic synovitis, lack of coordination, facial palsy, paralysis, and dementia. Tetracycline, penicillin, and ceftriaxone (Rocephin) help to relieve early symptoms and can possibly prevent later occurrences.
Nursing process step: Assessment

34. Which is true about dog bites?
[ ] **A.** Most dog bites occur in adults.
[ ] **B.** A large dog can exert a maximum of 100 lb of pressure per square inch (psi).
[ ] **C.** Osteomyelitis is a potential complication of dog bites.
[ ] **D.** Most dog bites occur in rural areas.

Correct answer—C. *Rationales:* Potential complications of dog bites include osteomyelitis, cellulitis, infection, and neurovascular compromise. Most dog bites occur in urban areas and in children. Large dogs can exert up to 400 lb psi.
Nursing process step: Assessment

35. Black widow spider bites can be identified by which sign?
[ ] **A.** A blue-red halo at the site of venom entry
[ ] **B.** Tiny red marks at the point of venom entry
[ ] **C.** Petechiae formation in the area of the bite
[ ] **D.** Wheal formation and edema

Correct answer—B. *Rationales:* Black widow bites can be identified by edema and tiny red fang marks at the point of venom entry. Brown recluse spider bites can be identified by a blue-red halo surrounding the area of venom entry. Petechiae formation is associated with Rocky Mountain spotted fever. Wheal formation and edema are associated with wasp and hornet stings.
Nursing process step: Assessment

36. Which statement about wood splinters as foreign bodies is true?
[ ] **A.** They can't be seen on radiologic examination.
[ ] **B.** The wounds should be soaked in Betadine to reduce the risk of infection.
[ ] **C.** Wood splinters don't need to be removed because scar tissue will encrust the object.
[ ] **D.** Wood splinters don't put the client at risk for developing tetanus.

Correct answer—A. *Rationales:* Wood splinters aren't radiopaque unless the wood has been painted. Paint creates a shadow. Wounds that involve wood shouldn't be soaked in liquid. The wood tends to absorb the liquid and disintegrates when removal is attempted. Occasionally, metal objects may be left in place if removal is difficult. Wood, however, should always be removed because of its tendency to swell. It can also carry *Clostridium tetani.* A tetanus immunization should be considered for any injury that breaks skin integrity.
Nursing process step: Evaluation

37. A client is treated for a laceration to his wrist from a human bite. Which *isn't* an appropriate treatment for the client's altered skin integrity?
[ ] **A.** The laceration is scrubbed and irrigated.
[ ] **B.** The site of injury is splinted.
[ ] **C.** Antibiotic therapy is prescribed.
[ ] **D.** The laceration is surgically closed and a sterile dressing is applied.

Correct answer—D. *Rationales:* Because human bites carry the highest rate of infection of all bite injuries, such a wound shouldn't be surgically closed. Intervention should include thorough cleansing of the site, antibiotic therapy, splinting of lacerations that occur over joints to minimize movement, and application of an appropriate dressing.
Nursing process step: Evaluation

38. Which is true about cat bite injuries?
[ ] **A.** The bacteria primarily associated with cat bites is *Bacillus cereus*.
[ ] **B.** Penicillin V potassium is the treatment of choice for cat bites.
[ ] **C.** Primary closure of lacerations from cat bites and scratches is always recommended.
[ ] **D.** Ciprofloxacin (Cipro) is the treatment of choice for cat bites.

Correct answer—B. *Rationales:* Prophylactic antibiotics should be prescribed for all extensive wounds from cats. Initially, penicillin V potassium is prescribed. Wounds that aren't initially seen and that develop infection after 24 hours should be treated with a first-generation cephalosporin. *Bacillus cereus* is associated with food poisoning. Primary closure of wounds from cat bites isn't recommended except in low-risk, cosmetically disfiguring facial bites. Ciprofloxacin is a fluoroquinolone and not indicated in the treatment of cat bites.
Nursing process step: Assessment

39. What's a symptom of rabies?

[ ] **A.** Hydrophobia
[ ] **B.** Headache
[ ] **C.** Depressed behavior
[ ] **D.** Increased salivation

Correct answer—D. *Rationales:* A client with rabies presents with dysphagia, excessive salivation, dyspnea, seizures, and extreme anxiety. Painful spasms occur whenever the client swallows; as a result, the client becomes hydrophobic. Additionally, the client develops irritability, fever, and sensitivity to light and noise. Headache isn't a symptom of rabies.
Nursing process step: Assessment

40. After airway, breathing, and circulation have been assessed, which intervention should be performed next for a client with an impaled object in the chest?

[ ] **A.** Obtain chest X-ray.
[ ] **B.** Remove the impaled object.
[ ] **C.** Administer tetanus toxoid.
[ ] **D.** Obtain arterial blood gas (ABG) analysis.

Correct answer—A. *Rationales:* After assessing airway, breathing, and circulation, the nurse should obtain a chest X-ray to help determine involvement of vital organs (heart and lungs). An impaled object shouldn't be removed until the client is in the surgical suite because any severed vessels temporarily tamponaded by the impaled object will need immediate clamping. Tetanus toxoid administration is recommended if the client's immunization history indicates a need, but this isn't the initial intervention in this scenario. ABG analysis should be obtained only after respiratory involvement is determined.
Nursing process step: Intervention

41. A puncture wound through the sole of a tennis shoe needs special attention because of which organism that happily lives in the soles of some tennis shoes?

[ ] **A.** *Eschericia coli*
[ ] **B.** *Staphylococcus aureus*
[ ] **C.** *Aeromonas*
[ ] **D.** *Pseudomonas*

Correct answer—D. Rationales: *Pseudomonas* lives in the soles of some tennis shoes and can be introduced into the tissues, muscles, tendons, or joint spaces of the foot by a puncture wound. *E. coli* is an organism found in the bowels. *S. aureus* is normal flora on the skin. *Aeromonas* is a bacterium that lives in lake water.
Nursing Process step: Analysis

42. A 12-year-old client comes to the emergency department after falling off his skateboard and striking his knee on concrete. The point of impact has tenderness, swelling, ecchymosis, and hematoma. On examination there's no loss of function of muscle and tendons. Which is the most appropriate intervention for this client?

[ ] **A.** Advise rest, immobilize the affected part, elevate, and apply cold (ice 10 to 20 minutes) every 1 hour for 24 hours.
[ ] **B.** Apply an elastic bandage to the middle of the limb to cause compression.
[ ] **C.** Contact a surgeon to see if the hematoma needs incision and drainage.
[ ] **D.** Instruct the client to apply heat and do light exercise to keep the limb mobile.

Correct answer—A. *Rationales:* Rest, immobilization, and elevation with ice to the affected limb every 1 hour for 10 to 20 minutes for 24 hours is the best method to manage a contusion. An elastic bandage could cause loss of circulation. The hematoma shouldn't be interfered with. Using the limb could increase the damage.
Nursing process step: Intervention

43. A young woman comes to the emergency department and states she was stung by either a bee or a wasp. How can the nurse differentiate which type of insect stung this client?

[ ] **A.** An ulcerating lesion forms following a wasp sting.

[ ] **B.** A wound with the insect's stinger within it is a honey bee sting.

[ ] **C.** A distinct, target-type lesion occurs around the sting from a honey bee.

[ ] **D.** Eschar will form around a wasp sting.

Correct answer—B. *Rationales:* Wasps don't leave a stinger in the wound, whereas honey bees do. Spider bites can leave an ulcerating lesion. Tick bites leave a target-type circle. Eschar is caused by an area of skin over a bony prominence where the circulation has been compromised and the tissue has died.

Nursing process step: Assessment

44. An emergency medical technician (EMT) calls the emergency department from a site at which a client has been shot in the leg with an arrow. What instructions should the nurse give the EMT to manage this foreign body in the leg?

[ ] **A.** Apply ice to the site to reduce swelling.

[ ] **B.** Attempt to remove the arrow by pulling it out.

[ ] **C.** Immobilize the leg with the arrow in it, and transport the client to the emergency department as soon as possible.

[ ] **D.** Apply moist heat to the area to reduce pain.

Correct answer—C. *Rationales:* The affected limb needs to be immobilized and the arrow left in place to reduce the risk of additional tissue and nerve damage as well as hemorrhage. Ice could be applied, but it isn't the best answer. Moist heat will only dilate vessels and increase the risk of hemorrhage.

Nursing process step: Intervention

18 Stabilization and transfer

1. Which level trauma center must have a trauma surgeon, trauma director, operating suite, and in-house operating room staff on duty 24 hours per day?
[ ] **A.** Level I trauma center
[ ] **B.** Level II trauma center
[ ] **C.** Both level I and II
[ ] **D.** Level IV trauma center

Correct answer—C. *Rationales:* Both level I and level II trauma centers must have a trauma surgeon, trauma director, and staffed operating room available around the clock. Level III trauma centers are excused from the staffed operating room requirement. Level IV trauma centers are excused from all the above requirements.
Nursing process step: Intervention

2. What advantage does ground transport have over helicopter transport?
[ ] **A.** Better radio communications with hospitals
[ ] **B.** More space inside
[ ] **C.** Faster speed
[ ] **D.** Fewer traffic and road factors

Correct answer—B. *Rationales:* Ground vehicles have more space inside. However, helicopter transport has the advantages of having better radio communication with hospitals, traveling at faster speeds, and contending with fewer traffic and road factors.
Nursing process step: Evaluation

3. Which specially trained personnel is the primary member of a transport team for critically ill or injured clients?
[ ] **A.** Registered nurse
[ ] **B.** Paramedic
[ ] **C.** Physician
[ ] **D.** Respiratory therapist

Correct answer—A. *Rationales:* A specially trained registered nurse is the primary member of all transport teams. The Emergency Nurses Association position statement holds that "clients should be transported at the same level of care needed within the hospital. If the client required specialized nursing care just before transport, he requires the same care during transport."
Nursing process step: Intervention

4. A multisystem trauma client is being transferred to a trauma center. The receiving physician has requested that the client be intubated before transfer. Who's legally responsible for ensuring that the client is intubated before transfer?
[ ] **A.** The receiving physician
[ ] **B.** The referring physician
[ ] **C.** The referring emergency department nurse
[ ] **D.** The transport team

Correct answer—B. *Rationales:* The transferring hospital is legally responsible for performing those treatment and diagnostic studies requested by the receiving facility. The referring physician is legally responsible for ensuring that tests and procedures are completed.
Nursing process step: Intervention

5. In-house, 24-hour surgeon availability isn't required in which center?
[ ] **A.** Level IV trauma center
[ ] **B.** Level III trauma center
[ ] **C.** Level II trauma center
[ ] **D.** Level I trauma center

Correct answer–A. *Rationales:* Immediate access to definitive care is the hallmark of excellent trauma care. Although surgical coverage is desirable, only level IV trauma centers are excused from the requirement of around-the-clock coverage.
Nursing process step: Intervention

6. Which device is considered unacceptable for interhospital transfers?
[ ] **A.** Plastic I.V. bags
[ ] **B.** Pneumatic antishock garment
[ ] **C.** Heimlich valves
[ ] **D.** Inflatable splints

Correct answer–D. *Rationales:* Inflatable air splints can change internal pressure (immobilization effectiveness) and are, therefore, unacceptable for air transport or ground transport over mountainous terrain. They're also subject to air leaks (decreasing pressure and immobilization effectiveness). Because there are other inexpensive alternatives for immobilization, air splints aren't recommended for transfer. Plastic I.V. bags, pneumatic antishock garment, and Heimlich valves are all acceptable for interhospital transfers.
Nursing process step: Intervention

7. Which intervention need not be completed before the transfer of a trauma client?
[ ] **A.** Closure of all lacerations
[ ] **B.** Gastric tube insertion
[ ] **C.** Indwelling urinary catheter insertion
[ ] **D.** Splinting fractures

Correct answer–A. *Rationales:* Suturing superficial lacerations is time-consuming and can be delayed until the client is stable. All of the other interventions should be completed before transfer.
Nursing process step: Intervention

8. A client has no medical insurance. The Emergency Medical Treatment and Active Labor Act (EMTALA) requires that:
[ ] **A.** the client be transferred to a teaching hospital that receives federal funds.
[ ] **B.** the initial hospital transfer to a level I trauma center as soon as possible.
[ ] **C.** the client be transferred if the receiving hospital can provide additional care.
[ ] **D.** the client be transferred as soon as an ambulance is available.

Correct answer–C. *Rationales:* EMTALA requires hospitals to provide a screening examination and stabilize clients. They are to be transferred only if the receiving hospital can provide additional resources for the client's care.
Nursing process step: Intervention

9. A client arrives at the emergency department with signs and symptoms consistent with a non-ST elevation myocardial infarction (MI). The client's vital signs are as follows: blood pressure, 100/68 mm Hg; pulse, 46 beats/minute; respirations, 24 breaths/minute. The hospital doesn't offer cardiac catheterization services, and the physician wishes to transfer the client to another facility by air. After stabilizing the client with oxygen, an arterial line, I.V. line placement, and appropriate medication therapy, which of the following should be considered prior to transport via aircraft?

[ ] **A.** Nothing; the client is ready to be transported
[ ] **B.** The effect of air transport on the arterial line pressure bag
[ ] **C.** The ability of the client's family to accompany the client
[ ] **D.** Ensuring that vital signs are documented just prior to departure

Correct answer—B. *Rationales:* Altitude changes will cause changes in air pressure, causing a hypobaric environment, whereby the pressure decreases as altitude increases. There will be enough of a pressure change to cause an arterial line pressure bag to lose some pressure, which may result in an inaccurate arterial blood pressure reading. The client isn't ready to be transported as of yet. Family can't accompany the client on board the aircraft. Documenting vital signs is important but only after the arterial line pressure bag is stabilized.
Nursing process step: Assessment

10. The client's airway, breathing, and circulation are stabilized. The nurse should document what as part of the initial assessment?

[ ] **A.** Neurologic assessment
[ ] **B.** Burn percentage calculation
[ ] **C.** Fluid volume infused
[ ] **D.** Head-to-toe assessment

Correct answer—A. *Rationales:* The initial assessment should always include airway, breathing, circulation, and disability. Disability, or the neurologic assessment, is the missing element in the initial assessment. The secondary survey comes after the primary survey and includes the burn percentage. Intakes and outputs should be documented, but they aren't part of the primary survey.
Nursing process step: Assessment

11. Which intervention is the highest priority before transporting this client?

[ ] **A.** Endotracheal intubation
[ ] **B.** Vascular access
[ ] **C.** Pneumatic antishock garment placed but not inflated
[ ] **D.** Blood administration

Correct answer—B. *Rationales:* The priority nursing diagnosis is fluid volume deficit. The highest priority intervention after airway, breathing, and circulation is vascular access followed by volume resuscitation.
Nursing process step: Intervention

12. What's an indication that a client's oxygenation has improved?

[ ] **A.** Capillary refill time decreases
[ ] **B.** Heart rate decreases
[ ] **C.** Respiratory rate decreases
[ ] **D.** SaO_2 increases to 95%

Correct answer—D. *Rationales:* A pulse oximeter value of 95% in a client who hasn't been exposed to products of combustion is a sign of improving oxygenation. Changes in capillary refill time are indicative of changes in perfusion. Changes in heart rate and respiratory rate are nonspecific to oxygenation.
Nursing process step: Evaluation

13. Who's responsible for ensuring that appropriate personnel and equipment are available to transport a critical client?
[ ] **A.** The referring hospital
[ ] **B.** The receiving hospital
[ ] **C.** The transport ambulance
[ ] **D.** The state ambulance regulators

Correct answer—A. *Rationales:* The referring hospital is responsible for ensuring that appropriate personnel and equipment are available to maintain care during transport. The receiving hospital should be involved in determining the mode of transport. The transport ambulance and the state ambulance regulators aren't responsible for ensuring that appropriate personnel and equipment are available to transport a critical client. The state ambulance regulators write broad-based guidelines for client care.
Nursing process step: Intervention

14. A pediatric client is intubated to treat increasing respiratory compromise. Which device should be used to ventilate the client optimally during transport?
[ ] **A.** Bag-valve-tube
[ ] **B.** T tube
[ ] **C.** Oxygen-powered, manually triggered breathing device
[ ] **D.** Transport ventilator

Correct answer—D. *Rationales:* A transport ventilator will best control ventilation. Bag-valve-tube devices allow for significant changes in respiratory rate and volume. Oxygen-powered, manually triggered breathing devices have the same limitations. A T tube will ensure high-flow oxygen but not ventilation.
Nursing process step: Analysis

15. Which factor should determine the composition of the intrahospital transport team?
[ ] **A.** Client's acuity level
[ ] **B.** Medications needed
[ ] **C.** Client's weight
[ ] **D.** Unit receiving client

Correct answer—A. *Rationales:* The client's needs for continuous monitoring, assessment, and interventions vary. The acuity level, complexity of care, and potential needs during the intrahospital transport will determine the combination of personnel needed on the transport team. The client's acuity will also dictate the treatment plan during the transport, which may include medications. The client's weight may add to the overall transport issues as far as manpower.
Nursing process step: Intervention

16. Which *isn't* a component of the transfer system?
[ ] **A.** Communications with the receiving hospital
[ ] **B.** Policies and procedures
[ ] **C.** Transportation resources
[ ] **D.** Cost of the transfer

Correct answer—D. *Rationales:* The components of a transfer system are communications, transport resources, and policies and procedures. Although financial issues may influence where and how the client is transferred, this should be addressed in the facility's policies and procedures.
Nursing process step: Intervention

17. The transfer process has begun when which entity has been notified?
[ ] **A.** Ambulance service
[ ] **B.** Family
[ ] **C.** Receiving hospital
[ ] **D.** Client's primary care provider

Correct answer—C. *Rationales:* The transfer process can't begin until the referring hospital contacts the receiving hospital. The client must be accepted for admission at the receiving hospital before a transfer can take place. Notification of an ambulance service would occur when transportation needs have been decided. The family should be informed as soon as possible of the client's condition and treatment plan, as well as the client's primary care provider as appropriate.
Nursing process step: Intervention

18. What's the primary factor to consider when making the decision to transfer a client to another facility?
[ ] **A.** Risks and benefits to the client
[ ] **B.** Mode of transportation
[ ] **C.** Consent of client or family
[ ] **D.** Client's insurance status

Correct answer—A. *Rationales:* The benefits must always outweigh the risks involved to the client when deciding to transfer a client. After risks and benefits have been discussed with the client or family, including the risks of mode of transportation, consent may be sought. The client's insurance status shouldn't be the first concern.
Nursing process step: Analysis

19. Which factor places a client at risk for instability during an intrahospital transport?
[ ] **A.** An organized transport
[ ] **B.** Monitoring the client
[ ] **C.** Long distance between facilities
[ ] **D.** Appropriate transport personnel

Correct answer—C. *Rationales:* The client is at greater risk when being transported in the hospital between treatment areas that are long distances apart, such as radiology, operating room, and so forth. That risk can be diminished with an organized transport of appropriate transport team members monitoring, assessing, and intervening for the client throughout the transport.
Nursing process step: Analysis

20. Which *isn't* an appropriate nursing action for the family of a client being transferred?
[ ] **A.** Provide maps to the receiving hospital.
[ ] **B.** Have the family see the client prior to transfer.
[ ] **C.** Caution the family to observe the traffic laws.
[ ] **D.** Send the family ahead to the receiving hospital before the client is transferred.

Correct answer—D. *Rationales:* Providing maps, reinforcing the need to observe the traffic laws for their safety, and allowing the family to see the client prior to transfer are all appropriate nursing actions. If the client deteriorates before leaving the referring hospital, they may not survive the transfer and the family will miss the opportunity to be with their loved one.
Nursing process step: Intervention

19 Client and community education

1. A client comes to the emergency department and complains of tremors, headache, and confusion. The nurse detects a fruity odor about the client. The client reports having diabetes controlled by diet and an oral agent. When physical assessment has been completed, which question should the nurse ask the client to determine his learning needs concerning nutrition and the disease process?

[ ] **A.** "When was the last time you ate?"
[ ] **B.** "What have you had to eat and drink in the past 24 hours?"
[ ] **C.** "Have you been using alcohol?"
[ ] **D.** "Have you been sticking to your diet?"

Correct answer–B. *Rationales:* The confused client may have difficulty understanding and responding to general questions. Specific time periods and specific information may be easier for the client to recall. Confusion blurs the client's ability to think and remember.
Nursing process step: Assessment

2. "I was afraid of getting low sugar so I ate some cereal and drank vodka and coke yesterday." This response indicates to the nurse that the client has some knowledge about low blood sugar. What conclusion should the nurse draw?

[ ] **A.** This client has some knowledge but not enough to realize that hypoglycemia and hyperglycemia mimic each other.
[ ] **B.** The client has a knowledge deficit related to the complications and control of diabetes.
[ ] **C.** The client's significant other should be monitoring the client's diet better.
[ ] **D.** The client is an alcoholic.

Correct answer–B. *Rationales:* The client has some knowledge but not enough to fully control the disease condition. Knowledge of hyperglycemia and hypoglycemia and the impact of diet on diabetes is important if the client is to remain in control. Unless the client is mentally incompetent, it isn't the spouse's responsibility to monitor the client. Not enough information has been presented to determine whether the client is an alcoholic.
Nursing process step: Evaluation

3. Which factor influences a client's readiness to learn?

[ ] **A.** Client's sex
[ ] **B.** Culture
[ ] **C.** Education level
[ ] **D.** Personality

Correct answer–B. *Rationales:* Education is best integrated when instruction occurs with consideration to the client's culture, including the client's primary language and culture-mediated values. Some anxiety is necessary for learning to occur, but too high a level interferes with learning. Personality, the client's sex, and the client's education level don't influence the client's readiness to learn.
Nursing process step: Assessment

4. After an acute episode of illness, a client has resolved to improve self-care actions. How can the nurse take advantage of this resolve?
[ ] **A.** Encourage the client to sign up for educational classes immediately.
[ ] **B.** Give the client a list of classes offered by the health care organization.
[ ] **C.** Provide the client with pamphlets and brochures.
[ ] **D.** Have the nurse educator talk to the client.

Correct answer—C. *Rationales:* Educational classes or one-on-one instruction by the nurse educator don't offer the client hard data. To augment the client's resolve, printed educational information, such as pamphlets and brochures, can be rapidly provided and reread as often as the client finds necessary. Encouraging the client to sign up for classes requires current action with future results. The client may or may not sign up for classes, and even if the client signs up, the client may not attend when the time arrives. Talking to the nurse educator after reading pamphlets and brochures allows for immediate confirmation of information learned or clarification of new information.
Nursing process step: Intervention

5. Learning goals and objectives should be written in measurable terms and describe whose behavior?
[ ] **A.** Nurse
[ ] **B.** Client
[ ] **C.** Client's significant other
[ ] **D.** Client's family

Correct answer—B. *Rationales:* Learning goals and objectives should be established by the client and nurse to meet the client's needs. They should describe the client's learning behavior. Although the client's significant other, his family, and the nurse may be involved in establishing goals, ultimately goals must focus on the client. Only in this way will the client have learning goals that meet his own learning needs.
Nursing process step: Intervention

6. A client on sublingual nitroglycerin tablets is discharged from the emergency department. Which adverse effect of nitroglycerin should be explained to the client?
[ ] **A.** Flushing
[ ] **B.** Hot flashes
[ ] **C.** Blurred vision
[ ] **D.** Headache

Correct answer—D. *Rationales:* The headache that can result from taking nitroglycerin tablets can be disconcerting and frightening for the client. Although the flushing and hot flashes may be uncomfortable, they aren't as frightening as the headache. Nitroglycerin doesn't usually cause blurred vision.
Nursing process step: Assessment

7. One of the Standards of Emergency Nursing Practice explicitly incorporates client education as an expectation. The expectation of client education is found in all of the following *except*?
[ ] **A.** Most state nurse practice acts
[ ] **B.** Accrediting criteria (The Joint Commission)
[ ] **C.** Quality assurance criteria
[ ] **D.** Health Insurance Portability and Accountability Act (HIPAA)

Correct answer—D. *Rationales:* The HIPAA doesn't deal with the expectation of client education. The need for client education is recognized and stated in all other documents cited. Client education is the responsibility of the emergency department nurse, especially when the client is discharged.
Nursing process step: Evaluation

8. The ability to assess a client's motivation for learning is important in order to use available opportunities for teaching. The nurse looks for clues to the client's motivational level in all areas *except*?

[ ] **A.** In what the client says (verbal)
[ ] **B.** In what the client doesn't say (nonverbal)
[ ] **C.** In what the client does (behavioral)
[ ] **D.** The client's education level

Correct answer—D. *Rationales:* Consideration of the behavioral, verbal, and nonverbal clues given by the client enables the nurse to accurately assess the client's motivation for learning. The client's education level may affect how he learns, but not his motivation.
Nursing process step: Assessment

9. Because of the relationship and time frame commonly available for client education in the emergency department (ED), which kind of learning goals are best established with the client in this setting?

[ ] **A.** Long-term
[ ] **B.** Short-term
[ ] **C.** Middle-range
[ ] **D.** Long-term goals and short-term objectives

Correct answer—B. *Rationales:* The relationship between nurse and client as well as the time the client spends in the emergency department is short term. Short-term learning goals or objectives are most appropriate in this setting. Long-term and middle-range goals are best met in a setting other than the ED.
Nursing process step: Assessment

10. Teaching a client with diabetes the symptoms of hyperglycemia and hypoglycemia is an example of which type of learning?

[ ] **A.** Cognitive
[ ] **B.** Affective
[ ] **C.** Psychomotor
[ ] **D.** Social

Correct answer—A. *Rationales:* Teaching a client the signs and symptoms of a disease process involves the client's use of cognitive learning skills. These skills require thinking and reasoning in order to integrate the learning. Affective learning involves feelings and attitudes. Psychomotor learning requires the coordination of the brain and extremities to complete a task. Social learning requires the ability to interact with others in a social setting.
Nursing process step: Assessment

11. In which situation is a potential nursing diagnosis of deficient knowledge most likely?

[ ] **A.** Acute dehydration resulting from participation in a walking event
[ ] **B.** Digoxin toxicity
[ ] **C.** Chronic renal failure
[ ] **D.** Bacterial pneumonia

Correct answer—A. *Rationales:* Clients who participate in amateur events for the sake of supporting a cause probably aren't athletes; therefore, their knowledge of potential illness may be lacking. A client can become digoxin toxic, have chronic renal failure, or acquire bacterial pneumonia without having a knowledge deficit.
Nursing process step: Analysis

12. What should the nurse tell the client with diabetes to do to prevent hypoglycemia?

[ ] **A.** Monitor glucose levels more closely.
[ ] **B.** Increase caloric intake by twice the normal amount.
[ ] **C.** Increase water intake.
[ ] **D.** Urinate every 4 hours.

Correct answer—A. *Rationales:* Monitoring glucose levels more frequently helps prevent hypoglycemia from occurring by identifying a downward trend in the client's blood glucose. Increasing caloric intake without monitoring blood glucose levels can lead to other complications, such as hyperglycemia, diabetic ketoacidosis, or hyperglycemic hyperosmolar nonketotic acidosis. The client should increase water intake to assist adequate kidney function. The client should urinate every 2 hours to promote adequate kidney function.
Nursing process step: Intervention

13. Which action would best serve a client when providing discharge instructions about his diabetes?
[ ] **A.** Provide written instructions about which foods to eat and which to avoid, and suggest carrying an insulated container of water in the truck.
[ ] **B.** Discuss the interaction of food, fluid, and medication, and teach the client how to perform self-care while continuing to work.
[ ] **C.** Encourage the client to take several days off work until the symptoms clear.
[ ] **D.** Suggest several alternative careers to the client to prevent chronic urinary tract infections (UTIs).

Correct answer—B. *Rationales:* Interaction between nurse and client provides opportunities for learning. Clients need help in problem solving, but they still must make their own decisions. Encouraging the client to take off work doesn't educate him on how to prevent further occurrences of UTI. Providing written instructions is helpful and gives the client a reference, but without explanation, compliance is less likely. Alternative career options shouldn't be necessary if education is completed.
Nursing process step: Intervention

14. Which type of learning takes more time to accomplish?
[ ] **A.** Cognitive
[ ] **B.** Psychomotor
[ ] **C.** Social
[ ] **D.** Affective

Correct answer—D. *Rationales:* Changes in attitudes, beliefs, and values take place over time. Cognitive learning is mental activity to learn some knowledge. Although cognitive material may be complex, it doesn't necessarily require a change in attitude or values. Psychomotor learning is the accomplishment of a skill requiring physical and mental coordination. Social learning or learning by observing others may or may not involve change in attitude or values.
Nursing process step: Evaluation

15. Generally speaking, the content and the learning goal dictate which step in the teaching-learning process?
[ ] **A.** Audiovisual resources
[ ] **B.** Teaching method
[ ] **C.** Time frame
[ ] **D.** Teacher

Correct answer—B. *Rationales:* The goals established by the nurse and client as well as what is to be learned dictate the teaching method. For example, a client can't be taught a diet without learning about the food pyramid and which foods should be eaten and which foods should be avoided. Teaching methods include lecture, self-study, small-group discussion, guided learning manual, one-on-one, and so forth. Time frame is the amount of time required to teach the material. Audiovisual resources are teaching aids that the teacher may use to explain content. The teacher is the person doing the teaching.
Nursing process step: Analysis

Part II
Professional issues

20 Legal issues

1. Which source of law governing the practice of emergency nursing is the authority when other areas do not address a problem?
[ ] **A.** The U.S. Constitution
[ ] **B.** Federal and state statutes
[ ] **C.** Common law
[ ] **D.** Institutional

Correct answer–D. *Rationales:* Institutional policy is the authority if other legal venues haven't addressed the specific issue. All three of the options listed can govern the practice of emergency department nursing. The Constitution is the supreme law of the land and can't be overturned by state or federal statute. In order of hierarchy, the Constitution is first and then federal, state, and common law.

2. Cases involving medical or nursing negligence or malpractice fall into the legal category of tort. What's the definition of a tort?
[ ] **A.** An intentional criminal act that can be remedied with money paid to the plaintiff
[ ] **B.** A civil wrong committed against a person or person's property that can be remedied with money paid to the plaintiff
[ ] **C.** An unintentional criminal act that can be remedied with money paid to the plaintiff
[ ] **D.** An unintentional criminal act that can't be remedied with money

Correct answer–B. *Rationales:* A tort is defined as a civil wrong, whether intentional or accidental, that results in injury to a person or the person's property.

3. What's the best method for the emergency department staff to protect themselves against possible negligence or malpractice litigation?
[ ] **A.** Document their actions with a difficult client.
[ ] **B.** Document the nurse–client ratio on a daily basis.
[ ] **C.** Provide and document care within accepted standards.
[ ] **D.** Provide care to the best of one's abilities, and document what wasn't done for specific clients.

Correct answer–C. *Rationales:* Meeting the standards of care and documenting them may not prevent litigation, but these actions will certainly provide support that the standards of care were known and adhered to. Actions should be documented for all clients, not just for difficult ones. Documentation of nurse–client ratios doesn't relieve the nurse of the responsibility to provide care within accepted standards. Accepted practice is to document what was done for a client, not the opposite.

4. What does the plaintiff have to prove in litigation for negligence?
[ ] **A.** Intent to cause harm
[ ] **B.** Substandard care delivery
[ ] **C.** Mitigating circumstances
[ ] **D.** Lack of intent

Correct answer–B. *Rationales:* The plaintiff must prove that the care received was substandard; it isn't necessary to prove intent to cause harm. Mitigating circumstances are issues that would be brought up by the defendant, not the plaintiff. Negligence is by definition an unintentional tort or a civil wrong done without intent by the defendant; therefore, it isn't necessary to demonstrate lack of intent.

5. What's the most common unintentional tort involving health care personnel?
[ ] **A.** Malpractice
[ ] **B.** Negligence
[ ] **C.** Assault
[ ] **D.** Battery

Correct answer—B. *Rationales:* Negligence is the most common unintentional tort involving health care personnel. Malpractice is a more restricted, specialized kind of negligence, defined as a violation of professional duty to act with reasonable care and in good faith. Assault and battery are *intentional* torts.

6. Which action is most likely to lead to a claim of battery?
[ ] **A.** Leaving foreign objects in a client's body after surgery
[ ] **B.** Failing to obtain informed consent
[ ] **C.** Threatening a client
[ ] **D.** Treatment of nonemergency conditions without informed consent

Correct answer—D. *Rationales:* Battery is the touching of a person without that person's consent. A nurse who treats a client beyond what the client has consented to has committed battery (the theory of implied consent doesn't apply to nonemergency conditions). Leaving foreign objects in a client's body after surgery and failing to obtain informed consent are examples of negligence. Threatening a client is an example of assault.

7. What's breach of duty?
[ ] **A.** Willful violation of an oath or code of ethics
[ ] **B.** Failure to meet accepted standards in providing care for a client
[ ] **C.** Threatening a client
[ ] **D.** Confining a client to a psychiatric unit without a physician's order

Correct answer—B. *Rationales:* If a client sues a nurse for negligence, the client must prove that the nurse owed him a specific duty and that she breached this duty. A breach of duty in this case means that the nurse didn't provide the client with care within the accepted standard. A breach isn't always willful, as implied in option A. Threatening a client is assault, more accurately described as a direct invasion of a client's rights rather than a breach of duty. Confining a client to a psychiatric unit without a physician's order is false imprisonment, another example of direct invasion of a client's rights.

8. It's the plaintiff's responsibility to prove six elements in a negligence lawsuit. Which *isn't* one of the six elements?
[ ] **A.** A duty was owed to the client.
[ ] **B.** The defendant breached the duty.
[ ] **C.** The breach of duty was the cause of the plaintiff's injury.
[ ] **D.** The plaintiff was at risk for sustaining an injury as a result of the breach of duty.

Correct answer—D. *Rationales:* The plaintiff must prove that the injuries sustained were real or actual. The plaintiff must prove that the defendant owed him a specific duty; that the defendant breached this duty; that the plaintiff was harmed physically, mentally, emotionally, or financially; and that the defendant's breach of duty caused this harm. The plaintiff must also prove foreseeability and damages.

9. "The protective privilege ends where the public peril begins" indicates the duty of the emergency department (ED) nurse when a client threatens another person with bodily injury or harm. What does the quoted statement mean?
[ ] **A.** The confidentiality enjoyed between client and nurse or physician doesn't relieve the ED personnel of the duty to warn the threatened person and authorities.
[ ] **B.** Confidentiality between nurse or physician and client is as sacred as the attorney-client privilege.
[ ] **C.** ED personnel must weigh the seriousness of the threat to another person before breaking the confidentiality between client and nurse or physician.
[ ] **D.** Warning the client not to commit a felony is relief from the duty to warn.

Correct answer—A. *Rationales:* Confidentiality between client and nurse or physician should be breached to alleviate a threat to another person. Medical personnel have a duty to warn the intended victim (if known) and the authorities. Warning the client not to commit a felony or weighing the seriousness of the threat isn't sufficient grounds for relief from the duty to warn.

10. With regard to the phrase "The protective privilege ends where the public peril begins," which client situation would be subject to this quoted phrase?
[ ] **A.** The discharge of a child with his parents
[ ] **B.** The discharge of a single mother and her neonate
[ ] **C.** The discharge of a psychiatric client threatening to kill a family member
[ ] **D.** The discharge of a woman with a gunshot wound

Correct answer—C. *Rationales:* Confidentiality between client and nurse or physician should be breached to alleviate a threat to another person. The medical personnel have a duty to warn the intended victim (if known) and the authorities if there's potential for harm to others. Even though the medical personnel may not know who the victim might be, there's an obligation to tell the authorities about the condition of the client. The other options don't pose a threat to someone.

11. Which type of assessment data should be recorded in the emergency department record about every woman of childbearing age who presents to the emergency department?
[ ] **A.** Number of pregnancies and live births
[ ] **B.** Date of last menstrual period
[ ] **C.** Known sexual partners
[ ] **D.** Birth name

Correct answer—B. *Rationales:* The date of the last menstrual period provides information about the likelihood of a first-trimester pregnancy. This information may affect medications ordered and radiographic procedures performed. The number of pregnancies and live births is important information, but it has no impact on ordered medications or radiographic procedures. Information about known sexual partners is only important in the presence of a sexually transmitted infection.

12. A mother brings her 3-year-old to the emergency department (ED) because of blood in the child's underwear. A physical examination reveals sexual assault and felonious penetration. Which action should the nurse take?
[ ] **A.** No action is necessary because the mother is the child's legal guardian and her decisions are final.
[ ] **B.** Report the findings to Children's Protective Services and the police.
[ ] **C.** Encourage the mother to reconsider her decision and refer her to a child psychologist.
[ ] **D.** Have the ED physician talk to the mother.

Correct answer—B. *Rationales:* The nurse has a duty of care to the client and to the public to report the crime to the authorities. Regardless of the mother's wishes, the child has been harmed and a report to the authorities is necessary. Even though the ED physician may talk to the mother and the mother may be encouraged to reconsider her wishes, the fact remains that the crime must be reported and evidence must be collected.

13. Children's Protective Services has decided to remove the child from the mother's care pending further investigation of a sexual assault on the child. The mother becomes upset and is afraid the child's father will beat her. The nurse can refer the mother to several social service agencies. Which one would be most appropriate?
[ ] **A.** A women's shelter
[ ] **B.** The welfare bureau
[ ] **C.** A homeless shelter
[ ] **D.** A soup kitchen

Correct answer—A. *Rationales:* A women's shelter can provide services that are necessary for the mother. The welfare bureau is a state agency that provides money, food, or shelter for people who need it. Homeless shelters and soup kitchens are voluntary organizations for people in need of shelter and food. They don't necessarily have resources to accommodate clients at risk for abuse.

14. What does the Emergency Medical Treatment and Active Labor Act mandate for a client having labor contractions?
[ ] **A.** If the contractions are 5 or more minutes apart, the client can be referred to a hospital that offers maternity services.
[ ] **B.** All clients having contractions must be medically screened and stabilized before transport to another facility.
[ ] **C.** Only clients in obvious active labor need to be medically screened before transport to another facility.
[ ] **D.** The emergency department has the right to refuse clients for whom it doesn't offer the needed services.

Correct answer–B. *Rationales:* All clients experiencing contractions must be medically screened before transport. Whether it's obvious that the client is in labor or not, the client must be medically screened and examined before the decision is made to transport the client to another facility. The emergency department doesn't have the right to refuse treatment to a client before medically screening the client.

15. What does the Emergency Medical Treatment and Active Labor Act (EMTALA) mandate for a client presenting without insurance?
[ ] **A.** Medical screening of clients can't be delayed until insurance coverage or the ability to pay has been determined.
[ ] **B.** The client must present proof of ability to pay before services are rendered.
[ ] **C.** Every urban area must maintain hospital beds for clients who aren't able to pay for services.
[ ] **D.** The ability to pay for services shouldn't be part of the admission procedure.

Correct answer–A. *Rationales:* To ensure that clients aren't denied care based on their ability to pay, clients must be medically screened and stabilized before their ability to pay is determined. Failure of a hospital to comply may result in denial of Medicare funding. Only hospitals accepting Medicare funding are required to have some beds available for the indigent. EMTALA doesn't address payment for services as part of the admission procedure. It only addresses medical screening and stabilization of clients before transport or the determination of ability to pay for services rendered.

16. Several sources of law affect the emergency department nurse. Which source of law would Medicare laws fall under?
[ ] **A.** Ordinances
[ ] **B.** Common law
[ ] **C.** Constitutional law
[ ] **D.** Statutory law

Correct answer–D. *Rationales:* Statutory law is law made by federal and state legislatures. Medicare law is an example of federal statute. Ordinances are laws passed by cities or local jurisdictions such as parking regulations. Common law is the body of law formed by judicial decisions in a courtroom setting. Constitutional law is the supreme law of the land.

17. A 44-year-old female with a broken right ankle refuses morphine for pain and takes two Tylenol. The nurse notices that the client continues to grimace after a cast has been applied. The client still refuses the morphine, but the nurse decides it's in the client's best interest and gives the I.V. morphine without telling the client. This is an example of:
[ ] **A.** assault.
[ ] **B.** breach of duty.
[ ] **C.** proximate cause.
[ ] **D.** battery.

Correct answer–D. *Rationales:* Battery is the nonconsensual, offensive touching of another person. Assault is the intention to cause harm with the ability to carry through with it. A breach of duty occurs when care falls below the standards or is omitted. Proximate cause is proof that a breach of duty caused injury to an individual.

18. A client goes into ventricular tachycardia after a nurse accidentally administers potassium. The client ends up on a ventilator with a hypoxic injury. The hospital settles with the client's family out of court. Which legal concept underlies the hospital's requirement of the nurse to repay the money they lost?

[ ] **A.** *Respondeat superior*
[ ] **B.** Indemnification
[ ] **C.** Captain of the ship
[ ] **D.** Vicarious liability

Correct answer—B. *Rationales:* If an employee is found liable for negligence, vicarious liability requires the employer to pay a settlement. The employer then has the option to require indemnification from the employee for the losses incurred to the hospital. *Respondeat superior* is a term that describes the vicarious liability that the employer has for negligent acts of employees who act within the scope of the hospital's employment. The captain of the ship rule says any negligence that occurs would be attributed to the physician because of his role as "captain of the ship."

19. A client who slashed his wrist wants to leave the emergency department. The physician orders a 48-hour hold, and security is called to watch the client. What type of consent would cover keeping this client and providing treatment?

[ ] **A.** Implied consent
[ ] **B.** Informed consent
[ ] **C.** Involuntary consent
[ ] **D.** Express consent

Correct answer—C. *Rationales:* Involuntary consent applies when an individual refuses treatment but a physician or police issues orders for care to be provided for up to 48 hours. When an individual in a life- or limb-threatening situation is unable to provide consent, it's assumed that consent is present to save the limb or life; this is known as implied consent. Informed consent is obtained when a physician has explained a procedure, risk, and alternate treatment options to a client. Expressed consent is a voluntary consent for treatment from a competent person.

20. A 33-year-old client who took an overdose of Valium requests that the incident not be reported because he could lose his job. It's a mandatory reportable situation. The physician states that he won't report it this time, but if it occurs again he will. What should the emergency department nurse do?

[ ] **A.** Confront the physician as to whether he's reporting the incident.
[ ] **B.** Assume the physician will report it because it's mandatory.
[ ] **C.** Report the incident regardless of the physician's promise to the client.
[ ] **D.** It's none of the nurse's business.

Correct answer—C. *Rationales:* If the nurse believes that the incident is a mandatory reportable incident, even if the physician disagrees, it's the nurse's responsibility to report it to the designated authority. The nurse shares equally with the physician in this legal responsibility.

21 Organizational issues and quality improvement

1. When conflict arises among the staff, which response by a nurse-manager is the most helpful?
[ ] **A.** To delegate the issue to assistants or clinical specialists
[ ] **B.** To invite an outside mediator to assist
[ ] **C.** To bring all conflicting parties together to resolve the problem with ample notification for each side to build coalitions
[ ] **D.** To help the staff clarify the issues and confront one another assertively and respectfully

Correct answer—D. *Rationales:* Assisting the staff to resolve conflicts falls within the role of a nurse-manager. Encouraging confrontation and clarifying issues are the most helpful interventions. A response that overemphasizes the problem or leads to increased conflict and division of staff isn't helpful. For most staff conflicts, the resolution of a problem best lies with the people who identified it. Nothing in the question suggests the need for a mediator.
Nursing process step: Intervention

2. To arrive at an appropriate nursing staff pattern in an emergency department, the manager must:
[ ] **A.** know the client volume and acuity levels by hour of the day, and take into consideration variability according to day of the week or time of year.
[ ] **B.** be aware of The Joint Commission (TJC) standard that emergency services shall be appropriately integrated with other units and departments within the organization.
[ ] **C.** realize that client visits are so unpredictable that a different staffing pattern will have to occur every day according to need.
[ ] **D.** for the sake of standardization, arrange staffing so that it closely corresponds with the rest of the organization.

Correct answer—A. *Rationales:* Although exact volume and acuity levels can be somewhat unpredictable, the manager should track both over time so that numbers and type of staff are appropriately placed. Staffing patterns are unit-specific and standardization is irrelevant. TJC's standard for integrating emergency services isn't directly related to the question.
Nursing process step: Assessment

3. A team of nurses, physicians, and registration clerks met to address a departmental goal of decreasing total client time in the department. First, they collected data (sorted by triage category) on the length of time clients wait to be seen. The activity described above is an early step in:
[ ] **A.** descriptive research.
[ ] **B.** indicator relevance testing.
[ ] **C.** collaborative research.
[ ] **D.** quality improvement process.

Correct answer—D. *Rationales:* The situation describes a quality improvement process. This reflects an interdisciplinary approach to process improvement for better client experience or outcome. It isn't intended to generate or validate a scientific knowledge base. The element of data collection is found in research also. In the research process, however, data collection occurs later (after a literature review and after decisions have been made regarding conceptual or theoretical framework and research design). Indicator relevance testing isn't a recognized entity in either process.
Nursing process step: Analysis

4. Which should the manager or peer recruitment team be certain to do when interviewing a prospective staff member?
[ ] **A.** Ascertain whether the applicant has health problems that have ever resulted in a workers' compensation claim
[ ] **B.** Verify experience and qualifications by checking references
[ ] **C.** Ask primarily open-ended questions
[ ] **D.** Verify that the applicant has appropriate child-care arrangements

Correct answer—B. *Rationales:* Checking references and verifying experience and education are common ways of ensuring that an applicant has the background for the job. Ascertaining whether the applicant has health or child-care problems is prohibited by federal laws addressing gender bias and disabled workers. Open-ended questions are useful for gleaning clues to personality and style. Direct questions, which have specific answers, are an efficient means of learning whether an applicant has the knowledge, experience, and attitude being sought.
Nursing process step: Assessment

5. An emergency department lobbies for a departmental pharmacist to function as a resource and consultant in toxicology and medication issues. What's the correct budget for such a request?
[ ] **A.** Operational
[ ] **B.** Capital
[ ] **C.** Manpower or personnel
[ ] **D.** Overhead

Correct answer—C. *Rationales:* Manpower or personnel budgets cover wages and benefits for regular and temporary workers. An operational budget covers supplies, unit equipment, repairs, and overhead. Capital budgets cover land, buildings, and expensive durable equipment (usually costing more than $500).
Nursing process step: Analysis

6. A client classification system that's reliable, valid, and consistently used can be a management tool for determining:
[ ] **A.** staffing levels based on nursing workload.
[ ] **B.** quality of care rendered by nurses.
[ ] **C.** problem solving and conflict resolution.
[ ] **D.** mix of paying and nonpaying clients and thereby improving the budget.

Correct answer—A. *Rationales:* Client classification systems measure workload, thereby determining staffing needs. They don't measure comparative quality or relate to client payment and aren't part of conflict resolution.
Nursing process step: Analysis

7. Brainstorming is a problem-solving method whereby a group rapidly generates which type of solutions?
[ ] **A.** As many as possible
[ ] **B.** As practical as possible
[ ] **C.** As wild and crazy as possible
[ ] **D.** As high-quality as possible

Correct answer—A. *Rationales:* Brainstorming is a problem-solving method that rapidly generates a large number of alternatives. Quality and practicality are unimportant. Some wild and crazy solutions emerge and make the process fun; such unconventional ideas help participants unleash their creativity.
Nursing process step: Analysis

8. An emergency department nursing team found that clients whose discharge instructions were reviewed by a registered nurse had a much better understanding of their diagnosis and follow-up than clients whose discharge instructions weren't reviewed. The team had evaluated which element?
[ ] **A.** A structure element
[ ] **B.** A process element
[ ] **C.** An outcome element
[ ] **D.** A hierarchical element

Correct answer—C. *Rationales:* Improved client understanding of discharge instructions is an outcome and a goal of care. The process element in client discharge involves the nurse reviewing instructions with responsible family members and ascertaining by way of return demonstration or verbalization that the instructions are understood. The structure element in client discharge addresses environment, instrumentation, and qualification of personnel. For example, all clients must have instructions reviewed by a registered nurse, and the client must sign a written copy. Hierarchy refers to the placing of people or things in a rank order according to importance.
Nursing process step: Evaluation

9. What's a manager allowed to do in response to a collective bargaining initiative?

[ ] **A.** Prevent employees from engaging in recruiting activities during nonworking hours

[ ] **B.** Prevent employees from participating in informal union activities in client care areas

[ ] **C.** Withhold desirable assignments from union organizers

[ ] **D.** Provide wage increases or special considerations to discourage employees from joining the union

Correct answer—B. *Rationales:* Federal laws allow management to prevent employees from engaging in collective bargaining in client care areas. The same laws prohibit managers from preventing union activities during nonworking hours, from withholding desirable assignments from staff engaging in union activities, and from providing special favors to discourage union activity or membership.

Nursing process step: Intervention

10. An emergency nursing staff sought to reach a fair distribution of major holidays worked. The manager held meetings in which each staff member agreed to work half of the holidays. Although some weren't completely satisfied, they said they could "live with it." This type of decision making is known as:

[ ] **A.** consensus.

[ ] **B.** group vote.

[ ] **C.** minority poll dissension.

[ ] **D.** authoritative facilitative coaching.

Correct answer—A. *Rationales:* The scenario depicts the process of reaching consensus, whereby an agreeable best solution is negotiated in a group. Group vote and minority poll dissension refer to voting and polling (a more informal term) and are limited to merely counting responses: the winning option is the one with the most votes. Neither coaching nor authoritative actions were described.

Nursing process step: Evaluation

11. Many emergency departments have customer service committees whose charge is to improve customer relations. Effectiveness is most likely to occur in which of these scenarios?

[ ] **A.** An all-nurse committee because nurses have the most client contact

[ ] **B.** A committee that includes all disciplines and levels of staff and management

[ ] **C.** A small committee of managers who can respond most effectively to complaints

[ ] **D.** A multidisciplinary staff-level committee that monitors client complaints closely and tracks numbers and types of complaints against staff members

Correct answer—B. *Rationales:* Optimal customer service includes all staff, at all levels, in all disciplines. The committee works best when the problem is "owned" by those delivering service to customers as well as those in authority. An all-nurse committee places inappropriate emphasis on nursing. It's evident that nurses do have a great deal of client contact and, therefore, opportunity to set a customer-friendly tone. However, there are countless factors that aren't directly related to nursing, such as billing, medical diagnosis, and housekeeping. Waiting for complaints is passive, and an after-the-damage-is-done strategy, which is limited to monitoring, doesn't improve goals.

Nursing process step: Analysis

12. An applicant for an emergency department nursing position is qualified depending on personal qualities, education, experience, and credentials. An applicant's ENPC (Emergency Nursing Pediatric Course), TNCC (Trauma Nursing Core Course), ACLS (Advanced Cardiac Life Support), and CEN (Certified Emergency Nurse) certification as well as RN (Registered Nurse) licensure are examples of which qualifications?

[ ] **A.** Personal qualities

[ ] **B.** Experience

[ ] **C.** Educational preparation

[ ] **D.** Credentials

Correct answer—D. *Rationales:* Certifications, courses, and licenses are known as credentials. Experience is an applicant's work history. Educational preparation refers to degrees held as well as academic institutions and programs attended. Personal qualities are subjectively measured and include perceptions of voice, dress, sense of humor, and energy level.

Nursing process step: Evaluation

13. A department with a shared governance model would probably have which of these scheduling processes?
[ ] **A.** Self-scheduling of staff
[ ] **B.** Management scheduling of staff
[ ] **C.** Designated staff leader scheduling of staff
[ ] **D.** A centralized system that includes computer-generated scheduling

Correct answer—A. *Rationales:* Self-scheduling is the option usually found in shared governance models, which emphasize staff accountability and involvement in operating a unit. Management scheduling, or having a designated staff leader for scheduling, places the work of schedule preparation directly on the manager (or designee); it deemphasizes staff maturity and responsibility. A centralized system with computer-generated scheduling would provide little opportunity for staff input and is a poor fit with the decentralized approach underlying the shared governance model.
Nursing process step: Analysis

14. What's the purpose of research in emergency nursing?
[ ] **A.** To enhance the professional status of emergency nursing
[ ] **B.** To generate a scientific knowledge base for validating and improving practice
[ ] **C.** To evaluate new medical devices and drugs
[ ] **D.** To help nurses identify problems in their clinical setting

Correct answer—B. *Rationales:* The purpose of nursing research is to generate a scientific knowledge base for validating and improving practice. Although the professional status of emergency nursing may be incidentally enhanced by research, such enhancement isn't the focus or goal. Identification of new problems may be an outcome of nursing research, but most research depends on problem or question identification. Emergency nurses may have opportunities to participate in drug studies and product evaluation programs, but neither represents the purpose of nursing research.
Nursing process step: Assessment

15. Research that aims to examine the feelings and perceptions of emergency nurses working with battered female clients is probably which type of study?
[ ] **A.** Qualitative
[ ] **B.** Quasi-scientific
[ ] **C.** Quantitative
[ ] **D.** Experimental

Correct answer—A. *Rationales:* A study that examines thoughts and perceptions is one that lends itself to a qualitative design. Qualitative research is concerned with understanding human beings and the nature of their transactions with themselves and their surroundings. The process isn't quasi-scientific but, rather, a well-accepted mode of rigorous, systematic inquiry used in the social sciences. Quantitative research methods analyze data statistically while striving for precision and control over external variables. Experimental research involves doing something to some of the subjects and not doing something to others; in it, subjects are randomly assigned to either group.
Nursing process step: Evaluation

16. A registered nurse is the preceptor for a new graduate nurse. The graduate nurse tells the nurse that his client has an order for a urinary catheter insertion but he doesn't know how to do the procedure. What action is best for the preceptor nurse?
[ ] **A.** Refer him to the policy and procedure book.
[ ] **B.** Do the procedure for him but require him to chart it.
[ ] **C.** Tell him to call the clinical nurse educator.
[ ] **D.** Perform the procedure with him.

Correct answer—D. *Rationales:* Doing the procedure for him or referring him to an outside resource (book or person) won't enhance the graduate nurse's technical skills to fulfill this client needs now. In addition, he may need assistance in physically locating the urethra (beyond a description). Documentation of a procedure should be done only by the nurse completing the procedure.
Nursing process step: Intervention

17. The emergency department staff is conducting a group interview with a nurse applicant. What's the most appropriate question for the staff to ask?
[ ] **A.** "This position requires being on-call every fourth weekend. Can you do that?"
[ ] **B.** "Tell us about your child-care arrangements."
[ ] **C.** "Do you have any religious requirements that we need to accommodate?"
[ ] **D.** "I see you live in another suburb. How will you get to work?"

Correct answer—A. *Rationales*: Job interview questions must be specifically job-related. It can be considered discrimination to ask about child care, religion, or transportation prior to the job being offered.
Nursing process step: Assessment

18. A registered nurse read a journal's research study. The study taught fever control measures to first-time parents. What information is most important to determine before attempting to apply the same project in the nurse's emergency department?
[ ] **A.** Was the study approved by an Institutional Review Board (IRB)?
[ ] **B.** What was the content that the researcher taught?
[ ] **C.** Are the researcher's and nurse's settings similar enough for transferability?
[ ] **D.** Did the researcher statistically verify the data results with an analysis of variance (ANOVA)?

Correct answer—C. *Rationales:* To apply the study, the two settings need to be similar enough to allow transferability. It wouldn't be as effective, for instance, if the emergency department population had a low population of neonatal/pediatric clients. IRBs are one method of ensuring protection of human rights, but the study would have to go through appropriate channels at her facility. It's essential to know the content of the teaching so it can be implemented, but transferability needs to be determined first. ANOVA is just one statistical option for testing differences among three or more group means.
Nursing process step: Assessment

19. A nurse delegates the responsibility of taking and recording a client's blood pressure to the unlicensed assistive personnel (nurse's aide). Later, the nurse notes that there's no blood pressure recorded on the client's chart. What's the best way for the nurse to handle this situation?
[ ] **A.** Take the blood pressure now herself and speak to the UAP at the end of the shift.
[ ] **B.** Talk to the involved UAP now.
[ ] **C.** Ask the client whether anyone took his blood pressure today.
[ ] **D.** Discuss the matter with the charge nurse.

Correct answer—B. *Rationales:* The unlicensed assistive personnel may have taken the blood pressure and forgotten to chart it. Even if the task wasn't done, it is important to follow up to reinforce responsibility for the future. Taking the blood pressure himself may be duplication of work, and the matter should be cleared up now, not at the end of the shift. The client could be mistaken about the blood pressure being taken if asked, and it still doesn't give the results even if it was done. More information should be clarified and the UAP dealt with directly prior to bringing in management. Management can be brought in if there's a repetitive pattern.
Nursing process step: Analysis

20. A client in the triage area is yelling and becoming increasingly agitated; he throws his bottle of water on the floor. The family states this agitated and aggressive behavior is new over the past few hours. What's the best response for the triage nurse at this time?
[ ] **A.** Approach the client and directly confront him to control him through authority.
[ ] **B.** Inform the client that this isn't acceptable behavior in the emergency department.
[ ] **C.** Reassure the client that the nurse is here to help him.
[ ] **D.** Shout for security to call the police.

Correct answer—C. *Rationales:* The client is exhibiting excessive agitation, which has a potential for violence; therefore, reassuring the client and his family is the most therapeutic response. The nurse should avoid being within the client's physical reach to reduce her risk for the client striking her. Taking an authoritative stance is likely to further agitate the client. He may not be able to cognitively take verbal cueing or instructions because of an underlying pathological process. Emotionally reacting and indicating to the client that outside authorities are being called will also likely incite further agitation.
Nursing process step: Intervention

Part III
Sample tests

Sample test 1

Questions

1. What's the best unit of measure for identifying early shock in a trauma client?
[ ] **A.** Hemoglobin (Hb) and hematocrit (HCT)
[ ] **B.** Central venous pressure (CVP)
[ ] **C.** Blood pressure
[ ] **D.** Heart rate

2. Immediately after delivery of a neonate's head, the nurse should:
[ ] **A.** suction the airway.
[ ] **B.** feel for the umbilical cord around the neonate's neck.
[ ] **C.** stimulate the baby to cry.
[ ] **D.** deliver the upper shoulder.

3. Which statement regarding the outcome of reimplantation is true?
[ ] **A.** Reimplantation is less successful in guillotine injuries than in crush injuries.
[ ] **B.** The more distal the amputation, the more successful the chance of reimplantation.
[ ] **C.** Amputation reimplantation is more successful in adults than in children.
[ ] **D.** The outcome of reimplantation is the same whether the injury occurred on an oil-coated machine or a shard of glass.

4. What's the treatment for a client who has inhaled cyanide?
[ ] **A.** Administration of naloxone
[ ] **B.** Administration apomorphine (Apokyn) to perform gastric emptying
[ ] **C.** Administration of hydroxocobalamin
[ ] **D.** Administration of activated charcoal

5. What does the Consolidated Omnibus Budget Reconciliation Act of 1989 (COBRA) mandate for a client who comes to a hospital that doesn't offer the services required?
[ ] **A.** The client must be medically screened and stabilized before transport to another health care agency.
[ ] **B.** The client can be transferred to another facility, regardless of condition, before admission to the emergency department.
[ ] **C.** The COBRA mandate has no requirements regarding this situation.
[ ] **D.** The emergency department has the right to refuse clients whenever necessary.

6. Hypertensive crisis secondary to monoamine oxidase inhibitor use also results in:
[ ] **A.** hypothermia.
[ ] **B.** bradycardia.
[ ] **C.** hyperthermia.
[ ] **D.** heart block.

7. Neuroleptic malignant syndrome is characterized by:
[ ] **A.** hypothermia related to dopaminergic hypoactivity in the hypothalamus.
[ ] **B.** muscular rigidity, akinesia, agitation.
[ ] **C.** hyperpyrexia, bradycardia, hypotension.
[ ] **D.** hyperpyrexia, diaphoresis, hypotension.

8. Continuous nitroglycerin infusion is indicated for the management of which condition?
[ ] **A.** Increased intracranial pressure (ICP)
[ ] **B.** Cerebral hemorrhage
[ ] **C.** Head trauma
[ ] **D.** Pulmonary edema

9. Which communication technique is most effective when interacting with an anxious client?
[ ] **A.** Silence
[ ] **B.** Active listening
[ ] **C.** Questioning
[ ] **D.** Verbalizing support

10. What should be given to the client who has taken an overdose of a beta-adrenergic blocker?
[ ] **A.** Lidocaine
[ ] **B.** Glucagon
[ ] **C.** Dextrose 50% in water ($D_{50}W$)
[ ] **D.** Bretylium

11. Triage is effective when an infant with a glassy stare is classified as:
[ ] **A.** acutely ill and categorized emergent.
[ ] **B.** not acutely ill and categorized nonurgent.
[ ] **C.** acutely ill and categorized urgent.
[ ] **D.** acutely ill and categorized nonurgent.

12. Increased intracranial pressure (ICP) can occur in the presence of a head injury, brain lesion, stroke, or other neurological disorder. What can be done to help reduce ICP?
[ ] **A.** Place the client in Trendelenburg's position.
[ ] **B.** Encourage the client to use a pillow to splint coughing.
[ ] **C.** Place a pillow under the client's legs.
[ ] **D.** Elevate the head of the bed by 40 degrees.

13. What are the expected compensatory cardiovascular mechanisms in response to shock?
[ ] **A.** Increased pulse rate and increased contractility of the heart
[ ] **B.** Decreased pulse rate and increased contractility of the heart
[ ] **C.** Increased pulse rate and decreased contractility of the heart
[ ] **D.** Decreased pulse rate and decreased contractility of the heart

14. What's the most commonly reported physical abnormality resulting from critical incident stress?
[ ] **A.** Appetite loss
[ ] **B.** Sleep disturbance
[ ] **C.** Intimacy loss
[ ] **D.** Fatigue

15. Successful fluid replacement in a 2-year-old child is evidenced by which urine output level?
[ ] **A.** 0.5 to 1 mL/kg/hour
[ ] **B.** 0.75 to 1.5 mL/kg/hour
[ ] **C.** 1 to 2 mL/kg/hour
[ ] **D.** 3 to 5 mL/kg/hour

16. Turner's sign, found on physical assessment, is indicative of:
[ ] **A.** retroperitoneal hemorrhage.
[ ] **B.** mediastinal bleeding.
[ ] **C.** increased intracranial pressure (ICP).
[ ] **D.** splenic injury.

17. A client who has suffered brain death with neurogenic diabetes insipidus will develop:
[ ] **A.** hypernatremia, hyperkalemia, hyperosmolar serum, hyposmolar urine.
[ ] **B.** hypernatremia, hypokalemia, hyperosmolar serum and urine.
[ ] **C.** hyponatremia, hyperkalemia, hyposmolar serum and urine.
[ ] **D.** hypernatremia, hypokalemia, hyperosmolar serum, hyposmolar urine.

18. A 4-year-old child with severe respiratory distress requires intubation and mechanical ventilation. Which endotracheal (ET) tube is the appropriate size for a child this age?
[ ] **A.** 3 mm
[ ] **B.** 4 mm
[ ] **C.** 5 mm
[ ] **D.** 6 mm

19. An electrocardiogram is performed and shows ST elevation in leads II, III, and aV_f. The myocardial infarction (MI) is occurring in which part of the heart?
[ ] **A.** Anterior wall
[ ] **B.** Inferior wall
[ ] **C.** Posterior wall
[ ] **D.** Lateral wall

20. After heart transplantation, what's the usual presenting sign or symptom of acute myocardial infarction?
[ ] **A.** Substernal chest pain
[ ] **B.** Heart failure
[ ] **C.** Tachycardia
[ ] **D.** Jaw pain

21. After an industrial accident, a client with a laceration to the hand and wrist comes to the triage area. Assessment priority should be directed toward:
[ ] **A.** tetanus immunization status.
[ ] **B.** time of last oral intake.
[ ] **C.** presence of industrial contaminants.
[ ] **D.** neurovascular status of injured extremity.

22. The physician orders a continuous infusion of epinephrine 1 mg in 250 mL of dextrose 5% in water (D_5W) by way of infusion pump at 125 mcg/minute. What's the infusion rate in milliliters per hour (assuming the use of microdrip 60 gtt/mL tubing)?
[ ] **A.** 15 mL/hour
[ ] **B.** 19 mL/hour
[ ] **C.** 23 mL/hour
[ ] **D.** 31 mL/hour

23. A client comes to the emergency department complaining of rapid heartbeat, shortness of breath, and syncope. Cardiac monitoring shows supraventricular tachycardia. Vital signs reveal pulse, 164 beats/minute; blood pressure, 80/50 mm Hg; and respirations, 28 breaths/minute. I.V. access is established and oxygen is administered. The emergency department nurse should anticipate an order for:
[ ] **A.** digoxin (Lanoxin).
[ ] **B.** diltiazem (Cardizem).
[ ] **C.** bretylium.
[ ] **D.** adenosine (Adenocard).

24. Classic signs of increased intracranial pressure (ICP) include all of the following *except:*
[ ] **A.** widening pulse pressure.
[ ] **B.** tachycardia.
[ ] **C.** altered level of consciousness (LOC).
[ ] **D.** bradycardia.

25. A client comes to the emergency department complaining of left calf pain that occurs during his morning walk each day. He states that the pain disappears with rest. Which condition should the emergency department nurse suspect?
[ ] **A.** Claudication
[ ] **B.** Compartment syndrome
[ ] **C.** Muscle cramps
[ ] **D.** Deep vein thrombosis

26. Which nursing intervention is appropriate for a sudden cardiac death survivor?
[ ] **A.** Notifying the client's support system, including family, friends, and clergy
[ ] **B.** Making decisions for the client and encouraging the client to rest
[ ] **C.** Providing the client with privacy so that he can reflect on the situation
[ ] **D.** Discussing advance directive information immediately after the event

27. Rhabdomyolysis is caused by muscle damage and the subsequent release of myoglobin into the circulatory system. Which of the following results would you expect to see in rhabdomyolysis?
[ ] **A.** Dark brown urine, decreased serum creatine kinase, and hyperkalemia
[ ] **B.** Elevated serum creatine kinase, dark brown urine, and positive Kernig's sign
[ ] **C.** Hyperkalemia, dark brown urine, and elevated serum creatine kinase
[ ] **D.** Hyperkalemia, decreased serum creatine kinase, and dark brown urine

28. Which device best ensures continued correct placement of an endotracheal tube for a client being transported to the emergency department by helicopter?
[ ] **A.** Cardiac monitor
[ ] **B.** Electronic end-tidal carbon dioxide detector
[ ] **C.** Pulse oximeter
[ ] **D.** Laryngoscope

29. Bradycardia and atrioventricular (AV) node conduction disturbances are most commonly associated with:
[ ] **A.** cardiogenic shock.
[ ] **B.** anterior wall infarction.
[ ] **C.** inferior wall infarction.
[ ] **D.** heart failure.

30. Which tissue pressure measurement is indicative of compartment syndrome?
[ ] **A.** 5 to 10 mm Hg
[ ] **B.** 10 to 20 mm Hg
[ ] **C.** 20 to 30 mm Hg
[ ] **D.** 30 to 40 mm Hg

31. Parkinson's disease occurs because of degeneration of which part of the brain?
[ ] **A.** Temporal lobe
[ ] **B.** Pituitary gland
[ ] **C.** Basal ganglia
[ ] **D.** Medulla

32. The following clients come to the emergency department for treatment after a building explosion and collapse. Which client should receive priority care?
[ ] **A.** A 17-year-old with an open head injury, a Glasgow Coma Scale of 3, fixed and dilated pupils, a pulse rate of 140 beats/minute, and a blood pressure of 60 mm Hg on palpation
[ ] **B.** A 32-year-old with several facial lacerations who's otherwise stable with a Glasgow Coma Scale of 15
[ ] **C.** A 43-year-old with a severed left leg, controlled bleeding at the severance site, a pulse rate of 138 beats/minute, a respiratory rate of 32 breaths/minute, and a blood pressure of 88/64 mm Hg
[ ] **D.** An unresponsive 68-year-old who arrives with third-degree burns over 95% of her body and a blood pressure of 60 mm Hg on palpation

33. A nitroprusside (Nitropress) drip is prepared by mixing 50 mg of the drug in 250 mL of dextrose 5% in water (D_5W). The nurse is instructed to administer 3 mcg/kg/minute. The client weighs 89 kg. Which drip rate is correct (the drip factor of the pump tubing is 60 gtt/mL)?
[ ] **A.** 10 mL/hour
[ ] **B.** 32 mL/hour
[ ] **C.** 75 mL/hour
[ ] **D.** 80 mL/hour

34. Which statement about the principles of disaster documentation is true?
[ ] **A.** Always use small disaster tags so that they can remain with the client throughout his stay in the emergency department.
[ ] **B.** Have as many carbon copies as possible on the tag so that they can be used to update the command post instead of verbally communicating.
[ ] **C.** Maintain record-keeping and charting as close to day-to-day operations as possible.
[ ] **D.** Documentation on forms specific for disaster situations should be used.

35. Which statement by a client indicates an understanding of genital herpes treatment?
[ ] **A.** "As long as I am taking the acyclovir (Zovirax) I can continue sexual activity."
[ ] **B.** "I'll share my prescription for acyclovir with my partner."
[ ] **C.** "I know that lesions may be getting ready to erupt if I have itching and a tingling sensation in the vaginal area."
[ ] **D.** "I need to douche twice a day for the next week with Betadine and water."

36. Kawasaki disease is manifested by which sign?
[ ] **A.** Erythema of the palms and soles
[ ] **B.** Butterfly rash
[ ] **C.** Exophthalmos
[ ] **D.** Koplik's spots

37. A 13-year-old male enters the emergency department after waking up with sudden onset of abdominal pain. His mother reports that the pain is so bad that it has caused the client to vomit. On physical examination, he is noted to have redness and edema in his scrotum. What diagnosis should be ruled out as soon as possible?
[ ] **A.** Epididymitis
[ ] **B.** Testicular torsion
[ ] **C.** Priapism
[ ] **D.** Chlamydia

38. Expected outcomes for a family after a sudden infant death syndrome (SIDS) diagnosis include all of the following *except:*
[ ] **A.** verbalizing positive memories of the infant.
[ ] **B.** accepting a referral for a SIDS support group.
[ ] **C.** verbalizing concerns about the cause of death.
[ ] **D.** verbalizing that the baby may have smothered or choked to death.

39. Which isn't indicative of a positive peritoneal lavage?
[ ] **A.** Aspiration of 10 mL of gross blood
[ ] **B.** Presence of intestinal contents
[ ] **C.** Return of fluid that doesn't contain blood or white blood cells
[ ] **D.** Return of cloudy fluid

40. A client comes to the emergency department (ED) complaining of substernal chest pain. Cardiac monitoring reveals sinus bradycardia with uniform premature ventricular contractions. After a saline lock has been started, the client becomes unresponsive. The monitor reveals ventricular fibrillation. The ED nurse defibrillates the client at 200 joules, 300 joules, and 360 joules. The client remains in ventricular fibrillation. Cardiopulmonary resuscitation is initiated. The client is intubated by the physician. What's the next action?
[ ] **A.** Defibrillate at 360 joules.
[ ] **B.** Administer epinephrine 1 mg I.V.
[ ] **C.** Administer lidocaine 15 mg/kg I.V.
[ ] **D.** Administer sodium bicarbonate 1 mEq/kg I.V.

41. The decision to transfer a client should be based on all of the following *except:*
[ ] **A.** written policies of the emergency department.
[ ] **B.** medical insurance approval.
[ ] **C.** need for a specialized unit.
[ ] **D.** need for a specialized procedure.

42. A client who's experiencing a situational crisis comes to the emergency department (ED). The ED nurse should:
[ ] **A.** obtain an order to administer anti-anxiety medication such as diazepam (Valium).
[ ] **B.** encourage verbalization of feelings, give emotional support, and initiate health-related teaching.
[ ] **C.** orient the client to reality (person, place, and time) and apply safety restraints.
[ ] **D.** insist that the client identify the precipitating factors and his emotional response to the event.

43. Tetany results when pathogenic organisms are introduced into human tissue. Which bacteria are responsible for this disease?
[ ] **A.** *Pasteurella multocida*
[ ] **B.** *Clostridium*
[ ] **C.** *Enterobacter*
[ ] **D.** *Streptococcus*

44. When evaluating the care of a client with bipolar disease in the emergency department (ED), what's the priority determination?
[ ] **A.** The client's thought process was organized before discharge.
[ ] **B.** The client was safe in the ED environment and was able to verbalize the appropriate use of lithium (Lithonate) on discharge.
[ ] **C.** The client's nutritional status was evaluated.
[ ] **D.** The client's auditory hallucinations had subsided before discharge.

45. After falling 20′ (6 m) from a platform, a client is admitted to the emergency department. He's complaining of chest pain that radiates to the back. Chest X-rays show widening of the mediastinum. What do these symptoms probably represent?
[ ] **A.** Ruptured hemidiaphragm
[ ] **B.** Pneumothorax
[ ] **C.** Ruptured trachea
[ ] **D.** Ruptured aorta

46. A client arrives in the emergency department and is placed on the electrocardiograph. Identify the rhythm.

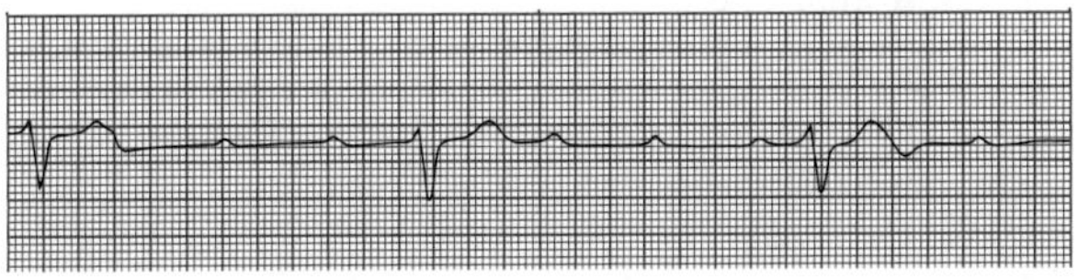

[ ] **A.** Idioventricular
[ ] **B.** Third-degree heart block
[ ] **C.** Sinus bradycardia
[ ] **D.** Wenckebach

47. Which of the following may cause a child to become fatigued during increased work of breathing?
[ ] **A.** Increased residual capacity
[ ] **B.** Increased tidal volumes
[ ] **C.** Lower glucose stores than an adult
[ ] **D.** Decreased metabolic demands

48. What's the most common cause of retinal detachment?
[ ] **A.** Degenerative changes in elderly clients
[ ] **B.** Direct trauma associated with sports activities
[ ] **C.** Blunt trauma from assault to the eye
[ ] **D.** Hereditary factors

49. Which equipment will be prepared for use before the transport of a conscious burn client?
[ ] **A.** An ice container for irrigation saline
[ ] **B.** A cooling blanket
[ ] **C.** An end-tidal carbon dioxide detector
[ ] **D.** An I.V. infusion pump

50. Which symptom distinguishes myocardial contusion from angina?
[ ] **A.** Chest pain that isn't affected by coronary vasodilators
[ ] **B.** Arrhythmias
[ ] **C.** Hypotension, distended jugular veins, and muffled heart sounds
[ ] **D.** Electrocardiogram (ECG) changes

51. A dystonic reaction can be caused by which medication?
[ ] **A.** Diazepam (Valium)
[ ] **B.** Haloperidol
[ ] **C.** Amitriptyline
[ ] **D.** Clonazepam (Klonopin)

52. A 3-year-old child weighing 15 kg is brought to the emergency department after being found floating in a pond. Initially, the child's electrocardiogram shows ventricular fibrillation. What's the appropriate initial energy level for defibrillation of this client?
[ ] **A.** 15 joules
[ ] **B.** 30 joules
[ ] **C.** 100 joules
[ ] **D.** 200 joules

53. Before administering a chelating drug to a client with heavy metal poisoning, the nurse should include which priority nursing assessment?
[ ] **A.** Level of consciousness (LOC)
[ ] **B.** Respiratory status
[ ] **C.** Urine output
[ ] **D.** Blood pressure

54. During an unusually busy day in the emergency department, the following clients come to the triage nurse within a 6-minute period. One bed is available for examinations. Which client should take priority?
[ ] **A.** A 13-year-old male with groin pain that was more severe $1\frac{1}{2}$ hours ago
[ ] **B.** A 58-year-old male with urgency and hesitancy to urinate; onset was 6 hours ago
[ ] **C.** A 27-year-old female with severe bilateral lower abdominal pain
[ ] **D.** A 42-year-old female with flank pain, fever, nausea, and vomiting

55. A client comes to the emergency department (ED) complaining of a sudden onset of chest pain that increases with deep breathing and when lying flat. The pain decreases somewhat when sitting up and leaning forward. Vital signs are blood pressure, 100/60 mm Hg; pulse, 100 beats/minute; respirations, 22 breaths/minute; and temperature, 103.4° F (39° C). Which condition should the ED nurse suspect?
[ ] **A.** Myocardial infarction (MI)
[ ] **B.** Pleurisy
[ ] **C.** Pericarditis
[ ] **D.** Endocarditis

56. Why should Allen's test be performed before the insertion of an arterial line?
[ ] **A.** To ensure that the monitor has been zeroed correctly
[ ] **B.** To ensure that collateral circulation to the hand is adequate
[ ] **C.** To ensure that no phlebitis is present in the radial artery
[ ] **D.** To ensure that the transducer is at the level of the right atrium

57. An 80-kg hypertensive client is ordered nitroprusside (Nitropress) to infuse at 5 mcg/kg/minute by way of an infusion pump. The concentration is 100 mg in 250 mL of dextrose 5% in water. What's the infusion rate in milliliters per hour (assuming the use of microdrip 60 gtt/mL tubing)?
[ ] **A.** 53 mL/hour
[ ] **B.** 56 mL/hour
[ ] **C.** 60 mL/hour
[ ] **D.** 70 mL/hour

58. Prolonged seizure activity can result in:
[ ] **A.** hyperglycemia.
[ ] **B.** alkalosis.
[ ] **C.** hypothermia.
[ ] **D.** acidosis.

59. A client with an insect in his left ear comes to the emergency department. What's the most effective way to remove the insect?
[ ] **A.** Irrigate the ear with copious amounts of water.
[ ] **B.** Using an ear speculum to visualize the insect, gently grasp and remove it using forceps.
[ ] **C.** Instill mineral oil or alcohol into the ear canal.
[ ] **D.** Instill hydrogen peroxide into the ear.

60. At which point is the client owed a duty of care?
[ ] **A.** At the time of arrival at the emergency department (ED)
[ ] **B.** After admission to the ED
[ ] **C.** After the physician has examined the client and found an emergency condition
[ ] **D.** At the time a treatment plan has been established

61. Which are the most common early systemic signs of septic shock?
[ ] **A.** Hyperthermia, tachycardia, wide pulse pressure, tachypnea, respiratory alkalosis, and mental obtundation
[ ] **B.** Hypothermia, bradycardia, narrow pulse pressure, tachypnea, respiratory acidosis, and coma
[ ] **C.** Hypothermia, tachycardia, narrow pulse pressure, tachypnea, respiratory alkalosis, and confusion
[ ] **D.** Hyperthermia, bradycardia, wide pulse pressure, tachypnea, respiratory acidosis, and mental obtundation

62. Hyperflexion of the upper extremities and hyperextension of the lower extremities are described as:
[ ] **A.** decortication.
[ ] **B.** hypotonia.
[ ] **C.** spasticity.
[ ] **D.** decerebration.

63. Which injury is most consistent with shaken baby syndrome?
[ ] **A.** Bilateral arm fractures
[ ] **B.** Basilar skull fractures
[ ] **C.** Retinal hemorrhages
[ ] **D.** Petechiae on the trunk

64. Achieving which prothrombin time (PT) is the goal of warfarin (Coumadin) therapy?
[ ] **A.** Equal to that of the control
[ ] **B.** Less than that of the control
[ ] **C.** $1\frac{1}{2}$ times that of the control
[ ] **D.** Three times that of the control

65. What's an appropriate treatment for a client with a diagnosis of herpes?
[ ] **A.** Decrease fluid intake.
[ ] **B.** Insert an indwelling urinary catheter.
[ ] **C.** Keep lesions moist.
[ ] **D.** Apply tight-fitting Dacron undergarments.

66. Irritation of the vagal centers in the medulla produces:
[ ] **A.** vomiting.
[ ] **B.** headache.
[ ] **C.** papilledema.
[ ] **D.** restlessness and irritability.

67. When an error in documentation is made in the medical record, how should the error be corrected?
[ ] **A.** Tear out the sheet with the error and recopy all the information on a new sheet, make the correct entry, and initial the sheet to indicate that it's a copy.
[ ] **B.** Apply correction fluid over the error and record the correct information over it.
[ ] **C.** Draw a single line through the incorrect entry, date the error and initial it, and give the reason for the error.
[ ] **D.** Scribble through the incorrect information as well as possible and then make the correct entry.

68. During cardiopulmonary resuscitation (CPR), it is suggested that the end-tidal carbon dioxide ($ETCO_2$) be maintained at what level to ensure adequate placement of the endotracheal tube?
[ ] **A.** Less than 10 mm Hg
[ ] **B.** Between 10 mm Hg and 20 mm Hg
[ ] **C.** Between 20 mm HG and 30 mm Hg
[ ] **D.** Greater than 40 mm Hg

69. What's the antidote for heparin overdose?
[ ] **A.** Fresh frozen plasma
[ ] **B.** Dimercaprol (BAL In Oil)
[ ] **C.** Naloxone
[ ] **D.** Protamine sulfate

70. What's the primary treatment for a client who complains of back pain?
[ ] **A.** Rest
[ ] **B.** Cold applications
[ ] **C.** Weight loss
[ ] **D.** Stretching exercises

71. Which diagnostic finding indicates the need for mechanical ventilation?
[ ] **A.** A partial pressure of arterial oxygen (PaO_2) of 80 mm Hg on room air
[ ] **B.** A vital capacity less than 10 mL/kg
[ ] **C.** A normal work of breathing
[ ] **D.** A partial pressure of arterial carbon dioxide ($PaCO_2$) of 42 mm Hg

72. What's an essential part of the emergency department record for the client discharged home?
[ ] **A.** Remarks of other personnel caring for the client
[ ] **B.** Discharge instructions and follow-up instructions
[ ] **C.** The client's comments regarding the care received
[ ] **D.** The apparent intellectual level of the client

73. An 18-year-old male arrives at the emergency department via EMS after being struck by a car while riding his motorcycle without a helmet. He was reported to have lost consciousness at the scene, but he is now awake and asking repetitive questions. Suddenly he loses consciousness and requires endotracheal intubation. A computed tomography (CT) scan shows diffuse blood located between the skull and dura mater with apparent shift. What is the likely differential diagnosis for this client?
[ ] **A.** Subdural hematoma
[ ] **B.** Concussion
[ ] **C.** Diffuse axonal injury
[ ] **D.** Epidural hematoma

74. What's a true statement about the responsibilities of the disaster committee?
[ ] **A.** The committee should review the disaster plan only after a disaster occurs.
[ ] **B.** The committee may disband after the disaster plan is developed or revised.
[ ] **C.** The committee needs to continually reevaluate and revise the disaster plan.
[ ] **D.** The committee should plan disaster exercises at times of low census to ensure maximum staff attendance.

75. After a motor vehicle accident, a client comes to the emergency department with an injury to the right leg. On physical assessment, the nurse notices that the client is unable to raise his leg when it is straightened and lacks sensation to the anterior thigh. Assessment of the left leg is normal. What's the possible cause of this finding?
[ ] **A.** Damage to the median nerve
[ ] **B.** Damage to the femoral nerve
[ ] **C.** Damage to the tibial nerve
[ ] **D.** Damage to the peroneal nerve

76. What's the earliest and most common respiratory alteration in a client with an intracranial injury?
[ ] **A.** Apneustic breathing
[ ] **B.** Biot's respirations
[ ] **C.** Cheyne-Stokes respirations
[ ] **D.** Cluster breathing

77. Preoperative antibiotic therapy in a client with an open fracture to the distal tibia will:
[ ] **A.** allow systemic prophylaxis in the event the wound is deeper than initially believed.
[ ] **B.** not do any good because the open wound is easily cleaned and debrided during surgery.
[ ] **C.** reach an effective blood concentration before or at the time of wound closure and, thus, limit the threat of infection.
[ ] **D.** work equally effectively if administered orally or I.V.

78. During a physical examination, which is the most characteristic finding in diagnosing asthma?
[ ] **A.** Dark circles under the eyes
[ ] **B.** Bluish, boggy nasal turbinates
[ ] **C.** Expiratory wheezing
[ ] **D.** Moist crackles

79. Initial treatment for the adult client with a severe anaphylactic reaction includes:
[ ] **A.** administration of diphenhydramine (Benadryl) 25 mg I.M.
[ ] **B.** administration of epinephrine .01 to .05 mg of a 1:1,000 solution.
[ ] **C.** administration of epinephrine .01 to .025 mg of a 1:10,000 solution.
[ ] **D.** administration of cimetadine (Tagamet) 300 mg I.V.

80. The nurse should seek clarification of which order for a 5-year-old child who has ingested a large amount of paint thinner?
[ ] **A.** Ipecac
[ ] **B.** Activated charcoal
[ ] **C.** Gastric lavage
[ ] **D.** Oxygen delivered at 2 L/minute

81. It's important to assess which of the following in the client receiving magnesium sulfate?
[ ] **A.** Urine output, respirations, reflexes
[ ] **B.** Urine output, reflexes, vaginal bleeding
[ ] **C.** Urine output, reflexes
[ ] **D.** Vaginal bleeding and reflexes

82. Honeybees and bumblebees cause a painful wound with swelling and intense itching. What's true about the treatment of these stings?
[ ] **A.** Heat should be applied to the sting area.
[ ] **B.** Removal of the stinger is done by scraping the area with a dull object.
[ ] **C.** Removal of the stinger is accomplished by grasping the stinger and pulling it away from the skin.
[ ] **D.** Ice should be applied and the extremity lowered below the heart.

83. During client assessment, the nurse finds the client's pupils to be pinpoint. What might this indicate?
[ ] **A.** Opioid overdose
[ ] **B.** Midbrain damage
[ ] **C.** Severe anoxia
[ ] **D.** Previous cataract surgery

84. Symptoms suggesting a scabies infestation include:
[ ] **A.** raised, scaly, round patches with relatively flat centers on the hands, feet, trunk, and groin.
[ ] **B.** pink macular rash over palms, soles, hands, feet, wrists, and ankles.
[ ] **C.** pruritus that intensifies at night.
[ ] **D.** generalized urticaria.

85. Which statement indicates a lack of understanding of long leg cast and extremity care?
[ ] **A.** "I'll keep the cast dry."
[ ] **B.** "If a foreign object drops into the cast, I'll attempt to retrieve it before calling my follow-up care provider."
[ ] **C.** "I'll wiggle my toes at least once each hour."
[ ] **D.** "I'll keep my leg elevated above the level of my heart for the next 24 hours."

86. A client with heavy vaginal bleeding after a spontaneous abortion is started on an oxytocin (Pitocin) infusion. Which of the following would indicate that the medication was effective?
[ ] **A.** Increased urine output
[ ] **B.** Cessation of bleeding
[ ] **C.** Increased abdominal cramping
[ ] **D.** Increased heart rate

87. What's the initial biologic response to new wounds?
[ ] **A.** Inflammation
[ ] **B.** Hemostasis
[ ] **C.** Cell proliferation
[ ] **D.** Scar formation

88. A 33-year-old client is dropped off at the front door of the emergency department with a single gun shot wound to his back. On physical examination, the client reports ipsilateral paresis and loss of motor function on the right side and decreased sensation on the left. What's the most likely diagnosis for this client?
[ ] **A.** Brown-Sequard syndrome
[ ] **B.** Central cord syndrome
[ ] **C.** Anterior cord syndrome
[ ] **D.** Posterior cord syndrome

89. Priority treatment for a client with suspected blunt abdominal trauma includes:
[ ] **A.** inserting two large-bore I.V. lines, administering 2 units of blood, and inserting an indwelling urinary catheter.
[ ] **B.** securing the airway, obtaining a toxicologic screen, and administering tetanus toxoid.
[ ] **C.** obtaining chest and cervical spine X-rays and inserting two large-bore I.V. lines.
[ ] **D.** securing the airway, inserting two large-bore I.V. lines, and obtaining a type and crossmatch for 6 units of blood.

90. What's the priority nursing intervention in a client presenting with a suspected pelvic fracture?
[ ] **A.** Placing and inflating the pneumatic antishock garment
[ ] **B.** Administering pain medication
[ ] **C.** Preparing for an X-ray
[ ] **D.** Administering high-flow oxygen

91. A client receiving beta-adrenergic blockers shows which responses to a shock state?
[ ] **A.** Increased pulse rate and hypotension
[ ] **B.** Bradycardia, hypotension, and decreased renin secretion
[ ] **C.** Increased pulse rate and hypertension
[ ] **D.** Bradycardia and hypertension

92. A client is admitted to the emergency department complaining of blurred vision and moderate left eye pain. Physical examination reveals a hazy cornea and a small, irregular pupil with sluggish reaction on the left. Which ocular impairment is the most likely?
[ ] **A.** Conjunctivitis
[ ] **B.** Glaucoma
[ ] **C.** Iritis
[ ] **D.** Central retinal artery occlusion

93. A client comes to the emergency department after slicing his wrist on a piece of steel while at work. How is extensor tendon function assessed?
[ ] **A.** Instructing the client to push downward and upward against resistance with all five digits
[ ] **B.** Instructing the client to abduct and adduct his fingers without finger flexion
[ ] **C.** Instructing the client to oppose his thumb to his little finger
[ ] **D.** Testing sensation over the dorsal surface of the thumb and index, second, and middle fingers

94. The client is provided discharge instructions regarding corneal abrasions. Which statement would assure the nurse that the client understands the instructions?
[ ] **A.** "I should be able to remove the eye patch after 1 hour."
[ ] **B.** "I should return to be checked in 1 week."
[ ] **C.** "The pain should be relieved within a few hours without medications."
[ ] **D.** "I'll need to see a physician tomorrow."

95. Which signs make up Beck's triad in cardiac tamponade?
[ ] **A.** Hypotension, dyspnea, and tracheal deviation
[ ] **B.** Hypotension, muffled heart sounds, and distended neck veins
[ ] **C.** Muffled heart sounds, dyspnea, and hypotension
[ ] **D.** Distended neck veins, dyspnea, and tracheal deviation

96. What's the minimum acceptable oxygen delivery mode for an unconscious multisystem trauma client under the influence of alcohol?
[ ] **A.** Simple face mask delivering 50% oxygen at 8 to 10 L/minute
[ ] **B.** Nasal cannula delivering 44% oxygen at 6 L/minute
[ ] **C.** Endotracheal intubation with bag valve mask device delivering oxygen at 100%
[ ] **D.** Nonrebreather mask delivering 90% oxygen at 15 L/minute

97. Which measure should the nurse focus on in a client with esophageal varices?
[ ] **A.** Recognizing hemorrhage
[ ] **B.** Controlling blood pressure
[ ] **C.** Encouraging nutritional intake
[ ] **D.** Teaching the client about esophageal varices

98. Therapeutic hypothermia has been shown to improve neurological outcomes in clients after cardiac arrest. Which of the following clients would be excluded from the therapeutic hypothermia protocol?
[ ] **A.** A 19-year-old who has experienced sudden cardiac arrest after complaining of dizziness while playing basketball
[ ] **B.** A 57-year-old male who was witnessed by family to have facial droop and difficulty speaking prior to his cardiac arrest
[ ] **C.** A 68-year-old female who collapsed after reporting to coworkers that she was having severe chest pain
[ ] **D.** A 62-year-old male who had sudden cardiac arrest and is known to be a two-pack-per-day smoker with a history of hypertension

99. A client involved in a motor vehicle accident complains of right shoulder pain when lying flat. Examination reveals right upper quadrant guarding. Vital signs are blood pressure, 90/50 mm Hg; pulse, 130 beats/minute; respirations, 26 breaths/minute; and temperature, 98° F (36° C). Chest X-ray reveals rib fractures in the lower right chest. The nurse should suspect injury to which organ?
[ ] **A.** Spleen
[ ] **B.** Colon
[ ] **C.** Pancreas
[ ] **D.** Liver

100. What isn't a physical finding consistent with acute cholecystitis?
[ ] **A.** Fever
[ ] **B.** Right upper quadrant tenderness
[ ] **C.** Positive Murphy's sign
[ ] **D.** Kehr's sign

101. A client arrives at the emergency department after falling from a horse. The computed tomography scan reveals a fracture at C6 with transection of the cord. Which of the following symptoms would you expect?
[ ] **A.** Hypotension and bradycardia
[ ] **B.** Hypertension and bradycardia
[ ] **C.** Hypotension and tachycardia
[ ] **D.** Hypertension and tachycardia

102. What's the initial intervention in caring for a child with pertussis?
[ ] **A.** Control fever with antipyretics.
[ ] **B.** Institute isolation measures.
[ ] **C.** Administer antibiotics.
[ ] **D.** Initiate seizure precautions.

103. A woman who's 30 weeks pregnant is brought to the emergency department after a motor vehicle accident. She's complaining of constant, severe abdominal pain. Examination reveals a rigid uterus and no vaginal bleeding. Vital signs are blood pressure, 90/58 mm Hg; pulse, 140 beats/minute; respirations, 32 breaths/minute; temperature, 99.2° F (37.3° C); and fetal heart sounds, 190 beats/minute. The nurse should suspect:
[ ] **A.** placenta previa.
[ ] **B.** abruptio placentae.
[ ] **C.** premature labor.
[ ] **D.** ruptured uterus.

104. A teenager is brought to the emergency department by his parents, who state that he has been smoking "ice" (the smokable form of methamphetamine). Which assessment finding indicates recent ingestion of an amphetamine?
[ ] **A.** Extreme self-confidence
[ ] **B.** Hypotension
[ ] **C.** Flushed skin
[ ] **D.** Fatigue

105. A client with acute angle-closure glaucoma is admitted to the emergency department. Signs and symptoms include acute eye pain, a fixed and slightly dilated pupil, a hard globe, a foggy-appearing cornea, nausea, vomiting, severe headache, halos around lights, and diminished peripheral vision. Which initial therapy is most appropriate for this client?
[ ] **A.** Instillation of pilocarpine eyedrops every 15 minutes
[ ] **B.** Preparation of client for an iridectomy
[ ] **C.** Preparation of client for an emergency trabeculectomy
[ ] **D.** Monitoring of intraocular pressure (IOP) and administration of cyclopegic eyedrops

106. The nurse should prepare to administer which cofactor to a client with methanol poisoning?
[ ] **A.** Folic acid
[ ] **B.** Thiamine
[ ] **C.** Pyridoxine
[ ] **D.** Calcium

107. A young adult comes to the emergency department triage desk complaining of blurred vision. Lid ptosis is present, and the nurse notes that ocular movement is limited. The client also complains of having some difficulty swallowing. Based on these findings, the nurse should specifically question the client about:
[ ] **A.** recent viral illnesses.
[ ] **B.** use of home-canned foods.
[ ] **C.** presence of numbness or tingling.
[ ] **D.** recent travel.

108. A client with a history of alcohol abuse and cirrhosis comes to the emergency department (ED). The client is vomiting large amounts of bright red blood and is poorly responsive. Vital signs are blood pressure, 80/50 mm Hg; pulse, 140 beats/minute; respirations, 36 breaths/minute; and temperature, 99.8° F (37.7° C). What should the ED nurse do first?
[ ] **A.** Suction blood from the airway.
[ ] **B.** Insert two large-bore I.V. lines.
[ ] **C.** Insert a nasogastric tube.
[ ] **D.** Administer fresh frozen plasma.

109. Labetalol (Normodyne) is ordered for a client with acute cocaine overdose. The nurse should evaluate the client's response to the drug by observing for which sign?
[ ] **A.** Normalization of temperature
[ ] **B.** Lowering of blood pressure
[ ] **C.** Absence of seizures
[ ] **D.** Increase in pupil size

110. A client with multiple facial injuries and suspected cervical spine injuries develops severe respiratory distress. Jaw thrust maneuvers are unsuccessful in improving the client's respiratory effort. What's the least desirable method for establishing an airway in this client?
[ ] **A.** Orotracheal intubation
[ ] **B.** Nasotracheal intubation
[ ] **C.** Needle cricothyrotomy
[ ] **D.** Surgical cricothyrotomy

111. A woman is admitted to the emergency department with a 2-hour history of right lower quadrant pain, which is increasing in severity. She is nauseous and has been vomiting. She also has a 7-day history of moderate vaginal bleeding. Which of the following indicates a strong suspicion for an ovarian cyst?
[ ] **A.** Elevated white blood cell (WBC) count
[ ] **B.** Decreased hemoglobin (Hb)
[ ] **C.** Elevated human chorionic gonadotropin (HCG) levels
[ ] **D.** Decreased calcium level

112. What's the main priority in the care of the client with acute pancreatitis?
[ ] **A.** Pain control
[ ] **B.** Nutritional support
[ ] **C.** Causal correction
[ ] **D.** Fluid resuscitation

113. A client is diagnosed with influenza A (H1N1). Which type of precautions should be taken when caring for this client?
[ ] **A.** Airborne isolation precautions
[ ] **B.** Contact precautions
[ ] **C.** Neutropenic precautions
[ ] **D.** Universal precautions

114. A client who experiences hypothermia will have a decrease in oxygen consumption and an increase in the production of carbon dioxide. The respiratory response to hypothermia would include which of the following?
[ ] **A.** Bronchodilatation to allow an increase in oxygen consumption
[ ] **B.** Decrease in ciliary function
[ ] **C.** Decrease in the rate and depth of respirations
[ ] **D.** Oxyhemoglobin dissociation curve shifts to the right

115. The Emergency Medical Treatment and Active Labor Act (EMTALA) was passed in 1986 to ensure access to emergency care regardless of an individual's ability to pay. Before a client is transferred to another facility, all of the following must occur *except*:
[ ] **A.** identification of the client's primary physician.
[ ] **B.** triage by a nurse.
[ ] **C.** a medical screening exam by an independent practitioner.
[ ] **D.** registration.

116. A 12-year-old child is brought to the emergency department by his mother. The child has had a rash over his entire body and inside his mouth for 1 day. The client also has a sore throat, headache, cough, and a low-grade fever of 100.8° F (38.2° C). Based on these findings, the physician makes a preliminary diagnosis of:
[ ] **A.** scarlet fever.
[ ] **B.** fifth disease.
[ ] **C.** rubella.
[ ] **D.** roseola infantum.

117. Which treatment is appropriate for a client with central retinal artery occlusion?
[ ] **A.** Performing the Valsalva maneuver
[ ] **B.** Surgical decompression
[ ] **C.** Avoiding ocular massage
[ ] **D.** Monitoring closely until symptoms present, followed by surgical intervention

118. Which lung sound requires immediate nursing intervention?
[ ] **A.** Crackles
[ ] **B.** Rhonchi
[ ] **C.** Stridor
[ ] **D.** Wheezing

119. A client involved in a motor vehicle accident arrives in the emergency department complaining of severe abdominal pain. Vital signs are blood pressure, 100/50 mm Hg; pulse, 120 beats/minute; respirations, 28 breaths/minute; and temperature, 98.9° F (37.2° C). Chest X-ray reveals right rib fractures. The nurse should most strongly suspect:
[ ] **A.** splenic injury.
[ ] **B.** perforated stomach.
[ ] **C.** pancreatic injury.
[ ] **D.** lacerated liver.

120. Chemical burns constitute a true ocular emergency. Which assessment finding is consistent with a chemical burn?
[ ] **A.** Corneal whitening
[ ] **B.** Dilated, nonreactive pupils
[ ] **C.** Redness with purulent discharge
[ ] **D.** Corneal irregularity with luster

121. A 64-year-old male presents to the triage nurse with shortness of breath and productive cough; he's using pursed-lip breathing. The client states that he has smoked $2\frac{1}{2}$ packs of cigarettes per day for the past 44 years and has been told that he has chronic obstructive pulmonary disease (COPD). Which diagnosis is considered a COPD?
[ ] **A.** Asthma
[ ] **B.** Emphysema
[ ] **C.** Bronchiectasis
[ ] **D.** Heart failure

122. Septic shock frequently causes which condition in children?
[ ] **A.** Hyperglycemia
[ ] **B.** Metabolic alkalosis
[ ] **C.** Hypoglycemia
[ ] **D.** Hypercalcemia

123. A woman arrives in the emergency department complaining of a 2-week history of lower abdominal and pelvic pain and a yellowish, foul-smelling vaginal discharge. Her pain is increasing. Vital signs are blood pressure, 94/60 mm Hg; pulse, 120 beats/minute; respirations, 28 breaths/minute; temperature, 101° F (38° C); pulse oximetry, 94% (on room air). Her white blood cell count is 16×10^3, hemoglobin level is 122 g/dL, and hematocrit is 38%. Which procedure shouldn't be performed?
[ ] **A.** Nasogastric (NG) tube insertion
[ ] **B.** Pelvic examination
[ ] **C.** Culdocentesis
[ ] **D.** Administration of I.V. fluids

124. Which X-ray finding is evident in a client with pancreatitis?
[ ] **A.** Free air under the diaphragm
[ ] **B.** Dilated loops of bowel
[ ] **C.** Sentinel loops of bowel
[ ] **D.** Abnormal air fluid levels in the bowel

125. Treatment for hyperkalemia includes:
[ ] **A.** administration of 10% glucose infusion with regular insulin.
[ ] **B.** administration of stored blood.
[ ] **C.** administration of calcium gluconate.
[ ] **D.** increasing the dose of a potassium-sparing diuretic in the client with impaired renal function.

126. A client with a sexually transmitted disease (STD) may have pain related to all of the following *except:*
[ ] **A.** dysuria.
[ ] **B.** discharge.
[ ] **C.** lesions.
[ ] **D.** pruritus.

127. Which of the following is associated with intestinal obstruction?
[ ] **A.** Distention, vomiting, and visible peristalsis
[ ] **B.** Right upper quadrant tenderness, fever, and jaundice
[ ] **C.** Abdominal free air, distention, and rebound tenderness
[ ] **D.** Nausea, abdominal mass, and bruit

128. Cellular function is abnormal during a shock state and results in which type of metabolism?
[ ] **A.** Aerobic metabolism
[ ] **B.** Metabolic alkalosis
[ ] **C.** Anaerobic metabolism
[ ] **D.** Metabolic acidosis

129. A trauma client who's in shock and has been diagnosed with a fractured pelvis and a lacerated spleen requires immediate blood replacement. Which type of blood should be administered?
[ ] **A.** O-positive packed red blood cells (RBCs)
[ ] **B.** O-negative packed RBCs
[ ] **C.** Type-specific, uncrossmatched packed RBCs
[ ] **D.** Typed and crossmatched packed RBCs

130. Arterial blood gas measurements for a trauma client are pH, 7.48; $PaCO_2$, 30 mm Hg; PaO_2, 84 mm Hg; HCO_3^-, 22 mEq/L. The client is in which metabolic state?
[ ] **A.** Metabolic acidosis
[ ] **B.** Respiratory alkalosis
[ ] **C.** Respiratory acidosis
[ ] **D.** Metabolic alkalosis

131. Which of the following determines whether reimplantation can occur?
[ ] **A.** Availability of a reimplantation team
[ ] **B.** Whether the amputated part is an upper or a lower extremity
[ ] **C.** Occupation of the client
[ ] **D.** Client's insurance status

132. Which drug should be administered when a client in septic shock develops bilateral pulmonary crackles and a third heart sound?
[ ] **A.** Nitroprusside
[ ] **B.** Nitroglycerin
[ ] **C.** Dopamine
[ ] **D.** Dobutamine

133. Which fracture type leads to severe complications in the pediatric client?
[ ] **A.** Open fracture
[ ] **B.** Closed fracture
[ ] **C.** Dislocation fracture
[ ] **D.** Epiphyseal growth plate fracture

134. An important intervention in treating open pneumothorax is covering the wound. This is accomplished with:
[ ] **A.** sterile saline-moistened gauze.
[ ] **B.** porous dressing taped on all four sides.
[ ] **C.** transparent nonporous dressing.
[ ] **D.** nonporous dressing taped on three sides.

135. Which of the following is associated with hepatitis A?
[ ] **A.** Left upper quadrant pain
[ ] **B.** Right upper quadrant pain
[ ] **C.** Dark, tarry stools
[ ] **D.** Hematuria

136. An emergency department nurse has made a serious medication error on a pediatric client. The nurse-manager spoke promptly with the nurse privately, asked for her version of the story, reviewed medication error prevention strategies, and helped the nurse inform peers of the problem that led to the error. The nurse-manager has provided:
[ ] **A.** constructive feedback.
[ ] **B.** emotional support.
[ ] **C.** recognition.
[ ] **D.** goal setting.

137. Major risk factors for developing a pulmonary embolus include all of the following *except*:
[ ] **A.** long bone fractures.
[ ] **B.** immobility.
[ ] **C.** pregnancy.
[ ] **D.** high cholesterol.

138. Which statement about applying a splint is true?
[ ] **A.** The splint must immobilize the joint above and below the injury.
[ ] **B.** A traction splint is used only for femur fractures.
[ ] **C.** The extremity must be readjusted so that it is in a neutral position before applying the splint.
[ ] **D.** Air splints are ideal for clients being transported by air because they cushion the client during the bumpy air ride.

139. The emergency department nurse should expect a client with severe burn injuries to have which electrolyte abnormalities in the immediate postburn phase?
[ ] **A.** Increased potassium, decreased sodium
[ ] **B.** Increased potassium, increased sodium
[ ] **C.** Decreased potassium, decreased sodium
[ ] **D.** Decreased potassium, increased sodium

140. What's a true statement about pelvic fractures?
[ ] **A.** Pelvic fractures usually involve only one fracture site.
[ ] **B.** Pelvic fractures are always stable.
[ ] **C.** Bleeding associated with a pelvic fracture is usually arterial.
[ ] **D.** Open pelvic fractures are associated with high mortality.

141. When introducing change to an emergency department, which tactic would increase acceptance?
[ ] **A.** Don't burden the staff with the responsibility for input in the planning phase.
[ ] **B.** Make several changes at once followed by a longer quiet phase with no changes.
[ ] **C.** Always explain the reason for change.
[ ] **D.** After carefully eliciting input from all staff, be firm and confident in presenting a final plan that should endure for the long term.

142. An adult is brought to the emergency department with a burn injury. He has partial-thickness burns to his entire chest, right arm, and right thigh. Which of the following is a fairly accurate estimate of the body surface area (BSA) that has been burned?
[ ] **A.** 18%
[ ] **B.** 27%
[ ] **C.** 36%
[ ] **D.** 45%

143. A client comes to the triage desk and complains of feeling like he's hungover. The symptoms have occurred for several mornings and go away as the day progresses. The client also states that other family members have similar symptoms. Which assessment question is most appropriate for the triage nurse to ask?
[ ] **A.** Has anyone at work had similar symptoms?
[ ] **B.** Do you own a car?
[ ] **C.** Do you use gas heat or appliances?
[ ] **D.** Have you had any numbness or tingling?

144. A 63-year-old male arrives at the triage desk complaining of severe pain in his left foot and ankle for several hours duration. There's no history of trauma, and upon examination, the foot and ankle are observed to be dusky, swollen, and extremely tender to touch. The client's vital signs reveal a temperature of 100.2° F (38.9° C) orally; pulse, 20 beats/minute; respirations, 24 breaths/minute; and blood pressure, 140/90 mm Hg. The client is evaluated for a diagnosis of gout. All of the following laboratory findings are consistent with a diagnosis of gout *except:*

[ ] **A.** serum uric acid level: 8 mg/dL.
[ ] **B.** white blood cell (WBC) count: 17,000/μL.
[ ] **C.** erythrocyte sedimentation rate (ESR): 18 mm/hour.
[ ] **D.** urine uric acid level: 900 mg/24-hour specimen.

145. Which drug would the nurse expect to be prescribed to treat a client's acute gout?

[ ] **A.** Colchicine
[ ] **B.** Allopurinol (Zyloprim)
[ ] **C.** Acetylsalicylic acid (ASA)
[ ] **D.** Probenecid

146. A client is diagnosed with acute pancreatitis. Which drug can be used to treat the severe pain?

[ ] **A.** Meperidine (Demerol)
[ ] **B.** Codeine
[ ] **C.** Morphine
[ ] **D.** Hydromorphone (Dilaudid)

147. Which of the following is synonymous with laceration (physical injury that results in an opening or break in the skin)?

[ ] **A.** Gash
[ ] **B.** Cut
[ ] **C.** Avulsion
[ ] **D.** Abrasion

148. What's a correct application of the client confidentiality requirements under the Health Insurance Portability Accountability Act (HIPAA)?

[ ] **A.** Only clients can pick up their filled prescriptions at a pharmacy if the order is called in.
[ ] **B.** Past medical records for clients must be stored in a secured place.
[ ] **C.** A client's name may not be called out loud in a public waiting room.
[ ] **D.** Triage sign-in sheets for the client's name and time of arrival breach confidentiality.

149. A client has been diagnosed with iritis. His discharge instructions should include:

[ ] **A.** normal saline irrigations.
[ ] **B.** cold eye compresses.
[ ] **C.** patching the affected eye.
[ ] **D.** the correct way to administer eye drops to prevent contamination and minimize systemic effects.

150. A client in the emergency department has been diagnosed with central renal artery occlusion (CRAO), after a sudden painless loss of vision in his right eye. What's the goal of treatment?

[ ] **A.** To regain light perception
[ ] **B.** To rule out risk factors for stroke
[ ] **C.** To administer thrombolytics to dissolve the clot
[ ] **D.** To dislodge the embolus by increasing the intravascular pressure in the artery and decreasing the intraocular pressure

151. Arterial and venous structures are most commonly injured in penetrating vascular trauma with the higher incidence in which type of injury?

[ ] **A.** Gunshot wound
[ ] **B.** Blunt trauma
[ ] **C.** Stab injury
[ ] **D.** Crushing injury

152. It's generally accepted that nerve repair in cases of missile injuries should be delayed especially in war times because:

[ ] **A.** the facility may not have enough trained staff to perform the procedure.
[ ] **B.** these injuries usually involve multiple contaminated wounds.
[ ] **C.** the procedure is too lengthy to perform during wartime.
[ ] **D.** military health coverage doesn't reimburse for this surgery.

153. A 54-year-old male with chest pain is brought to the emergency department. An electrocardiogram indicates the client is having an anterior myocardial infarction. Vital signs are blood pressure, 100/52 mm Hg; pulse, 80 beats/minute; respiratory rate, 20 breaths/minute; oxygen saturation, 100% on 2 L/nasal cannula. The decision is made to transfer him to a nearby hospital 10 miles away for cardiac catheterization. Based on the initial assessment of the client, which intervention is most important prior to transfer?
[ ] **A.** Intubation
[ ] **B.** I.V. access
[ ] **C.** Thrombolytic therapy
[ ] **D.** Chest X-ray

154. A client with an anterior myocardial infarction (MI) is being transferred to another hospital for a cardiac catheterization. In anticipation of the client's needs during transfer, which medication is the most useful to have available?
[ ] **A.** Calcium chloride
[ ] **B.** Morphine
[ ] **C.** Diazepam
[ ] **D.** Dextrose 50%

155. The emergency department (ED) nurses believe that they have inadequate staff for their current client census. What would be the most appropriate data for them to consider in preparing their request for additional staff?
[ ] **A.** ED client acuity and length-of-stay
[ ] **B.** Consensus of the physicians' and the nurses' opinions
[ ] **C.** Amount of nursing staff overtime and unfilled positions
[ ] **D.** Number and frequency of client complaints

156. A staff nurse is setting up a quality improvement project for the emergency department to have 100% compliance in consistent, thorough documentation of pain assessment after analgesic administration. What would be the best criterion for the nurse to choose as an outcome indicator?
[ ] **A.** The mandatory in-service is attended by 100% of the nursing staff.
[ ] **B.** An audit of department charts one month later reveals a 20% improvement in documentation.
[ ] **C.** Random selection from one nurse's charts showed complete documentation for that client.
[ ] **D.** The emergency department physicians unanimously agree that the documentation has improved.

157. While in the emergency department, a 65-year-old male client complains of increased shortness of breath, is diaphoretic, and states that he feels as if he's going to die. His vital signs are as follows: respiratory rate, 40 breaths/minute; pulse, 122 beats/minute; blood pressure, 170/100 mm Hg. He begins to expectorate pink frothy sputum from his lungs. Which of the following medications would be beneficial to this client?
[ ] **A.** Levophed
[ ] **B.** Dopamine
[ ] **C.** Dobutamine
[ ] **D.** Diltiazem (Cardizem)

158. What are the signs and symptoms of a wound infection?
[ ] **A.** Skin pale, white-blue in color, cool-to-cold to touch with swelling in the tissues
[ ] **B.** Skin red, hot-to-touch, with cordlike streak
[ ] **C.** Edema, erythema, exudate, induration, systemic fever
[ ] **D.** Skin black and cold

159. An infected wound is often closed by which of the following?
[ ] **A.** Primary intention
[ ] **B.** Secondary intention
[ ] **C.** Never closed, left open
[ ] **D.** Tertiary intention

160. Discharge instructions for the client with gastritis would include all of the following *except*:
[ ] **A.** recommendation to limit caffeine intake.
[ ] **B.** smoking cessation.
[ ] **C.** use of nonsteroidal anti-inflammatory drugs (NSAIDs) for discomfort.
[ ] **D.** ranitidine (Zantac) 150 mg twice per day.

161. Gastritis—inflammation of the stomach lining—may be caused by:
[ ] **A.** shigella infection.
[ ] **B.** aplastic anemia.
[ ] **C.** alcohol abuse.
[ ] **D.** enzyme deficiencies.

162. The five-level emergency severity index (ESI) triage system sorts clients based on:
[ ] **A.** acuity of the client.
[ ] **B.** client complaint.
[ ] **C.** vital signs.
[ ] **D.** resources needed and risk.

163. To what emergency severity index level would the nurse assign a 40-year-old woman who's on chemotherapy and presents with nausea, vomiting, and a fever?

[ ] **A.** Level 1
[ ] **B.** Level 2
[ ] **C.** Level 3
[ ] **D.** Level 4

164. What's the most commonly occurring sexually transmitted disease in the United States with symptoms that include lower abdominal pain and foul-smelling vaginal discharge that's clear and stringy?

[ ] **A.** Chlamydia
[ ] **B.** Gonorrhea
[ ] **C.** Trichomonas
[ ] **D.** Syphilis

165. The client who comes to the emergency department with a sexually transmitted disease becomes increasingly hemodynamically unstable with a blood pressure of 70/30 mm Hg, a heart rate of 130 beats/minute, a respiratory rate of 22 breaths/minute, and a temperature of 97° F (36.1° C). She has an oxygen saturation of 97% on room air. She's awake and talking but restless. What's the priority intervention for this client?

[ ] **A.** Intubation and mechanical ventilation
[ ] **B.** Large-bore I.V. access and infusion of a 500 cc bolus of crystalloid solution
[ ] **C.** Large-bore I.V. access and infusion of a 500 cc bolus of 5% dextrose solution
[ ] **D.** Reassessment of the client's abdomen for rigidity, guarding, and rebound tenderness

166. What's considered a hallmark assessment finding for clients with pelvic inflammatory disease (PID)?

[ ] **A.** Vaginal discharge
[ ] **B.** External irritation of the genitalia
[ ] **C.** Cervical motion tenderness on bimanual examination
[ ] **D.** Vaginal bleeding

167. A 17-year-old high school student comes to the emergency department (ED) with complaints of weakness, severe fatigue, and depression. She's 5′7″, attractive, and weighs 102 lb (46 kg). She's accompanied by her mother, who states that her daughter has been preoccupied with dieting and has lost over 40 lb (18 kg) during the last 7 months. The mother also reports that her daughter has missed her period for the last 3 months, although she has been regular for the last 2 years. Her mother states she has always been the "model daughter," has made straight A's throughout school, and is socially active and popular. The mother can't understand why this is happening. Laboratory work shows that the client is in severe metabolic acidosis. What would the ED nurse suspect in this case?

[ ] **A.** Possible drug abuse
[ ] **B.** Severe reactive depression
[ ] **C.** Possible metabolic or hormonal disturbance
[ ] **D.** Possible eating disorder

168. A 72-year-old widow of 10 years complains of insomnia, poor appetite, and depression. She has a history of growing up in an alcoholic home, but reports she doesn't drink. There's no suicidal ideation. She fights back tears as she tells her story: Ten years ago, following outpatient chemotherapy treatments, her husband's health improved significantly, and he began to work around the house. Unfortunately, while he was mowing the lawn, a large abdominal aneurysm burst, and he died within minutes. She continues to believe to this day that she could have prevented his death had she been more protective and prevented him from engaging in physical activity. What's most likely true concerning this client?

[ ] **A.** She has moved to an acceptance phase regarding his death.
[ ] **B.** She's angry with her husband for dying suddenly.
[ ] **C.** She has difficulty accepting emotion and hasn't sufficiently processed her grief.
[ ] **D.** She's concerned her emotions may lead her to drink alcohol and, eventually, alcoholism.

169. A client comes to the emergency department with a blood pressure of 80/40 mm Hg and a strong central pulse of 126 beats/minute. Peripheral pulses aren't palpable. His skin is pale, cool, and moist. Which type of shock is the client most likely experiencing?

[ ] **A.** Cardiogenic
[ ] **B.** Hypovolemic
[ ] **C.** Obstructive
[ ] **D.** Distributive

170. Which intervention should the nurse prepare to perform immediately on a client with hypotension, tachycardia, and a distended, firm abdomen with bruising and adhesions?

[ ] **A.** Draw blood specimen for type and Rh and infuse type O-negative packed red blood cells (RBCs) while awaiting type-specific blood products.

[ ] **B.** Draw blood specimen for hemoglobin and hematocrit, decrease normal infusion to 15 mL/ hour, and await hematocrit determination before proceeding with further volume replacement.

[ ] **C.** Initiate infusion of dopamine at 15 mcg/kg/ minute to increase the blood pressure to 120 mm Hg systolic.

[ ] **D.** Gather supplies for immediate pericardiocentesis.

171. Which abdominal injury would most likely cause hypotension, tachycardia, firm abdomen to palpation, absent bowel sounds, and abdominal distention with bruising and adhesions across the upper quadrants?

[ ] **A.** Complete aortic rupture

[ ] **B.** Hepatic or splenic laceration

[ ] **C.** Small-bowel contusion

[ ] **D.** Diaphragmatic rupture

172. Neurologic assessment reveals a client who's unresponsive and intubated. His pupils are equal and react sluggishly to light. There's no extremity movement. The nurse suspects that the client's decreased level of consciousness (LOC) is due to:

[ ] **A.** hypotension and decreased perfusion.

[ ] **B.** increased intracranial pressure (ICP).

[ ] **C.** head injury.

[ ] **D.** central venous pressure (CVP) elevation.

173. The physician performs an ultrasound evaluation of the abdomen, which indicates free fluid in the abdomen. The nurse knows that the free fluid most likely represents:

[ ] **A.** hepatic failure with ascites.

[ ] **B.** intra-abdominal hemorrhage.

[ ] **C.** retroperitoneal bleeding.

[ ] **D.** hemothorax.

174. Nitroprusside (Nitropress) is commonly used in the treatment of hypertensive crisis. What's the usual initial dosage?

[ ] **A.** 10 mcg/kg/min

[ ] **B.** 10 to 50 mcg I.V.

[ ] **C.** 50 to 100 mcg I.V. bolus every 5 to 10 minutes

[ ] **D.** 0.3 mcg/kg/min I.V. and then titrate

175. A client who's 34 weeks pregnant comes to the emergency department in traumatic arrest. The nurse knows that:

[ ] **A.** fetal death is certain.

[ ] **B.** the mother and the infant have a greater chance of survival if an emergency cesarean delivery is performed.

[ ] **C.** the infant has a greater chance of survival if allowed to go to term.

[ ] **D.** the mother's chances of survival are greater if the infant isn't immediately delivered.

Answer sheet

	A	B	C	D		A	B	C	D		A	B	C	D		A	B	C	D
1.	○	○	○	○	25.	○	○	○	○	49.	○	○	○	○	73.	○	○	○	○
2.	○	○	○	○	26.	○	○	○	○	50.	○	○	○	○	74.	○	○	○	○
3.	○	○	○	○	27.	○	○	○	○	51.	○	○	○	○	75.	○	○	○	○
4.	○	○	○	○	28.	○	○	○	○	52.	○	○	○	○	76.	○	○	○	○
5.	○	○	○	○	29.	○	○	○	○	53.	○	○	○	○	77.	○	○	○	○
6.	○	○	○	○	30.	○	○	○	○	54.	○	○	○	○	78.	○	○	○	○
7.	○	○	○	○	31.	○	○	○	○	55.	○	○	○	○	79.	○	○	○	○
8.	○	○	○	○	32.	○	○	○	○	56.	○	○	○	○	80.	○	○	○	○
9.	○	○	○	○	33.	○	○	○	○	57.	○	○	○	○	81.	○	○	○	○
10.	○	○	○	○	34.	○	○	○	○	58.	○	○	○	○	82.	○	○	○	○
11.	○	○	○	○	35.	○	○	○	○	59.	○	○	○	○	83.	○	○	○	○
12.	○	○	○	○	36.	○	○	○	○	60.	○	○	○	○	84.	○	○	○	○
13.	○	○	○	○	37.	○	○	○	○	61.	○	○	○	○	85.	○	○	○	○
14.	○	○	○	○	38.	○	○	○	○	62.	○	○	○	○	86.	○	○	○	○
15.	○	○	○	○	39.	○	○	○	○	63.	○	○	○	○	87.	○	○	○	○
16.	○	○	○	○	40.	○	○	○	○	64.	○	○	○	○	88.	○	○	○	○
17.	○	○	○	○	41.	○	○	○	○	65.	○	○	○	○	89.	○	○	○	○
18.	○	○	○	○	42.	○	○	○	○	66.	○	○	○	○	90.	○	○	○	○
19.	○	○	○	○	43.	○	○	○	○	67.	○	○	○	○	91.	○	○	○	○
20.	○	○	○	○	44.	○	○	○	○	68.	○	○	○	○	92.	○	○	○	○
21.	○	○	○	○	45.	○	○	○	○	69.	○	○	○	○	93.	○	○	○	○
22.	○	○	○	○	46.	○	○	○	○	70.	○	○	○	○	94.	○	○	○	○
23.	○	○	○	○	47.	○	○	○	○	71.	○	○	○	○	95.	○	○	○	○
24.	○	○	○	○	48.	○	○	○	○	72.	○	○	○	○	96.	○	○	○	○

	A	B	C	D		A	B	C	D		A	B	C	D
97.	○	○	○	○	126.	○	○	○	○	155.	○	○	○	○
98.	○	○	○	○	127.	○	○	○	○	156.	○	○	○	○
99.	○	○	○	○	128.	○	○	○	○	157.	○	○	○	○
100.	○	○	○	○	129.	○	○	○	○	158.	○	○	○	○
101.	○	○	○	○	130.	○	○	○	○	159.	○	○	○	○
102.	○	○	○	○	131.	○	○	○	○	160.	○	○	○	○
103.	○	○	○	○	132.	○	○	○	○	161.	○	○	○	○
104.	○	○	○	○	133.	○	○	○	○	162.	○	○	○	○
105.	○	○	○	○	134.	○	○	○	○	163.	○	○	○	○
106.	○	○	○	○	135.	○	○	○	○	164.	○	○	○	○
107.	○	○	○	○	136.	○	○	○	○	165.	○	○	○	○
108.	○	○	○	○	137.	○	○	○	○	166.	○	○	○	○
109.	○	○	○	○	138.	○	○	○	○	167.	○	○	○	○
110.	○	○	○	○	139.	○	○	○	○	168.	○	○	○	○
111.	○	○	○	○	140.	○	○	○	○	169.	○	○	○	○
112.	○	○	○	○	141.	○	○	○	○	170.	○	○	○	○
113.	○	○	○	○	142.	○	○	○	○	171.	○	○	○	○
114.	○	○	○	○	143.	○	○	○	○	172.	○	○	○	○
115.	○	○	○	○	144.	○	○	○	○	173.	○	○	○	○
116.	○	○	○	○	145.	○	○	○	○	174.	○	○	○	○
117.	○	○	○	○	146.	○	○	○	○	175.	○	○	○	○
118.	○	○	○	○	147.	○	○	○	○					
119.	○	○	○	○	148.	○	○	○	○					
120.	○	○	○	○	149.	○	○	○	○					
121.	○	○	○	○	150.	○	○	○	○					
122.	○	○	○	○	151.	○	○	○	○					
123.	○	○	○	○	152.	○	○	○	○					
124.	○	○	○	○	153.	○	○	○	○					
125.	○	○	○	○	154.	○	○	○	○					

Sample test 1

Answers and rationales

1. Correct answer—B.

Rationales: CVP is the best unit of measure for identifying shock in a trauma client. CVP measures right-sided heart pressure, which reflects blood and fluid status. A normal CVP measurement is 4 to 10 cm H_2O pressure. A value less than 4 cm H_2O may indicate hypovolemia or vasodilation. Hb and HCT aren't the best indicators of early shock in a trauma client because they may be normal in the early phase of shock unless there has been massive blood loss. It normally takes 4 to 6 hours for the actual blood loss to be reflected in the Hb level and HCT.
Nursing process step: Assessment

2. Correct answer—B.

Rationales: The nurse should look and feel around the neonate's neck to determine whether the umbilical cord is wrapped around it. If the umbilical cord is present, the nurse should attempt to slip it over the neonate's head. If the cord is too tight, the nurse should clamp it in two places and cut between the clamps, after which the airway may be suctioned. The neonate may need to be stimulated to cry after delivery. The shoulders aren't delivered until the nurse has checked for the umbilical cord.
Nursing process step: Intervention

3. Correct answer—B.

Rationales: Parts that are distally positioned, such as fingers and toes, have less muscle tissue involvement and, therefore, have a good reimplantation rate. Because of extensive damage to blood vessels and the increased risk of debris-contaminated tissue, crush injuries have a less successful reimplantation rate than guillotine injuries (those that are severed with an extremely sharp cutting edge rather than a twisted or torn type of injury). A clean injury (caused by sharp glass or a sharp knife, for example) has less need for debridement than contaminated injuries such as those sustained in a crush from a surface that's coated with soil, rust, or oil. Other factors that affect reimplantation success include the client's age (children have more successful implantations due to generally healthier vascular systems) and care of the amputated part before reattachment (amputated parts should be kept cool and reattached within 6 hours of the injury).
Nursing process step: Analysis

4. Correct answer—C.

Rationales: Ingestion or inhalation of cyanide produces an intracellular anoxic poisoning by preventing oxidative phosphorylation; the result is anaerobic metabolism, lactic acidosis, and decreased adenosine triphosphate production. Cyanide ingestion quickly results in apnea, seizures, and coma. Hydroxocobalamin injection is used to treat cyanide inhalation. Naloxone is used in the treatment of opioid analgesic overdose. Apomorphine is an antiparkinsonian drug and isn't used to treat cyanide poisoning. Activated charcoal is used in a variety of toxic poisonings, although it isn't commonly used in clients who have ingested ethanol, hydrocarbon, or cyanide.
Nursing process step: Intervention

5. Correct answer—A.

Rationales: This rule prohibits unstable, critical clients from being diverted to hospitals farther away rather than being transported to the closest emergency department. Even though the hospital may not offer the needed services, the client must be medically stable before transport to another facility, as specifically mandated in COBRA. The emergency department can't refuse critical or unstable clients for any reason.

6. Correct answer—C.

Rationales: Hypertensive crisis secondary to psychotropic drug therapy is characterized by hyperthermia, chest pain, tachycardia, and palpitations.
Nursing process step: Assessment

7. Correct answer–B.

Rationales: Neuroleptic malignant syndrome is thought to occur as a result of dopaminergic blockade at receptor sites secondary to administration of neuroleptic agents. Classic signs include hyperthermia, muscle rigidity, diaphoresis, tachycardia, hypertension, akinesia, and agitation.

Nursing process step: Assessment

8. Correct answer–D.

Rationales: Nitroglycerin reduces preload and is, therefore, beneficial in the management of acute pulmonary edema. Nitroglycerin's vasodilator properties prevent its use in the management of cerebral hemorrhage, head trauma, and increased ICP.

Nursing process step: Intervention

9. Correct answer–B.

Rationales: Interacting with an anxious client requires that the nurse be an active listener and provide an environment in which the client can maintain self-control. Questioning an anxious client tends to increase his anxiety, and verbalizing support takes away his self-control. Silence may imply doubt on the part of the listener.

Nursing process step: Analysis

10. Correct answer–B.

Rationales: After a beta-adrenergic blocker or calcium channel blocker overdose, glucagon is administered in a dose of 50 to 150 mcg/kg to reverse the effects of beta-blockade. Glucagon enhances myocardial contractility and increases heart rate and atrioventricular conduction in a separate cellular pathway distinct from the adrenergic receptor pathway. Therefore, it can stimulate the myocardium in the presence of beta-adrenergic blockade. Lidocaine and bretylium are used in the treatment of ventricular tachyarrhythmias. $D_{50}W$ is used in the treatment of hypoglycemia.

Nursing process step: Intervention

11. Correct answer–A.

Rationales: The ability to respond and focus in children is comparable to adult orientation to person, place, and time. A glassy stare (indicating an inability to focus) in an infant may result from serious central nervous system derangement, necessitating emergent treatment.

Nursing process step: Evaluation

12 Correct answer–D.

Rationales: Normal ICP is between 0 to 10 mm Hg. By elevating the head of the bed by 40 degrees, the body uses gravity to help promote intracranial drainage, thus decreasing pressure. If elevated ICP persists, ischemia and necrosis of brain tissue may occur. Placing a client in Trendelenburg's position has the opposite effect and can raise ICP. The client's legs shouldn't be elevated greater than 90 degrees. Coughing is discouraged because it can raise ICP.

Nursing process step: Intervention

13. Correct answer–A.

Rationales: Initial response to low perfusion states results in increased secretion of catecholamines (epinephrine and norepinephrine). Vasoconstriction of the peripheral vessels shunts blood to the vital organs (heart and brain). The heart rate and contractility increase in an effort to increase preload. When compensatory mechanisms fail, peripheral vessels dilate and peripheral and splanchnic pooling occur.

Nursing process step: Evaluation

14. Correct answer–B.

Rationales: Sleep disturbances (nightmares, insomnia) are the earliest and most frequently reported physical symptom after critical incident stress. Loss of appetite, loss of intimacy, and fatigue may also be seen but are less common.

Nursing process step: Assessment

15. Correct answer–C.

Rationales: A 2-year-old child receiving adequate fluid replacement has a normal urine output of 1 to 2 mL/kg/hour.

Nursing process step: Evaluation

16. Correct answer–A.

Rationales: Turner's sign is a discoloration of the flank area as a result of a retroperitoneal bleed. Blood in the mediastinum is indicative of an aortic disruption and is best seen on an upright chest X-ray. Increased ICP is exhibited by alterations in mental status, blood pressure, heart rate, and respirations. Splenic injury produces referred pain to the left shoulder and neck and is known as *Kehr's sign.*

Nursing process step: Assessment

17. Correct answer—D.

Rationales: Neurogenic diabetes insipidus occurs after insult to the hypothalamus or the posterior pituitary gland, resulting in an alteration in antidiuretic hormone (ADH) secretion. After traumatic injury to the brain, ADH levels can decrease, resulting in high urine output. Classic signs include high serum sodium, hypokalemia, and low urine osmolality due to excessive urine output.
Nursing process step: Assessment

18. Correct answer—C.

Rationales: The nurse should anticipate the use of a 5 mm ET tube. ET tube size is estimated using the following formula:
(16 + age in years) divided by 4 = ET tube size in millimeters
In this situation, the equation would be: (16 + 4) divided by 4 = 5 mm.
Nursing process step: Analysis

19. Correct answer—B.

Rationales: The presence of ST elevation in leads II, III, and aV_f indicate that the client is having an inferior wall MI. An anterior wall MI will show ST elevation in leads V_1 through V_6. A lateral wall MI will show ST elevation in leads I, aV_l, V_5, and V_6. Posterior wall infarctions are indicated by ST depression in leads V_1 to V_4 as well as by reciprocal changes of the anterior wall, the portion of the heart opposite of the posterior wall.
Nursing process step: Analysis

20. Correct answer—B.

Rationales: Heart failure is the most common presenting symptom after heart transplantation. Because of the lack of vagal innervation of the transplanted heart, tachycardia, chest pain, and jaw pain related to ischemia aren't possible.
Nursing process step: Assessment

21. Correct answer—D.

Rationales: Of primary importance in a client with an orthopedic injury is the determination of neurovascular status. Impaired neurovascular status may be limb-threatening or life-threatening. Tetanus immunization, last oral intake, and the presence of contaminants are secondary concerns.
Nursing process step: Assessment

22. Correct answer—D.

Rationales: The concentration of epinephrine is 1 mg divided by 250 mL = 0.004 mg/mL or 4 mcg/mL. To infuse 125 mcg/minute, the nurse should infuse 31 mL/hour. Use the following formula: Dosage in micrograms per minute multiplied by 60 minutes divided by the concentration of drug = pump setting: 125 mcg/minute × 60 minutes = (7,500) divided by 4 mcg/mL = 1,875 divided by 60 = 31.25 mL/hour. Round to 31 mL/hour.
Nursing process step: Analysis

23. Correct answer—D.

Rationales: Adenosine is the drug of choice for paroxysmal supraventricular tachycardia; 6 mg is given rapid I.V. push over 1 to 3 seconds. If there's no response in 1 to 2 minutes, 12 mg may be given. Bretylium is used to treat refractory ventricular fibrillation. Digoxin and diltiazem are considered third-line drugs in the treatment of supraventricular tachycardia.
Nursing process step: Intervention

24. Correct answer—B.

Rationales: Tachycardia isn't an indicator of increased ICP. The earliest and most sensitive indicator of increased ICP is a change in LOC. A compensatory mechanism that attempts to provide adequate cerebral perfusion pressure as ICP increases is Cushing's triad. Signs of the triad include widening pulse pressure, bradycardia, and increased systolic blood pressure.
Nursing process step: Assessment

25. Correct answer—A.

Rationales: Extremity pain that's regularly produced by the same of degree of exercise and is relieved by rest is probably claudication. The other conditions aren't immediately relieved by rest and aren't consistent in presentation.
Nursing process step: Assessment

26. Correct answer—A.

Rationales: Survivors of sudden death need the support of loved ones. Therefore, the emergency department nurse should ensure that the family has been notified. The survivor needs to participate in decision making regarding the treatment plan. Providing opportunities for decision making decreases the client's feelings of powerlessness. When possible, have someone stay with the client to promote feelings of security. Advance directive information should be discussed prior to the event so that the client's wishes can be carried out.
Nursing process step: Intervention

27. Correct answer—C.

Rationales: Hyperkalemia and an increase in serum creatine kinase are predominant findings in rhabdomyolysis. Dark brown urine results from the myoglobinuria that accompanies rhabdomyolysis. A positive Kernig's sign may indicate subarachnoid hemorrhage or meningitis, but not rhabdomyolysis.
Nursing process step: Analysis

28. Correct answer—B.

Rationales: During helicopter transfer, assessment of breath sounds is difficult. An electronic end-tidal carbon dioxide detector best ensures that the client is ventilating. Cardiac monitors show rate changes, but a rate change is a nonspecific finding. Pulse oximetry isn't accurate in the presence of vibrations such as those experienced during transfer. A laryngoscope allows visual assessment of tube placement, but isn't useful for constant monitoring.
Nursing process step: Evaluation

29. Correct answer—C.

Rationales: A client with inferior wall infarction may experience bradycardia and AV conduction disturbances. Anterior wall infarction may lead to tachycardia and heart block. Tachycardia is also a sign of heart failure and cardiogenic shock, both complications of myocardial infarction.
Nursing process step: Assessment

30. Correct answer—D.

Rationales: Normal tissue pressure is less than 20 mm Hg. Tissue pressures in excess of 30 mm Hg with suspicious clinical findings are usually indicative of compartment syndrome and require further intervention.
Nursing process step: Analysis

31. Correct answer—C.

Rationales: Parkinson's disease is a degenerative condition of the basal ganglia. It can also be induced as a result of drug therapy. Such drugs include neuroleptics, antihypertensives, and antiemetics.
Nursing process step: Assessment

32. Correct answer—C.

Rationales: The client with a severed leg has a serious injury that requires immediate attention and is amenable to medical intervention. Therefore, that client should receive priority in this situation. The client with an open head injury and the client with severe burns are hemodynamically compromised and have grave prognoses. In addition, the resources to treat them during a disaster are inadequate. The client with facial lacerations is stable and the injuries are relatively minor; therefore, that client's care can be delayed.
Nursing process step: Assessment

33. Correct answer—D.

Rationales: First determine the concentration:

$$\frac{50 \text{ mg}}{250 \text{ mL}} = 0.2 \text{ mg/mL}$$

then, because the dose is ordered mcg/kg/min, convert to mcg/mL:

$$0.2 \times 1{,}000 = 200 \text{ mcg/mL}$$

Then set up the following equation:

$$\frac{\text{Dosage} \times \text{client's weight (in kg)} \times 60}{\text{Infusion concentration}}$$

$$\frac{3 \text{ mcg/kg/min} \times 89 \text{ kg} \times 60}{200 \text{ mcg/mL}} = 80.1$$

Round off to 80 mL/hour.
Nursing process step: Analysis

34. Correct answer—C.

Rationales: During times of increased stress, confusion, and overwhelming client volumes, the use of familiar forms and medical records increases compliance with documentation of client care. Disaster tags can minimize and standardize documentation. They're most useful if they have multiple copies, and these copies are distributed to the command post, public relations, or admissions.
Nursing process step: Analysis

35. Correct answer—C.

Rationales: Prodromal symptoms, which include itching, tingling, and paresthesia, may occur a few hours to 2 days before actual eruption of herpes lesions. Acyclovir reduces the duration of viral shedding, which begins just before lesion appearance and continues for about 12 days, but sexual activity should cease until lesions are healed or a posttreatment examination is done. All partners should have their own examination and treatment regimen. Douching isn't recommended because it disturbs the normal flora that assists with preventing infection.
Nursing process step: Evaluation

36. Correct answer—A.

Rationales: Kawasaki disease is a form of vasculitis that attacks multiple body systems. Signs and symptoms include elevated temperature, conjunctivitis, "strawberry" tongue and lips, cervical lymphadenopathy, erythema of the palms and soles, and periungual desquamation. A butterfly rash (malar erythema) is associated with lupus erythematosus. Exophthalmos is associated with Graves' disease, a thyroid disorder. Koplik's spots, which are associated with rubeola, are reddened areas with gray-blue centers on the buccal mucosa.
Nursing process step: Assessment

37. Correct answer—B.

Rationales: Testicular torsion is the sudden twisting of the spermatic cord, causing vascular compromise to the affected testicle. Emergent surgical intervention or manual detorsion under local anesthesia is needed within 2 to 6 hours, depending on the severity of the torsion. Epididymitis is an inflammatory, nonemergent infection that can be associated with a sexually transmitted infection. Although an emergency, priapism (painful persistent erection) doesn't affect the testes.
Nursing process step: Assessment

38. Correct answer—D.

Rationales: Verbalizing that the baby may have smothered or choked demonstrates that they aren't well-informed or don't comprehend what they have been told about SIDS. It's normal for family members to be concerned about the cause of death and to verbalize positive memories about the child. Accepting a referral for a SIDS support group demonstrates that they are ready to move on.
Nursing process step: Evaluation

39. Correct answer—C.

Rationales: The return of cloudy fluid or the aspiration of gross blood or intestinal contents represents a positive peritoneal tap. The return of clear fluid indicates a negative tap.
Nursing process step: Evaluation

40. Correct answer—B.

Rationales: Following the advanced cardiac life support guidelines for ventricular fibrillation, the appropriate action is to administer epinephrine 1 mg I.V. The client may be defibrillated at 360 joules within 30 to 60 seconds. Lidocaine may then be administered in persistent ventricular fibrillation. Sodium bicarbonate isn't indicated at this point, and its use should be guided by arterial blood gas levels.
Nursing process step: Intervention

41. Correct answer—B.

Rationales: Decisions regarding client transfer must be based on need for additional or specialized care. Lack of insurance isn't a reason to prevent transfer of a client to a specialized facility.
Nursing process step: Assessment

42. Correct answer—B.

Rationales: Immediate psychosocial interventions should focus on getting the client to identify the cause of the distress and to identify coping behaviors successfully used in the past. The ED nurse must support the client and initiate health-related teaching. Giving anti-anxiety medications won't address the underlying problem. These clients aren't disoriented and don't require restraints. Denial may be used as a coping mechanism before the client is ready to face the situation. The client shouldn't be pressured to talk about the crisis.
Nursing process step: Intervention

43. Correct answer—B.

Rationales: Clostridium tetani is a gram-positive anaerobic spore that produces bacteria that inhabit the intestinal tracts of humans and animals. The bacterium enters the bloodstream and travels to the central nervous system. *Clostridium* can survive in soil for years. *Pasteurella multocida, Enterobacter,* and *Streptococcus* are commonly associated with dog bites.
Nursing process step: Analysis

44. Correct answer—B.

Rationales: The client's safety is the first priority in the ED. A psychiatric client should be told how to take his medication, and he should be able to verbalize an understanding of the instructions. It's unrealistic to expect the client's thought process to be organized or the client's auditory hallucinations to subside completely before discharge. The ED isn't the place for a complete nutritional evaluation.
Nursing process step: Evaluation

45. Correct answer—D.

Rationales: The widened mediastinum along with clinical correlation represents a ruptured aorta. Blood leaking into the mediastinum increases intrathoracic pressure, resulting in pain and increased respiratory rate. A ruptured hemidiaphragm or pneumothorax is evident on chest X-ray and doesn't involve a widening of the mediastinum. A ruptured trachea could produce a pneumomediastinum on chest X-ray.
Nursing process step: Assessment

46. Correct answer—B.

Rationales: In third-degree heart block, there's no relation between P waves and QRS complexes. The atria and ventricles beat independently of one another. Idioventricular rhythms are wide complex and are usually slower and without P waves. Sinus bradycardia has a P wave for each QRS complex. Wenckebach has progressively longer PR intervals until a QRS complex is dropped. It has a regularly irregular rhythm.

Nursing process step: Assessment

47. Correct answer—C.

Rationales: Glucose is needed to sustain the work of the diaphragm in breathing. Because a child has small stores of glucose, he's likely to suffer respiratory distress more quickly than an adult. Decreased metabolic demands don't cause fatigue. Increased vital capacity and tidal volumes improve oxygenation and decrease the work of breathing.

Nursing process step: Analysis

48. Correct answer—A.

Rationales: Degenerative changes in the elderly, direct trauma, blunt trauma, and hereditary factors can all lead to retinal detachment. The most common cause, however, is degenerative changes in elderly clients. Minimal to moderate trauma to the eye may cause retinal detachment, but in such cases, predisposing factors play an important role. Severe trauma may cause retinal tears and detachment, even if there are no predisposing factors.

Nursing process step: Assessment

49. Correct answer—D.

Rationales: Monitoring I.V. infusion rates is commonly difficult in transport; therefore, an I.V. infusion regulating pump is helpful. Iced saline is important for initial burn cooling, but it could precipitate hypothermia during transport. Cooling blankets are similarly not warranted. Pain should be controlled with analgesics. An end-tidal carbon dioxide monitor is of no value unless the client is intubated.

Nursing process step: Analysis

50. Correct answer—A.

Rationales: The pain associated with myocardial contusion isn't affected by coronary vasodilators. Both myocardial contusion and angina may result in arrhythmias and ECG changes. Hypotension, distended jugular veins, and muffled heart sounds represent findings of cardiac tamponade.

Nursing process step: Assessment

51. Correct answer—B.

Rationales: Haloperidol is a phenothiazine and is capable of causing dystonic reactions. Diazepam and clonazepam are both benzodiazepines, and amitriptyline is a tricyclic antidepressant. Benzodiazepines and tricyclic antidepressants don't cause dystonic reactions. Benzodiazepines can cause drowsiness, lethargy, and hypotension. Tricyclic antidepressants can cause a decreased level of consciousness, tachycardia, dry mouth, and dilated pupils.

Nursing process step: Intervention

52. Correct answer—B.

Rationales: The initial defibrillation attempt would be 2 joules/kg ($2 \times 15 = 30$). If unsuccessful, double the energy level for the second and third attempts.

Nursing process step: Analysis

53. Correct answer—C.

Rationales: Chelating agents bind with a heavy metal, and the compound formed is primarily excreted in the urine. The client should have adequate urine output before administration of chelating agents. The nurse should monitor renal function and urine output during and after therapy. LOC, respiratory status, and blood pressure should be monitored, but they aren't specific to chelation therapy.

Nursing process step: Assessment

54. Correct answer—A.

Rationales: Testicular torsion occurs as a sudden onset of testicular pain and, possibly, nausea, vomiting, and swelling of testes. Pain that significantly decreases may be a detrimental sign pointing to testicular ischemia, which may occur from 2 to 4 hours past initial onset. The other clients are in pain and moderate distress, but they can wait if necessary.

Nursing process step: Assessment

55. Correct answer—C.

Rationales: Pericarditis is an inflammation of the pericardium. The symptoms described are indicative of pericarditis. The pain of MI generally doesn't change with deep breathing or a change in position. Pleurisy and endocarditis are usually gradual in onset.

Nursing process step: Assessment

56. Correct answer—B.

Rationales: Allen's test is performed to ensure that collateral circulation to the hand is adequate. The radial and ulnar arteries are compressed simultaneously. The client is then instructed to open and close his fist several times. The hand will become blanched. The radial artery is released, and the hand is observed for hyperemia. The procedure is repeated with the ulnar artery.
Nursing process step: Analysis

57. Correct answer—C.

Rationales: The concentration of nitroprusside is 0.4 mg/mL, or 400 mcg/mL (100 mg divided by 250 mL). To infuse 5 mcg/kg/minute, the nurse needs to infuse 60 mL/hour and should use this formula: Dosage in micrograms per kilogram per minute multiplied by the client's weight in kilograms multiplied by 60 minutes divided by the concentration of the drug in micrograms per milliliter:
5 mcg/kg/minute × 80 kg = (400) × 60 minutes = (24,000) divided by 400 mcg/mL = 60 mL/hour.
Nursing process step: Analysis

58. Correct answer—D.

Rationales: Status epilepticus is seizure activity that exceeds 30 minutes' duration or is a series of seizures that doesn't allow for full recovery between events. Prolonged seizure activity can result in loss of base reserve that will lead to metabolic acidosis. Other complications associated with status epilepticus include hyperthermia, hypoglycemia, cardiac arrhythmias, hypoxia, increased intracranial pressure, and airway obstruction.
Nursing process step: Evaluation

59. Correct answer—C.

Rationales: Insects are the most common foreign materials in the ears of adults. To remove an insect from a client's ear, the nurse should instill mineral oil or alcohol to fill the ear canal and then direct a light at the canal opening. The insect will crawl toward the light and out of the canal. Instilling water or hydrogen peroxide will cause the insect to swell and make removing it more difficult. Using forceps may cause the insect to break into pieces and necessitate further intervention.
Nursing process step: Intervention

60. Correct answer—A.

Rationales: On arrival at the ED, the client is owed a duty of care by the physician and hospital staff.

61. Correct answer—A.

Rationales: The early clinical indicators for septic shock include hyperthermia, tachycardia, wide pulse pressure, tachypnea (resulting in respiratory alkalosis), and mental obtundation ranging from mild disorientation to confusion, lethargy, agitation, and coma. While alive in the body, bacteria and other microorganisms release endotoxins. Endotoxins activate the mediators—tumor necrosis factor, interleukin-1, and interferon g—which elicit a febrile response, resulting in hyperthermia. (Note that clients who are elderly, very young, or immunocompromised may be unable to elicit a febrile response to the chemical mediators and may develop hypothermia). Tachycardia is initiated by the sympathetic response to the increase in body temperature and the decrease in cardiovascular insufficiency from the dilation of the ventricles and vasodilation of the vasculature. Tachypnea results from the direct effects of endotoxins or secondary to kallikreins, bradykinin, prostaglandins, or complement activation. The wide pulse pressure comes from decreases in systemic vascular resistance and vasodilation of the vasculature. The altered mental state is thought to be from an altered state of amino acid metabolism or a disruption of the blood–brain barrier.
Nursing process step: Assessment

62. Correct answer—A.

Rationales: Decorticate and decerebrate posturing are indicative of cerebral damage. In decortication, the upper extremities are abducted with obvious flexion of the arms, wrists, and fingers; the lower extremities are hyperextended with plantar flexion. Hypotonia (flaccidity) presents with decreased muscle tone and weakness. Spasticity is an increase in muscle resistance to passive movement and is followed by a sudden decrease in resistance. Decerebration presents as hyperextension of the upper and lower extremities.
Nursing process step: Analysis

63. Correct answer—C.

Rationales: Retinal hemorrhages result from a temporary obstruction of venous return and are consistent with being shaken. Bilateral arm fractures, basilar skull fractures, and petechiae on the trunk may result from other forms of child abuse.
Nursing process step: Assessment

64. Correct answer—C.

Rationales: The recommended therapeutic range is 1½ to 2½ times the control time. PT equal to or less than the control is of no therapeutic value. PT greater than three times the control has no added benefit and may be associated with a higher risk of bleeding.
Nursing process step: Evaluation

65. Correct answer—B.

Rationales: Many women present with distended bladders because of the intense, scalding pain from urine touching the lesions. These women can benefit from the use of an indwelling urinary catheter for bladder relief and continuous urine drainage. Fluid intake should be increased rather than decreased to dilute the acidic urine and to correct or prevent dehydration. Lesions should be kept dry, and loose-fitting cotton underwear is recommended. Other treatment regimens include the use of sitz baths and anesthetic ointments as well as acyclovir ointment for pain control.
Nursing process step: Intervention

66. Correct answer—A.

Rationales: Vomiting occurs secondary to increased intracranial pressure (ICP) as the vagal centers of the medulla become irritated. Headache is usually in response to increased ICP, localized swelling, and distortion of blood vessels. Papilledema occurs as the result of edema of the optic nerve. Restlessness and irritability (altered level of consciousness) are signs of increased ICP, not stimulation of the vagal center.
Nursing process step: Assessment

67. Correct answer—C.

Rationales: Anything other than a single line, date, initials, and reason is suspect to legal counsel, insurance examiners, and other responsible authorities.

68. Correct answer—D.

Rationales: Continuous waveform capnography is the most reliable method of confirming and monitoring correct placement of an endotracheal tube. Because blood must circulate through the lungs for carbon dioxide to be exhaled and measured, capnography can also serve as a physiologic monitor of the effectiveness of chest compressions. A reading of greater than 40 mm Hg is consistent with a substantial improvement of blood flow.
Nursing process step: Analysis

69. Correct answer—D.

Rationales: Protamine sulfate, when given alone, acts as an anticoagulant. When given in the presence of heparin, a stable salt is formed and the anticoagulant ability of both medications is lost. Fresh frozen plasma is the antidote for warfarin ingestion. Dimercaprol is used to promote the excretion of arsenic, gold, and mercury. Naloxone is effective in reversing the effects of opioids.
Nursing process step: Intervention

70. Correct answer—A.

Rationales: The primary treatment for a client with back pain is rest. Anti-inflammatory and antispasmodic medications will help the client rest. Applying heat, not cold, is recommended. Weight loss and stretching exercises are interventions that should be initiated after acute pain subsides.
Nursing process step: Intervention

71. Correct answer—B.

Rationales: The key rationale for initiation of mechanical ventilation is apnea, $PaCO_2$ greater than 50 mm Hg, pH less than 7.25, a gradient greater than 350 mm Hg, increased work of breathing, and a vital capacity of less than 10 mL/kg.
Nursing process step: Assessment

72. Correct answer—B.

Rationales: Discharge and follow-up instructions can serve as a defense in litigation if it can be demonstrated that the client was nonadherent to instructions and, therefore, furthered his or her own injury. The client's remarks, the remarks of other personnel, and the client's intellectual level should be included in the record only if the discharging nurse believes that the comments illustrate the client's ability or willingness to adhere to instructions.

73. Correct answer—D.

Rationales: Epidural hematoma, a result of bleeding between the skull and the dura mater, can follow a direct blow to the head. Signs and symptoms typically include a brief loss of consciousness, followed by a lucid period, then another loss of consciousness. Subdural hematoma, which is more common, results from bleeding into the subdural space between the dura mater and the arachnoid space. Diffuse axonal injuries are caused by blunt trauma resulting in shearing or disruption of the neuronal structures. Early CT scans may be unremarkable in a concussion.
Nursing process step: Analysis

74. Correct answer—C.

Rationales: Disaster preparedness planning is an ongoing process and shouldn't end with the revision or development of a plan. Plan revision may occur after a disaster, but this isn't the only time to make changes. Census fluctuations are too unpredictable to adequately plan a disaster exercise.

Nursing process step: Evaluation

75. Correct answer—B.

Rationales: Damage to the femoral nerve results in the client's inability to raise the affected leg when it's straight, extend the knee, or sense stimulus to the anterior thigh. Median nerve injuries are evidenced by inability to dorsiflex the affected wrist or extend the metacarpophalangeal joints. Sensory deviation with median nerve injury results in altered sensation to the dorsal web space between the thumb and index finger. Tibial nerve injuries result in altered plantar flexion of the foot and sensory changes to the sole. Peroneal nerve damage results in altered dorsiflexion of the foot and sensory changes to the web space between the great and second toes.

Nursing process step: Assessment

76. Correct answer—C.

Rationales: Cheyne-Stokes respirations are characterized by respirations of increasing depth and frequency followed by a period of apnea lasting for 10 to 60 seconds. The changes in rate and depth are in response to levels of carbon dioxide. Periods of apnea occur when the stimulation to respiratory centers diminishes. Apneustic breathing is characterized by a pause of 2 to 3 seconds after a full or prolonged inspiration. Biot's respirations are irregular and unpredictable with deep and shallow random breaths and pauses. Cluster breathing appears as a group of irregular breaths with periods of apnea at irregular intervals.

Nursing process step: Assessment

77. Correct answer—C.

Rationales: Antibiotic therapy should be administered as soon as possible after traumatic injury. Research indicates that antibiotics given preoperatively are most effective because the bacterial count is low and the bacteria are most amenable to antibiotics. The goal of early antibiotic therapy is to reach an effective blood concentration before or at the time of wound closure and, thus, limit the threat of infection. I.V. administration of antibiotics results in higher concentrations than oral dosing.

Nursing process step: Evaluation

78. Correct answer—C.

Rationales: The most characteristic finding of asthma is expiratory wheezing; however, absence of wheezing could indicate increased severity of the attack. The nurse should remember that not all wheezing signals asthma. Dark circles under the eyes, also known as *allergic shiners,* and bluish, boggy nasal turbinates are seen in clients with allergies as well as asthma. Therefore, these aren't significant findings for diagnosing asthma. Moist crackles indicate the presence of fluid in the lungs' small airways and are heard in clients with pneumonia and early stages of pulmonary edema.

Nursing process step: Assessment

79. Correct answer—C.

Rationales: The initial pharmacologic treatment for an anaphylactic allergic reaction is epinephrine. Epinephrine slows the release of cellular chemical mediators and causes vasoconstriction. This vasoconstriction improves hypotensive states and decreases edematous tissue. In severe anaphylaxis, a 1:10,000 epinephrine solution should be administered I.V. slowly in a .01 to .025 mg dose. The administration of .01 to .05 mg of 1:1,000 subcutaneous epinephrine is an appropriate intervention as treatment for allergic reactions that aren't true anaphylaxis. Diphenhydramine, a histamine receptor antagonist, can be administered in doses of 25 to 50 mg by way of oral, I.V., or I.M. routes. Cimetadine, also a histamine receptor antagonist, isn't a first-line drug in the treatment of anaphylactic reactions.

Nursing process step: Intervention

80. Correct answer—A.

Rationales: Ipecac is contraindicated in the ingestion of most petroleum distillates, such as paint thinner, because of the potential for aspiration. The risk of aspiration must be weighed against the toxicity of the petroleum product ingested. Activated charcoal may be ordered to absorb toxins in the petroleum product. Gastric lavage may be ordered to remove toxins if the airway is protected by endotracheal intubation. Oxygen may be ordered if aspiration has occurred.

Nursing process step: Intervention

81. Correct answer—A.

Rationales: Magnesium sulfate is used to control seizures in pregnancy-induced hypertension. Urine output of less than 30 mL/hour should be reported. The drug should be withheld if respirations are fewer than 16 breaths/minute, because it may cause respiratory depression. Hypermagnesemia may result in depressed patellar reflexes. Vaginal bleeding isn't associated with magnesium sulfate administration.

Nursing process step: Assessment

82. Correct answer–B.

Rationales: Removal of the stinger is best done by using a dull object to scrape the stinger from the surface of the skin. Cold packs, not heat, should be applied to the site. Grasping and pulling the stinger aren't recommended because those actions may release more venom from the sac. The area should be cleaned and cold packs applied to the site. Elevating the extremity reduces accompanying edema.
Nursing process step: Intervention

83. Correct answer–A.

Rationales: An opioid overdose or pontine hemorrhage produces pupils that can be described as "barely visible" or pinpoint. The client with midbrain damage has pupils that are nonreactive and midposition. Severe anoxia results in bilateral fixed and dilated pupils. Previous cataract surgery should be suspected in the client with keyhole-shaped pupils.
Nursing process step: Assessment

84. Correct answer–C.

Rationales: Symptoms associated with scabies infestation include red-brown linear markings on the wrists, between the fingers, at the belt and nipple line, and in the genital area. Pruritus is present and is accentuated at night when the activity of the mites increases. Raised, scaly, round patches with relatively flat centers on the hands, feet, trunk, and groin are associated with ringworm. A pink macular rash over the palms, soles, hands, feet, wrists, and ankles is associated with Rocky Mountain spotted fever. The rash later becomes petechial and mimics meningococcemia. Urticaria is rapidly appearing wheals or papules that are the result of a vascular allergic reaction that's commonly accompanied by severe itching.
Nursing process step: Assessment

85. Correct answer–B.

Rationales: A foreign object dropped into the cast may result in a wound or pressure ulcer to the skin. If a wound occurs, the risk of infection is great. Therefore, the client must be instructed not to attempt to retrieve the object and to call the follow-up care provider instead. Keeping the cast dry will maintain cast stability and prevent premature degradation. Having the client wiggle the toes at least once every hour assists with circulation and ensures distal neuromotor function. Elevating the extremity above the level of the heart promotes venous drainage and decreased extremity swelling and pain.
Nursing process step: Evaluation

86. Correct answer–C.

Rationales: Oxytocin causes uterine smooth muscle to contract and, therefore, increases abdominal cramping. It doesn't increase urine output or heart rate. Vaginal bleeding should slow down but doesn't cease completely.
Nursing process step: Evaluation

87. Correct answer–B.

Rationales: Normal healing consists of a series of steps: The first is hemostasis. In this step, vasoconstriction, coagulation, and platelet aggregation occur. The second step in wound healing is inflammation. This is caused by capillary dilation, which allows increased blood flow to the site of injury. During this stage, granulocytes, lymphocytes, neutrophils, and macrophages migrate to the injury. As the products of injury are removed, reconstructive cells proliferate and lead to scar formation.
Nursing process step: Assessment

88. Correct answer–A.

Rationales: Brown-Sequard syndrome is a rare injury typically due to hemisection of the spinal cord. This injury is commonly seen with penetrating trauma. Signs and symptoms include ipsilateral paresis or hemiparesis and loss of motor function, touch, pressure, and proprioception. Symptoms of central cord syndrome occur following trauma (most commonly, falls) and consist of upper- and lower-extremity weakness, with varying degrees of sensory loss; neck pain and urinary retention are common. Symptoms of anterior cord syndrome may include paralysis or loss of fine control of movements in the arms and hands, with relatively less impairment of leg movements. In posterior cord syndrome, muscle power, pain, and temperature sensation are preserved; however, the client may have trouble with limb coordination.
Nursing process step: Analysis

89. Correct answer–D.

Rationales: All the interventions may be appropriate for the client with suspected blunt abdominal trauma. However, the priority of care should always be airway stabilization and then I.V. access. Fluid resuscitation is begun as needed. A nasogastric tube and an indwelling urinary catheter should be inserted. Additional diagnostic tests are performed based on client stability.
Nursing process step: Intervention

90. Correct answer—D.

Rationales: The priority intervention for a trauma client is the administration of high-flow oxygen. The application of a pneumatic antishock garment, radiologic evaluation, and analgesic administration can occur when the priorities of airway, breathing, and circulation are complete.
Nursing process step: Intervention

91. Correct answer—B.

Rationales: Beta-adrenergic blockers may mask the signs of shock. The sympathetic stimulation causing an increase in heart rate is prevented by beta-adrenergic blockers. The client may present with bradycardia, hypotension, and decreased renin secretion.
Nursing process step: Analysis

92. Correct answer—C.

Rationales: Iritis produces blurred vision and unilateral pain that's moderate to severe. The cornea appears clear to hazy, and pupils are irregular and small with sluggish reaction. Conjunctivitis results in no change in vision, has a clear cornea, normal pupil size, and purulent or mucopurulent discharge. Glaucoma is marked by severe, sudden-onset pain; decreased visual acuity; hazy, lusterless cornea; and a semidilated, nonreactive pupil on the affected side. Central retinal artery occlusion is painless and causes a sudden unilateral loss of vision. The pupil in the affected eye is dilated and nonreactive.
Nursing process step: Assessment

93. Correct answer—A.

Rationales: Extensor tendons are prone to injury. The nurse should look for strength along with motor response when the client extends and flexes against resistance. Tendon lacerations that go unrecognized and thus untreated can lead to permanent deformity. The remaining tests are used to determine peripheral nerve damage.
Nursing process step: Assessment

94. Correct answer—D.

Rationales. A client with a corneal abrasion must receive daily outpatient follow-up care. If the injury is bilateral, the client is generally admitted to the hospital. Ophthalmologic consultation should be made if the corneal abrasion fails to resolve in 48 to 72 hours. The eye patch should be left in place until the eye is examined by a physician the next day. The pain is usually severe and requires medication for relief.
Nursing process step: Evaluation

95. Correct answer—B.

Rationales: Cardiac tamponade is identified by the three main signs known as Beck's triad. They include hypotension, muffled heart sounds, and distended neck veins. Dyspnea isn't associated with Beck's triad. Tracheal deviation is a late sign of a tension pneumothorax.
Nursing process step: Analysis

96. Correct answer—C.

Rationales: Because a client with alcohol intoxication is commonly unable to maintain an airway, the safest oxygen delivery mode is intubation. A client sustaining multisystem trauma should receive high concentrations of oxygen to maintain adequate cellular oxygenation. The nasal cannula is a passive device that requires the client to perform adequate minute ventilations (tidal volume × respiratory rate). The nasal cannula can deliver a maximum oxygen of 44%. The simple face mask can deliver up to 60% oxygen, but it often results in carbon dioxide accumulation and respiratory acidosis. The nonrebreather mask can deliver adequate oxygenation to clients who can protect their airway.
Nursing process step: Analysis

97. Correct answer—A.

Rationales: Recognizing hemorrhage is the focus of nursing care because the client could succumb quickly. Although controlling blood pressure is important to help reduce the risk of variceal rupture, it isn't the primary focus of care. It's also important to teach the client about esophageal varices and what foods he should avoid, such as spicy foods, but these aren't the primary focus.
Nursing process step: Assessment

98. Correct answer—B.

Rationales: The inclusion criteria for therapeutic hypothermia include any client older than 18 who's experiencing cardiac arrest with return of spontaneous circulation but remains unresponsive, respiratory support with endotracheal intubation, and a systolic blood pressure greater than 90 mm Hg. The exclusion criteria include any client who may have another reason for the collapse (such as stroke or overdose), is pregnant, has a temperature of less than 86° F (30° C) after the arrest, or has a do-not-resuscitate order.
Nursing process step: Analysis

99. Correct answer—D.

Rationales: Lower right rib fractures are commonly associated with liver injury. The nurse may also find decreased hematocrit from bleeding. Kehr's sign (pain in the left shoulder secondary to diaphragmatic irritation by blood) and Ballance's sign (fixed dullness to percussion in the left flank and dullness in the right flank that disappears with a change in position) may also be present. Injury to the spleen is associated with left upper quadrant pain and lower left rib fractures. Colon injuries are often associated with rectal bleeding and free air, which is detected by X-ray, under the diaphragm. Pancreatic injuries are associated with left upper quadrant or epigastric pain and Turner's sign (ecchymosis in the flank area suggesting retroperitoneal bleeding).
Nursing process step: Assessment

100. Correct answer—D.

Rationales: A client with acute cholecystitis presents with fever, right upper quadrant tenderness, and a positive Murphy's sign. Murphy's sign is pain in the right upper quadrant on inspiration; the pain prevents the client from taking a deep breath. Kehr's sign, which is associated with abdominal bleeding, is referred pain in the left shoulder and is caused by diaphragmatic irritation from blood.
Nursing process step: Assessment

101. Correct answer—A.

Rationales: In neurogenic shock, the vasomotor center of the medulla is inhibited, causing loss of sympathetic vasomotor regulation. Uncontested parasympathetic responses cause vasodilatation and loss of sympathetic tone. Inhibition of sympathetic innervation impedes release of norepinephrine and interferes with the body's ability to vasoconstrict, causing a decrease in venous return and cardiac output.
Nursing process step: Analysis

102. Correct answer—B.

Rationales: To prevent the possible spread of infection, respiratory isolation should be initiated when pertussis is suspected. Isolation is recommended to prevent the transmission of airborne infectious diseases. With respiratory isolation, gowns and gloves aren't indicated. Masks, however, are to be worn by any staff member who comes within arm's length of the client. Additional interventions should focus on the client's symptoms: control fever with antipyretics, administer antibiotics, and initiate seizure precautions as necessary.
Nursing process step: Intervention

103. Correct answer—B.

Rationales: The symptoms described are typical in a client with abruptio placentae, which is the separation of the placenta from the uterus before delivery. It's also commonly associated with blunt abdominal trauma. If the outer edges of the placenta remain attached, bleeding may be concealed. In placenta previa, the placenta develops in the lower part of the uterus, and it may cover the opening. The client presents with painless vaginal bleeding. The client in premature labor doesn't have a rigid uterus. A client with a ruptured uterus shows signs of shock and doesn't have fetal heart tones.
Nursing process step: Assessment

104. Correct answer—A.

Rationales: Amphetamines are stimulants. They cause increased energy, decreased appetite, extreme self-confidence, tachycardia, arrhythmias, hypertension, vasoconstriction, and insomnia. Fatigue is a sign of amphetamine withdrawal.
Nursing process step: Assessment

105. Correct answer—A.

Rationales: Miotic drops are given to decrease the pupil size and allow for aqueous humor drainage. Morphine is given to reduce pain, and acetazolamide or osmotic diuretics are given to reduce IOP. Surgery may be indicated if pharmacologic intervention is unsuccessful.
Nursing process step: Intervention

106. Correct answer—A.

Rationales: Folic acid is the cofactor necessary for metabolizing toxic metabolites of methanol to nontoxic metabolites in the liver. Thiamine and pyridoxine are the cofactors administered for ethylene glycol ingestion. Calcium may be administered if hypocalcemia occurs in ethylene glycol ingestion.
Nursing process step: Intervention

107. Correct answer—B.

Rationales: This client presents with classic signs of botulism poisoning. This toxin causes descending paralysis. The earliest signs are visual, followed by dysphagia and, later, respiratory paralysis. Improperly canned foods are the primary source of this toxin. A form of this toxin is found in honey and may cause signs of botulism poisoning in infants. It isn't a problem for adults. A history of recent viral infection and the presence of numbness or tingling are signs of Guillain-Barré syndrome. Recent travel isn't specific to the symptoms mentioned.
Nursing process step: Assessment

108. Correct answer—A.

Rationales: Establishing a clear airway is the first priority of care. Airway, breathing, and circulation are always included in the primary assessment and take precedence over other problems. The other interventions are a high priority after establishment of an airway.
Nursing process step: Intervention

109. Correct answer—B.

Rationales: Cocaine is a stimulant drug. It causes hyperthermia, tachycardia, hypertension, and seizures. Labetalol is an alpha- and beta-adrenergic blocking agent. Its effect is to slow tachycardia and lower blood pressure. It doesn't have a direct effect on temperature or pupils. The drug used for seizures is a benzodiazepine.
Nursing process step: Evaluation

110. Correct answer—B.

Rationales: Contraindications to nasotracheal intubation include suspected basilar skull fractures and nasal fractures. Nasotracheal intubation may also put the client at risk for developing encephalitis or meningitis. Orotracheal intubation is the most common method for establishing an airway. It isn't the method of choice in obvious cervical spine injuries, but 96% of clients with cervical spine injuries can be intubated safely. Cricothyrotomy is a surgical procedure used to establish an airway. Needle cricothyrotomy is generally performed on children younger than age 12 when an airway can't be obtained by other means. Surgical cricothyrotomy isn't recommended for children younger than age 12 because damage to the cricoid cartilage could harm the only structure supporting the larynx and the upper trachea.
Nursing process step: Analysis

111. Correct answer—B.

Rationales: Ovarian cysts, if they rupture, can cause hemorrhage and hypovolemic shock. Serial hematocrit and Hb level are helpful in the evaluation process. The WBC count isn't significantly elevated unless peritonitis has occurred. This client's pain is only of 2 hours' duration; therefore, the likelihood of peritonitis is low. An elevated HCG level indicates a possible ectopic pregnancy. A decreased calcium level isn't important to this diagnosis.
Nursing process step: Assessment

112. Correct answer—D.

Rationales: Although controlling pain, supporting nutrition, and treating the underlying cause are important aspects of care, fluid resuscitation is the priority. Severe hypovolemic shock may result in acute pancreatitis, and it must be treated with judicious fluid and electrolyte replacement.
Nursing process step: Analysis

113. Correct answer—A.

Rationales: Airborne isolation precautions should be used to prevent the spread of germs via tiny droplets in the air from the mouth or nose. These germs may stay suspended in the air and can spread to others. Clients are required to wear a mask if they need to leave their room. A negative-airflow room or machine should be provided. Client visitors should be limited; they should wear masks during the visit and be sure to wash their hands upon entering and leaving the room. Contact precautions are instituted when germs can be spread easily from direct and indirect contact. Neutopenic precautions are implemented for patients who are immunocompromised. Universal precautions are implemented for all patients regardless of their condition.
Nursing process step: Intervention

114. Correct answer—B.

Rationales: Hypothermia results in a decrease in the airway protective mechanisms (ciliary function), thus increasing the possibility of aspiration and pneumonia. Because of shivering and an increase in metabolic demand, the client may experience bronchospasm. The client will also increase respirations in an attempt to rid the lungs of excess carbon dioxide. The oxyhemoglobin dissociation curve will shift to the left, resulting in impaired oxygen delivery and tissue hypoxia.
Nursing process step: Analysis

115. Correct answer—A.

Rationales: The U.S. Congress enacted EMTALA to ensure care for those who can't pay and to keep hospitals from "dumping" or transferring clients to other hospitals. Identification of a client's primary physician isn't necessary because a portion of the population doesn't have one. The Centers for Medicare and Medicaid Services (CMS) has stated that triage is *not* considered a medical screening.
Nursing process step: Analysis

116. Correct answer—C.

Rationales: The symptoms are consistent with rubella, a childhood disease transmitted through droplets or direct contact with infected people. Scarlet fever is identified by a fine rash that's primarily found on the chest, neck, axillae, and inner thighs. The rash doesn't affect the face and is usually accompanied by high fever and vomiting. Fifth disease is distinguished by an intensely red rash that begins on the face and then develops on the trunk and extremities. The rash clears centrally, leaving a lacy appearance that can last for weeks. There's no accompanying fever. Roseola infantum is identified by a high fever (104° F [30° C]) that abruptly stops and is followed by a rash that fades on pressure.
Nursing process step: Analysis

117. Correct answer—B.

Rationales: Within 30 to 60 minutes after onset, an ophthalmologist should perform an anterior chamber paracentesis. Some centers have used tissue plasminogen activator and heparin for partial retinal artery occlusions with success. Gentle ocular massage may be performed by a physician before the arrival of an ophthalmologist. Breathing into a paper bag to increase carbon dioxide causes retinal arteriole vasodilation until definitive therapy can be performed.
Nursing process step: Intervention

118. Correct answer—C.

Rationales: Stridor is a loud, musical noise that can be heard without a stethoscope. It's usually the result of partial upper airway obstruction and is common in croup and epiglottiditis. Stridor requires immediate intervention. Crackles are popping noises heard most commonly during inspiration, and they indicate the presence of fluid, pus, or mucus in the smaller airways. When the nurse hears crackles, the client should be instructed to cough and breathe deeply and then the nurse should auscultate again since the crackles may have cleared. Rhonchi are snoring, low-pitched sounds produced by air passing through narrowed air passages. Wheezing is a high-pitched, musical sound that can be heard during inspiration and expiration. It usually accompanies an asthma attack or bronchospasm.
Nursing process step: Assessment

119. Correct answer—D.

Rationales: Liver injuries are commonly associated with lower right rib fractures. Lacerations of the liver may cause profuse bleeding and lead to hypovolemia. The client with blunt abdominal trauma should be evaluated for other abdominal injuries. Injuries to the spleen are more commonly associated with left rib fractures. Perforations of the stomach and pancreatic injury are less common.
Nursing process step: Analysis

120. Correct answer—A.

Rationales: The most significant assessment finding in a chemical burn to the eye, especially an alkaline burn, is corneal whitening. There's pain and variable visual loss. It's also difficult to define specific eye structures. There may be redness but no purulent discharge. A corneal abrasion presents with corneal irregularity without luster.
Nursing process step: Assessment

121. Correct answer—B.

Rationales: COPD includes emphysema and bronchitis. Asthma is no longer considered part of COPD because it's a restrictive airway disorder, not an obstructive one. Heart failure and bronchiectasis aren't considered obstructive airway disorders.
Nursing process step: Analysis

122. Correct answer—C.

Rationales: Septic shock typically causes hypoglycemia in pediatric clients. Infants have limited glycogen stores that are rapidly depleted during stress. During the resuscitative stage, all pediatric clients should have serum glucose levels monitored. Hypoglycemia should be treated with 2 to 4 mL/kg of 25% dextrose solution I.V. Septic shock results in a metabolic acidosis state from decreased cellular perfusion. Hypercalcemia doesn't occur. Hypocalcemia results from impaired tissue perfusion during septic shock and should be treated with calcium chloride 10% solution 10 to 20 mg/kg I.V. administered slowly.
Nursing process step: Assessment

123. Correct answer—C.

Rationales: Untreated pelvic inflammatory disease can create a tubo-ovarian cyst. If it ruptures, the client can develop peritonitis and become septic. Before any invasive procedure, such as a culdocentesis, the infection should be treated with I.V. antibiotics. Therefore, an I.V. line is necessary for antibiotics and for fluid resuscitation. An NG tube is inserted because of decreased peristalsis, which can occur with peritonitis or sepsis. A pelvic examination is performed to obtain cultures and assess the client.
Nursing process step: Intervention

124. Correct answer—C.

Rationales: In inflammatory conditions, such as pancreatitis, a loop of bowel adjacent to the inflammation may become distended with gas. This is known as a sentinel loop of bowel. Free air under the diaphragm is indicative of perforation. Dilated loops of bowel and abnormal air fluid levels in the bowel may be indicative of bowel obstruction.
Nursing process step: Assessment

125. Correct answer—A.

Rationales: An infusion of 10% glucose and regular insulin is administered to induce the transfer of potassium from the serum to the intracellular fluid. Clients with a potassium excess should receive only fresh blood because the cells in stored blood release potassium during storage. Calcium gluconate is used to reverse magnesium intoxication. A client with already impaired renal function shouldn't be given potassium-sparing diuretics.
Nursing process step: Intervention

126. Correct answer—B.

Rationales: A client with an STD may complain of painful urination. The pain may be from an associated urinary tract infection or from urine passing over lesions. The lesions themselves may also be painful, and itching can be so severe that it elicits pain (either from the desire to scratch or from actual scratching). A discharge doesn't produce pain.
Nursing process step: Analysis

127. Correct answer—A.

Rationales: Intestinal obstruction may be associated with distention, vomiting, visible peristalsis, localized tenderness, and altered bowel sounds. Right upper quadrant tenderness, fever, and jaundice are related to cholecystitis. Abdominal free air, distention, and rebound tenderness are found with a perforated viscous. Nausea, abdominal mass, and bruit are found in clients with a leaking abdominal aneurysm.
Nursing process step: Assessment

128. Correct answer—C.

Rationales: During normal cellular function, an aerobic environment exists. Adequate cellular perfusion of glucose and oxygen occurs, and waste products are removed. When cellular perfusion is reduced, tissue hypoxia ensues and results in an abnormal cellular metabolism, creating an anaerobic environment. A byproduct of anaerobic metabolism is lactic acid. Decreased tissue perfusion doesn't remove the byproduct, and metabolic acidosis occurs.
Nursing process step: Assessment

129. Correct answer—B.

Rationales: O-negative packed RBCs are recommended when blood replacement must occur immediately. In some institutions, O-positive packed RBCs are being administered to male clients without complications; however, the gender of this client wasn't mentioned. Type-specific, uncrossmatched packed RBCs take 15 to 20 minutes to process. Typed and crossmatched packed RBCs require 30 to 60 minutes to process. To prevent transfusion reactions, type-specific or typed and crossmatched blood should be administered as soon as possible.
Nursing process step: Analysis

130. Correct answer—B.

Rationales: During the initial phase of shock, respiratory alkalosis occurs as the body attempts to rid itself of the carbonic acid that accumulates as a result of inadequate tissue perfusion. Respiratory acidosis and metabolic acidosis result when fluid or blood loss continues and compensatory mechanisms fail to restore normal cellular function. Metabolic alkalosis occurs in clients who have lost hydrogen ions or have an accumulation of bicarbonate.
Nursing process step: Assessment

131. Correct answer–A.

Rationales: Having a reimplantation team available is an important factor. Other factors include the amount of damage to the attachment area or amputated part, length of time since amputation occurred, predicted outcome of reimplantation, and the general physical condition of the client. It makes no difference whether the amputated part is an upper or a lower extremity. The client's occupation, although important to consider, shouldn't determine whether attempts at reimplantation occur. The insurance status of the client should never be a factor in the provision of life- and limb-threatening interventions.

132. Correct answer–C.

Rationales: This client has pulmonary edema as a result of heart failure. In doses of 5 to 20 g/kg/minute, dopamine stimulates the beta-adrenergic and alpha-adrenergic receptors of the sympathetic nervous system and results in vasoconstriction of peripheral blood vessels, increased heart rate, increased contractility, and enhanced conduction through the atria and ventricles. Dobutamine stimulates the beta receptors of the heart to increase myocardial contractility and stroke volume and results in increased cardiac output. Clients in septic shock also suffer from peripheral vasodilation. Dobutamine doesn't act on the peripheral vascular beds and is used in conjunction with dopamine. Nitroprusside and nitroglycerin are vasodilators and have the ability to enhance perfusion through vasoconstricted vessels. The pharmacologic activity of vasodilation on the systemic vessels is unpredictable; therefore, the client should have a thermodilution catheter inserted for measuring systemic vascular resistance. Vasodilators are seldom used in the emergency department.
Nursing process step: Intervention

133. Correct answer–D.

Rationales: Fractures to the epiphyseal growth plate may result in early closure. As the child continues to grow, there may be no growth in the affected bone. If the growth plate fracture is partial, angulated growth may subsequently occur, leading to deformity. Open fractures, closed fractures, and dislocation fractures usually don't result in long-term problems, provided initial orthopedic care is appropriate.
Nursing process step: Analysis

134. Correct answer–D.

Rationales: The dressing of choice for a client with an open pneumothorax is a nonporous dressing taped on three sides. The dressing should be placed over the wound at the end of expiration. The client should be monitored closely for condition worsening. Saline-moistened gauze would increase the potential for infection. When a porous dressing is used, pieces of gauze can move into the chest. If the dressing is taped on all four sides, it predisposes the client to the development of tension pneumothorax.
Nursing process step: Intervention

135. Correct answer–B.

Rationales: The symptoms associated with hepatitis A include fever, anorexia, malaise, vomiting, nausea, light-colored stools, and dark-colored urine. Hepatitis is also associated with liver inflammation, which causes pain in the right upper quadrant. The spleen, not the liver, is located in the left upper quadrant. Dark, tarry stools are associated with GI bleeding. Hematuria is associated with trauma, anticoagulant therapy, renal tumors, and renal calculi.
Nursing process step: Assessment

136. Correct answer–A.

Rationales: The situation describes constructive feedback because the manager responded respectfully to the staff nurse promptly and privately. The manager also implemented a positive approach to preventing future errors. Emotional support and goal setting are irrelevant in the situation described. Recognition is feedback for a positive contribution, not an error.

137. Correct answer–D.

Rationales: About 90 percent of all pulmonary thromboemboli originate in the deep veins of the leg. Other risk factors include trauma, surgery, cancer, heart failure, and estrogen use. High cholesterol doesn't directly cause pulmonary embolus formation.
Nursing process step: Analysis

138. Correct answer–A.

Rationales: Proper application of a splint occurs when the splint immobilizes the joint above and below the injury. A traction splint is used for femur fractures as well as fractures of the proximal tibia. The extremity should be splinted in the position found if the neurovascular status is intact. Air splints are contraindicated for air transport of clients because altitude changes result in pressure changes within the splint, which may cause neurovascular compromise.
Nursing process step: Analysis

139. Correct answer—A.

Rationales: Potassium may increase in the early postburn period from hemolysis of red blood cells and loss of intracellular potassium. Sodium may decrease slightly because of extracellular body fluid loss and sodium trapped in the edema surrounding the burn wound.
Nursing process step: Assessment

140. Correct answer—D.

Rationales: Pelvic fractures always involve at least two fracture sites because of the bony ring structure of the pelvis. They can be stable or unstable; however, more than 66% of them are stable. A fracture of the pelvis can produce bleeding, which is usually venous and caused by the disruption of the pelvic veins. Open pelvic fractures are associated with injuries to the perineum, genitourinary structures, or rectum and have a significantly higher mortality.
Nursing process step: Assessment

141. Correct answer—C.

Rationales: Many people find it difficult to adjust to major changes in structure and ways of operating. Explaining reasons for change makes acceptance more likely. A manager's approach should also include the following: obtaining as much input from staff as possible, making no more than one major change at a time, and letting staff know that if the change doesn't work, adjustments can usually be made. The goal is to find a workable process.

142. Correct answer—C.

Rationales: The nurse should use the rule of nines to estimate the percentage of BSA. In an adult, the head compromises 9% BSA; the torso, 18% front and 18% back; arms, 9% each; legs, 18% each; and the perineum, 1%. In a child, the head comprises 18% and each leg is 14%; the other percentages are the same as for an adult.
Nursing process step: Assessment

143. Correct answer—C.

Rationales: Common signs of early carbon monoxide poisoning are headache and nausea or flulike symptoms. Because the symptoms improve during the day, an environmental cause, such as a faulty gas appliance or heating system, may be responsible. A car can also be a source of carbon monoxide poisoning, but unless the client leaves the car's motor running in an attached garage, it's unlikely that the car is the cause. If the client reported that symptoms occurred at work (rather than reporting that family members shared similar symptoms), then asking the client if anyone at work had similar symptoms would be appropriate.
Nursing process step: Assessment

144. Correct answer—C.

Rationales: Normal serum uric acid levels in males are 3.4 to 7 mg/dL. Serum uric acid levels are almost always elevated to 8 mg/dL in gout. A normal WBC count in an adult male is 4,500 to 11,000/µL and is expected to be elevated in the presence of an inflammatory process.
A Westergren ESR, or sed rate, is normally 1 to 20 mm/hour in men older than 50 and is elevated in inflammation or tissue injury. The normal value for urine uric acid is 250 to 750 mg/24-hour specimen. Increased urinary uric acid levels are seen in clients with a diagnosis of gout.
Nursing process step: Analysis

145. Correct answer—A.

Rationales: Acute gouty arthritis is treated with colchicine and nonsteroidal anti-inflammatory drugs (NSAIDs). Colchicine has known anti-inflammatory effects but no analgesic property. So, an NSAID is added to the treatment regimen primarily for pain management. Future attacks are prevented by a maintenance dose of allopurinol in combination with weight reduction, as needed, and avoidance of alcohol and foods high in purine. Aspirin inactivates the effect of the uricosurics, resulting in urine retention. Probenecid is ineffective when creatinine clearance is reduced, as can occur in clients over age 60.
Nursing process step: Intervention

146. Correct answer—A.

Rationales: Meperidine, a nonopioid analgesic, is the drug of choice for pain control in pancreatitis. Opioids can cause spasms of the sphincter of Oddi and exacerbate pain. The spasms block the normal flow of pancreatic enzymes and raise the levels of the enzymes in the pancreas. The increased enzyme levels worsen autodigestion in the pancreas and exacerbate pain.
Nursing process step: Intervention

147. Correct answer—B.

Rationales: Cut refers to a skin wound with separation of the connective tissue. The term *gash* is used for a dramatic effect. Avulsion refers to a wound where tissue is torn away from the body. Abrasion is a skin alteration caused by scraping or friction.
Nursing process step: Assessment

148. Correct answer–B.

Rationales: Only Protected Health Information (PHI) is affected by HIPAA. Medical records must be secured in a locked place such as a file cabinet or room. Someone other than the client may pick up a filled prescription. Calling out a client's name isn't a breach of HIPPA, and a sign-in sheet may be used as long as it doesn't report the client's diagnosis or reason for his visit.
Nursing process step: Analysis

149. Correct answer–D.

Rationales: The treatment for iritis is instillation of eye drops. It's important to teach proper handwashing and technique for instilling eye drops. Clients with iritis don't require patching, irrigation or cold compresses. Hot compresses may provide relief.
Nursing process step: Evaluation

150. Correct answer–D.

Rationales: Treatment for CRAO must begin immediately to have any chance of reversing the visual loss. The goal is to dislodge the embolus by vasodilatation techniques to increase vascular blood flow (breathing into a paper bag for 10 minutes) and decreasing intraocular pressure (massaging the eye, giving I.V. acetazolamide, or withdrawing aqueous humor from the anterior chamber). Treatment is frequently unsuccessful. Clients with CRAO usually don't lose light perception. CRAO is an embolic event; therefore, risk factors for stroke are the same, but this isn't a goal of treatment. Thrombolytic agent administration for this type of event has been studied, but no clear guidelines exist for the use of thrombolytics.
Nursing process step: Evaluation

151. Correct answer–A.

Rationales: Gunshot wounds cause more trauma to the tissues related to the bullet fragments. There's less exposure to tissues with stabbing injury, blunt trauma, and crushing injury.
Nursing process step: Analysis

152. Correct answer–B.

Rationales: Missile injuries usually involve multiple contaminated wounds, which must be treated before the refined work of nerve repair can be done. The military has adequately trained staff and time. The military health coverage will cover this procedure.
Nursing process step: Analysis

153. Correct answer–B.

Rationales: The initial assessment of the client includes airway, breathing, and circulation. The client's airway and breathing aren't compromised. The next step is to evaluate his circulation and establish I.V. access. The chest X-ray is a diagnostic tool that can be obtained after the initial assessment and interventions are completed. Thrombolytic therapy may be ordered upon consultation with the cardiologist in the catheterization laboratory.
Nursing process step: Intervention

154. Correct answer–B.

Rationales: Pain control is a high priority for the client experiencing an MI. It would be important to have morphine available in case the client develops chest pain during the transfer. Relieving the client's pain will help prevent further myocardial tissue damage. Diazepam may be helpful if the client is overly anxious. Calcium chloride is indicated if the client is hyperkalemic, and dextrose 50% would be indicated if the client was hypoglycemic. If indicated, these medications can be administered before transfer.
Nursing process step: Intervention

155. Correct answer–A.

Rationales: The new Emergency Nurses Association (ENA) Guidelines for Determining Emergency Department Nurse Staffing include client census, client acuity, client length-of-stay, nursing time for interventions, skill mix, and adjustment factor for the nonclient care time. Although the other factors may be supportive information, the objective criteria from the national professional organization, backed by research, is more meaningful. Factors other than staffing numbers could also be influences or causes such as inexperienced or rude staff members.
Nursing process step: Assessment

156. Correct answer–B.

Rationales: The best indicator that learning has taken place is a change in behavior. Evidence for that is an actual improvement in the desired requirement. Attending a class doesn't necessarily mean learning took place or that there's an ability to apply the new information. While one nurse is achieving the desired goal, as in option C, the rest of the staff may still be showing no improvement. It's also unclear whether the randomly selected nurse actually improved or was working effectively before the project even began. As for option D, opinions lack objectivity and can be wrong.
Nursing process step: Evaluation

157. Correct answer—C.

Rationales: Pulmonary edema occurs when increased pressure within the pulmonary capillaries pushes fluids into the surrounding tissues. In this case, dobutamine would help increase contractility while reducing peripheral vascular resistance. Dopamine would be contraindicated because it increases contractility while increasing peripheral vascular resistance. Levophed is vasoconstrictive and increases contractility, making the heart work harder. Cardizem isn't indicated for this client.
Nursing process step: Intervention

158. Correct answer—C.

Rationales: Edema, erythema, exudate, induration, and systemic fever are the textbook definition of a wound infection. Option A describes the signs and symptoms of an infiltration. Option B describes the signs and symptoms of phlebitis. Option D describes dead tissue.
Nursing process step: Analysis

159. Correct answer—D.

Rationales: An infected wound is left open to granulate and then closed by tertiary intention when the infection has resolved. Primary intention isn't possible because of the infection, and secondary intention would be just leaving it to granulate.
Nursing process step: Analysis

160. Correct answer—C.

Rationales: NSAIDs, aspirin products, and caffeine are irritating to the stomach's mucosal lining. Smoking impedes the healing of ulcers and increases secretion of gastric acid. Ranitidine inhibits the action of histamine at receptor sites of the parietal cells, which decreases gastric acid secretion.
Nursing process step: Evaluation

161. Correct answer—C.

Rationales: Gastritis may be the result of drinking too much alcohol. Nausea, vomiting, abdominal pain, and heartburn are common symptoms. They're caused by the inflammation and irritation of the stomach lining. Gastritis isn't caused by shigella, aplastic anemia, or enzyme deficiencies
Nursing process step: Assessment

162. Correct answer—D.

Rationales: The five-level ESI index is based on resources needed for the client and risk. In the old acuity system, there were clients who needed many resources yet their acuity might be assigned a lower level, which was not a valid reflection of the care the client needed.

163. Correct answer—C.

Rationales: Based on the Emergency Severity Index (ESI), this client would be triaged as level 3. This client needs quick attention but can wait as long as 30 minutes for assessment and treatment. Although the client may be immunocompromised, she doesn't need immediate intervention and may be given a mask while she waits. She'll need blood work, fluid replacement, and antibiotics.

164. Correct answer—A.

Rationales: Chlamydia is listed as the most commonly occurring sexually transmitted disease by the Centers for Disease Control and Prevention. While the others are present in the general population in the United States, the incidence of Chlamydia in females and males is higher. Females typically have symptoms, whereas males don't.
Nursing process step: Assessment

165. Correct answer—B.

Rationales: Based on her history and symptoms, this client is now exhibiting the beginning signs of hypovolemic shock. Appropriate as an intervention is large-bore venous access and resuscitation with a crystalloid solution, not a dextrose solution. Reassessment isn't a client intervention. The client is awake and talking with an adequate saturation; therefore, her airway is patent at this time.
Nursing process step: Intervention

166. Correct answer—C.

Rationales: Because of the irritation associated with PID, cervical motion tenderness is considered a diagnostic sign for it. Although vaginal discharge, spotting or bleeding, and external irritation of the genitalia may also be present with PID, they aren't considered diagnostic for the disease.
Nursing process step: Assessment

167. Correct answer—D.

Rationales: Individuals with eating disorders are typically young females who have a distorted self-image. They may avoid food or go through repeated episodes of bingeing and purging. Generally, there's a significant loss in body weight, although the client may persist in the belief of being overweight. In extreme cases, metabolic and fluid imbalances resulting from this behavior can lead to severe physical distress and even death. Other disorders, such as endocrine, thyroid, and psychiatric, should be ruled out.
Nursing process step: Analysis

168. Correct answer–C.

Rationales: Death of a loved one is a major life loss. Due to the client's history of having come from an alcoholic home, she's experiencing overwhelming emotions resulting both from the loss and from self-blame. She should be evaluated for depression.
Nursing process step: Assessment

169. Correct answer–B.

Rationales: Hypovolemic shock is the most common type of shock in injured clients. The client's hypotension and tachycardia are typical of hypovolemia. Cardiogenic shock is most common in clients after myocardial infarction or cardiac contusion. Cardiac contusion is a possibility in this client, but the emergency department nurse suspects intra-abdominal bleeding as the cause of the client's hypotension and tachycardia. Obstructive shock could occur in this client, but there are strong central pulses and no tension pneumothorax. Distributive shock would be more likely to result in warm skin with hypotension and bradycardia.
Nursing process step: Assessment

170. Correct answer–A.

Rationales: A blood specimen should be drawn and sent to the laboratory for immediate type and Rh. While awaiting type-specific blood products, the nurse may administer O-negative packed RBCs. The nurse wouldn't want to decrease the I.V. rate to 15 mL/hour, because the client has inadequate circulating volume and no peripheral pulses are palpable. Dopamine isn't indicated in a client with hypovolemic shock but may be used in distributive shock to promote vasoconstriction. Pericardiocentesis would be indicated if the client had signs of cardiac tamponade, but heart sounds are clear.
Nursing process step: Intervention

171. Correct answer–B.

Rationales: Hepatic or splenic rupture will result in bleeding into the abdominal cavity and commonly cause hypovolemic shock. Complete aortic rupture would cause very rapid exsanguinations and death, typically before the client reaches the hospital. Small-bowel contusions typically produce no symptoms initially and won't usually cause hypovolemic shock or blood in the abdomen. Diaphragmatic rupture is a possibility in this client because of the mechanism and upper abdominal injury, but there weren't any abdominal contents noted in the chest on the radiograph, nor were bowel sounds auscultated in the chest. If diaphragmatic rupture had been considered likely, the chest tube insertion might have been withheld until further diagnostics had confirmed the presence or absence of rupture.
Nursing process step: Assessment

172. Correct answer–C.

Rationales: Head injury is a possibility in this client given the mechanism of injury. Hypotension and decreased perfusion can cause changes in LOC but aren't as likely to result in prolonged unconsciousness. Decreases in ICP aren't likely in a client who has a head injury; rather, increased ICP is a danger. CVP wouldn't be elevated in a client in hypovolemic shock.
Nursing process step: Assessment

173. Correct answer–B.

Rationales: Free fluid in the abdomen in a trauma client is most likely due to intra-abdominal hemorrhage, and the client has bruising and abrasions over the upper abdomen. Hepatic failure with ascites wouldn't cause the abrupt vital sign deterioration seen in this client. Retroperitoneal bleeding isn't noted on abdominal ultrasound, nor does it cause fluid in the abdomen. Hemothorax is blood in the chest cavity, not in the abdomen.
Nursing process step: Assessment

174. Correct answer–D.

Rationales: Nitroprusside has a rapid onset of action. Initial dosage for hypertensive crisis is 0.3 mg/kg/minute I.V. and then titrate every few minutes until desired effect is achieved or maximum dose is reached.
Nursing process step: Implementation

175. Correct answer–B.

Rationales: In the instance of a trauma arrest, both the mother and the infant have a greater chance of survival if the baby is delivered by emergency cesarean delivery. A cesarean delivery is indicated when gestation is greater than 26 weeks and resuscitation attempts seem terminal.
Nursing process step: Analysis

Sample test 2

Questions

1. What's the primary adverse effect of thrombolytic therapy?
[ ] **A.** Reperfusion arrhythmias
[ ] **B.** Bleeding
[ ] **C.** Release of oxygen-free radicals
[ ] **D.** Hypotension

2. What's the nursing priority when caring for a suspected schizophrenic client who's delusional?
[ ] **A.** Obtain a psychiatric consult as soon as possible.
[ ] **B.** Assist with the medical workup because the behavior could be organic and medical causes need to be ruled out.
[ ] **C.** Anticipate an order for lithium (Lithobid).
[ ] **D.** Insist that the delusions aren't real.

3. Discharge instructions to the family of a client with a concussion should include:
[ ] **A.** aspirin (acetylsalicylic acid) 650 mg every 4 hours for complaints of mild discomfort.
[ ] **B.** oxycodone (Roxicodone) 30 mg every 4 hours for severe pain.
[ ] **C.** to return immediately if the client behaves in a way that isn't normal for the client.
[ ] **D.** reassurance that neurologic symptoms will subside in 4 to 8 hours.

4. Which document outlines a client's wishes regarding emergency treatment if the client can't speak for himself?
[ ] **A.** Durable power of attorney for health care
[ ] **B.** Last will and testament
[ ] **C.** Advance directive
[ ] **D.** Instructions for care after death

5. In addition to dietary restrictions, discharge instructions for a client with a diagnosis of acute gout include informing him of other factors that may precipitate an acute attack. These include all of the following *except:*
[ ] **A.** excessive caloric intake.
[ ] **B.** moderate alcohol use.
[ ] **C.** stress.
[ ] **D.** excessive vitamin A intake.

6. What's the most common underlying cause of pediatric cardiopulmonary arrest?
[ ] **A.** Genetic cardiac abnormalities
[ ] **B.** Electrolyte disturbances
[ ] **C.** Hypoxemia
[ ] **D.** Primary cardiac arrhythmias

7. A 2-year old is evaluated in the emergency department for "pulling at his right ear." Upon otoscopic examination, a bean is observed in his ear canal. Which method for removal is contraindicated?
[ ] **A.** Alligator forceps
[ ] **B.** Irrigation
[ ] **C.** Right-angled hook
[ ] **D.** Ear curette

8. A gardener is brought to the emergency department by his family after spilling insecticide on himself as he filled a sprayer. He developed symptoms including headache, ataxia, and difficulty breathing. Before assessing this client, the nurse should:
[ ] **A.** double glove.
[ ] **B.** identify the type of insecticide.
[ ] **C.** determine how much insecticide was spilled.
[ ] **D.** apply respiratory protection.

9. Successful repair of a renal pedicle injury should be evaluated by:
[ ] **A.** no extravasation of contrast on cystography.
[ ] **B.** visualization of kidney on excretory urography.
[ ] **C.** patency on retrograde urethrography.
[ ] **D.** normal kidney-ureter-bladder (KUB) X-ray.

10. A 49-year-old man presents to triage with complaints of mid-sternal chest pain. His 12-lead electrocardiogram shows ST elevation in leads V_2, V_3, and V_4. If an anterior myocardial infarction (MI) is suspected, in what leads will reciprocal ST depression be found?
[ ] **A.** Leads I, II, and aV_F
[ ] **B.** Leads II, III, and aV_F
[ ] **C.** Leads I and aV_L
[ ] **D.** Leads II and aV_L

11. What's a common finding in a client with an open pneumothorax?
[ ] **A.** A chest wound with sucking sounds
[ ] **B.** Increased breath sounds over the affected area
[ ] **C.** Resonance over the affected area
[ ] **D.** Hemoptysis

12. A multitrauma client has just arrived in the emergency department. Nasotracheal intubation was initiated at the scene by an emergency medical service unit. Which intervention must be done first?
[ ] **A.** Connect the nasotracheal tube to a volume ventilator.
[ ] **B.** Obtain arterial blood gas measurements to determine acid-base status.
[ ] **C.** Verify nasotracheal tube placement.
[ ] **D.** Attach the client to a cardiac monitor and pulse oximeter.

13. Which statement from a client discharged from the emergency department with acute otitis externa indicates an understanding of instructions?
[ ] **A.** "I should wear earplugs when swimming."
[ ] **B.** "I should make position changes slowly."
[ ] **C.** "I need to keep my home uncluttered to minimize the risk of falling."
[ ] **D.** "I should contact my physician if my ear aches and the pain increases when I lie down."

14. A treatment plan for a client in cardiogenic shock should produce which outcome?
[ ] **A.** Increased left ventricular end-diastolic pressure
[ ] **B.** Increased systemic vascular resistance
[ ] **C.** Decreased cardiac output
[ ] **D.** Decreased left ventricular end-diastolic (LVED) pressure

15. A client with a LeFort II fracture is transferred to the emergency department. The nurse looks for free-floating movement of:
[ ] **A.** unilateral periorbital area.
[ ] **B.** nose and dental arch.
[ ] **C.** teeth and lower maxilla.
[ ] **D.** all facial bones.

16. What's a true statement about epididymitis?
[ ] **A.** Elevation of the testes increases pain.
[ ] **B.** A child with epididymitis should be screened for possible molestation.
[ ] **C.** It isn't necessary to examine and treat sexual partners.
[ ] **D.** Fertility isn't affected in a client with epididymitis.

17. All of the following clients have an increased risk of liver injury after abdominal trauma *except:*
[ ] **A.** a 78-year-old male with a history of congestive heart failure.
[ ] **B.** a 25-year-old male with an injury to his left lower ribs.
[ ] **C.** a 20-year-old female with sickle cell anemia.
[ ] **D.** a 55-year-old male with cirrhosis.

18. What should be the treatment plan for a suicidal client who presents to the emergency department?
[ ] **A.** Notification of the family
[ ] **B.** Contracting for safety
[ ] **C.** Sedation
[ ] **D.** Involuntary commitment

19. A client is brought to the emergency department following a motor vehicle collision in which he was ejected from the car into a lake. His vital signs are as follows: blood pressure, 70/50 mm Hg; heart rate, 140 beats/minute; temperature, 95° F (35° C). He's orally intubated and currently receiving 100% oxygen through an Ambu bag. What interventions do you anticipate?
[ ] **A.** Stat of the computed tomography (CT) scan
[ ] **B.** Infusion of warmed fluid and warming blanket
[ ] **C.** Transfer to the intensive care unit (ICU)
[ ] **D.** Blood transfusion

20. All emergency department (ED) nurses are compelled to treat homeless clients with multiple minor complaints with dignity. What directive requires the nurses to respond in this manner?
[ ] **A.** Personal or religious beliefs
[ ] **B.** Code of ethics for ED nurses
[ ] **C.** Clinical expertise
[ ] **D.** State and federal laws

21. A 44-year-old female is brought to the emergency department with shortness of breath and persistent chest pain for 2 hours. Vital signs include blood pressure of 126/70 mm Hg, pulse rate of 88 beats/minute, and respiratory rate of 26/minute. What is the client's mean arterial pressure (MAP)?
[ ] **A.** 37 mm Hg
[ ] **B.** 63 mm Hg
[ ] **C.** 88 mm Hg
[ ] **D.** 107 mm Hg

22. The release of histamine in the antigen-antibody reaction during anaphylactic shock results in:
[ ] **A.** vasodilation.
[ ] **B.** vasoconstriction.
[ ] **C.** increased myocardial contractility.
[ ] **D.** decreased vascular permeability.

23. A client with known bipolar disorder (manic-depressive illness) is brought to the emergency department (ED) by friends who state that he hasn't been taking his medicine. The ED nurse should expect to find which symptoms?
[ ] **A.** Labile emotions, hyperactivity or hypoactivity, poor social judgment, and grandiose context to speech
[ ] **B.** An increase in heart rate, respiratory rate, and blood pressure
[ ] **C.** Normal thought process
[ ] **D.** Flat or inappropriate affect

24. Which of the following is the medication of choice for a client presenting with hypertensive crisis?
[ ] **A.** Nitroglycerin
[ ] **B.** Labetalol
[ ] **C.** Hydralazine
[ ] **D.** Nitroprusside

25. Which acid-base imbalance is most likely seen in a client with chronic obstructive pulmonary disease (COPD)?
[ ] **A.** Metabolic acidosis
[ ] **B.** Respiratory acidosis
[ ] **C.** Metabolic alkalosis
[ ] **D.** Respiratory alkalosis

26. Which amputation isn't favorable for successful reimplantation?
[ ] **A.** Multiple digits
[ ] **B.** Thumb
[ ] **C.** Pediatric extremity
[ ] **D.** Injuries at multiple levels on the same extremity

27. Which statement about ventricular fibrillation is correct?
[ ] **A.** Ventricular fibrillation is less likely to respond to countershock if the client is acidotic.
[ ] **B.** Ventricular fibrillation requires synchronized cardioversion.
[ ] **C.** Ventricular fibrillation can be distinguished from asystole by auscultation.
[ ] **D.** Ventricular fibrillation should be treated by an initial countershock at 360 joules.

28. What's the most serious adverse effect of vasopressin I.V. therapy in the client with bleeding esophageal varices?
[ ] **A.** Coronary vasoconstriction
[ ] **B.** Abdominal cramping
[ ] **C.** Water intoxication
[ ] **D.** Tissue damage due to infiltration

29. A client comes to the emergency department (ED) complaining of shortness of breath, dizziness, and chest pain after a diving trip with friends. Which condition should the ED nurse suspect?
[ ] **A.** Decompression sickness
[ ] **B.** Air embolism
[ ] **C.** Nitrogen narcosis
[ ] **D.** Spontaneous pneumothorax

30. Chemotherapeutic drugs appear to damage cardiac myofibrils, leading to hypertrophy of the heart muscle and decreased function. Resulting clinical manifestations may include:
[ ] **A.** increased systolic blood pressure.
[ ] **B.** decreased diastolic blood pressure.
[ ] **C.** epigastric pain.
[ ] **D.** bradycardia.

31. The client with carpal tunnel syndrome presents with all of the following symptoms *except:*
[ ] **A.** paresthesias of thumb, index finger, middle finger, and one-half the ring finger.
[ ] **B.** weakness.
[ ] **C.** worse pain at night.
[ ] **D.** swelling.

32. Cocaine-induced myocardial ischemia may be related to:
[ ] **A.** bradycardia.
[ ] **B.** coronary artery vasodilation.
[ ] **C.** increased myocardial oxygen consumption.
[ ] **D.** pulmonary emboli.

33. A client develops anaphylactic shock after receiving radiopaque dye. The client is currently taking atenolol (Tenormin) 100 mg by mouth daily for hypertension. Which intervention should be implemented?
[ ] **A.** Administer glucocorticoids.
[ ] **B.** Administer high doses of epinephrine and glucagon 5 to 15 mcg/minute I.V.
[ ] **C.** Administer diphenhydramine (Benadryl).
[ ] **D.** Administer high doses of inhaled bronchodilators.

34. A client's electrocardiogram reveals ST-segment changes in leads II, III, and aV_F. The emergency department nurse suspects damage to which wall of the myocardium?
[ ] **A.** Inferior
[ ] **B.** Lateral
[ ] **C.** Anterior
[ ] **D.** Apical

35. What's the strongest indication that a client may be violent?
[ ] **A.** A history of violence
[ ] **B.** Rapid, loud speech and heavy alcohol consumption
[ ] **C.** Clenched fists, pacing, and tense posture
[ ] **D.** Complaints of extreme pain from a client who has had to wait several hours

36. Which of the following best demonstrates the criteria necessary to assess the presence of psychosis?
[ ] **A.** Delusions of grandeur or persecution, anxiety, depression, and sleep disturbances
[ ] **B.** Preoccupation with egocentric ideas, defiance of authority, and a history of drug abuse
[ ] **C.** Disturbed affect, bizarre thinking, illogical speech, delusions, and relational withdrawal
[ ] **D.** Psychomotor abnormalities, self-mutilation, anorexia, and catatonia

37. The pumping ability of the heart depends on which four factors?
[ ] **A.** Contractility, preload, heart rate, and afterload
[ ] **B.** Contractility, heart rate, cardiac output, and cardiac index
[ ] **C.** Heart rate, cardiac output, left ventricular hypertrophy, and pulmonary venous congestion
[ ] **D.** Heart rate, preload, cardiac output, and cardiac index

38. What's an appropriate intervention for a trauma client with hypovolemic shock and a urine specific gravity of 1.050?
[ ] **A.** Withhold all I.V. fluids.
[ ] **B.** Administer a bolus of 40 mL/kg of crystalloid.
[ ] **C.** Insert an indwelling urinary catheter.
[ ] **D.** Administer furosemide (Lasix) 40 mg I.V.

39. A 79-year-old female comes to the emergency department complaining that she feels something moving in her ear. Upon otoscopic examination, the physician observes a live cockroach in the client's ear. Which irrigation would be most appropriate for this client?
[ ] **A.** Normal saline
[ ] **B.** Alcohol diluted with water
[ ] **C.** Tap water
[ ] **D.** Mineral oil

40. Ventricular shunts are used to treat which condition?
[ ] **A.** Pneumocephalus
[ ] **B.** Encephalopathy
[ ] **C.** Subdural empyema
[ ] **D.** Hydrocephalus

41. Which symptom is *not* related to cardiac tamponade?
[ ] **A.** Hypotension
[ ] **B.** Tracheal deviation
[ ] **C.** Muffled heart tones
[ ] **D.** Distended neck veins

42. Herpes zoster is an inflammatory condition with localized burning and shearing pain. Which term refers to herpes zoster lesions?
[ ] **A.** Papule
[ ] **B.** Vesicle
[ ] **C.** Bulla
[ ] **D.** Pustule

43. A client in sickle-cell crisis is brought to the emergency department in an ambulance. The nurse anticipates all of the following to be collaborative measures utilized to treat the client initially *except*:
[ ] **A.** frequent doses of opioid analgesics.
[ ] **B.** oxygen via nasal cannula.
[ ] **C.** oral or I.V. fluid and electrolyte administration.
[ ] **D.** transfusion therapy.

44. The emergency nurse notes an ST-segment elevation in leads II, III, and aV_F during assessment of a 12-lead electrocardiogram (ECG). Which coronary artery is most likely occluded?
[ ] **A.** Circumflex
[ ] **B.** Left anterior descending
[ ] **C.** Left coronary artery
[ ] **D.** Right coronary artery

45. What's a contraindication for lumbar puncture?
[ ] **A.** Increased intracranial pressure (ICP)
[ ] **B.** Allergy to local anesthetic (1% lidocaine)
[ ] **C.** Suspected blood in cerebrospinal fluid (CSF)
[ ] **D.** Presence of spinal cord lesion

46. A client with a severe posterior epistaxis of short duration is admitted to the emergency department. The client is pale, weak, slightly dizzy, and complains of a headache. Vital signs are blood pressure, 200/110 mm Hg; pulse, 104 beats/minute; respirations, 28 breaths/minute; and temperature, 98° F (36.7° C). Which laboratory test result is possible?
[ ] **A.** Markedly decreased hemoglobin
[ ] **B.** Decreased platelet count
[ ] **C.** Diminished prothrombin time
[ ] **D.** Increased creatinine level

47. The emergency department nurse knows that the most important principle in client education is:
[ ] **A.** providing the most up-to-date information available.
[ ] **B.** alleviating the client's guilt associated with not knowing appropriate self-care.
[ ] **C.** determining client readiness to learn new information.
[ ] **D.** building on previous information.

48. A client presents with an ankle injury. The ankle is moderately swollen, ecchymotic, and painful to palpation over the lateral and medial malleolus. What's the nursing priority for this client?
[ ] **A.** Applying ice and elevating the ankle
[ ] **B.** Teaching the principles of crutch walking
[ ] **C.** Getting an order for pain medication
[ ] **D.** Applying a traction splint with 15 lb of traction

49. Triage has been effective when the client presenting with heart failure is classified as:
[ ] **A.** urgent.
[ ] **B.** acute.
[ ] **C.** nonacute.
[ ] **D.** referable.

50. What's the most effective treatment of intrapulmonary shunt in the client with acute respiratory distress syndrome (ARDS)?
[ ] **A.** Administer a diuretic.
[ ] **B.** Increase the fraction of inspired oxygen (FIO_2).
[ ] **C.** Implement positive end-expiratory pressure (PEEP).
[ ] **D.** Decrease fluid intake.

51. Which type of learning is demonstrated when the nurse teaches a parent to change the sterile dressing on a child's arm?
[ ] **A.** Cognitive
[ ] **B.** Affective
[ ] **C.** Social
[ ] **D.** Psychomotor

52. When educating the client with tendinitis or bursitis, discharge instructions should include which of the following?
[ ] **A.** Take aspirin for severe pain or discomfort.
[ ] **B.** Take nonsteroidal anti-inflammatory drugs (NSAIDs) on an empty stomach.
[ ] **C.** Discontinue NSAIDs and call your physician if you have bright red, bloody, or dark, tarry stools.
[ ] **D.** Discontinue NSAIDs if you don't obtain relief from pain or inflammation in 48 hours.

53. When preparing to irrigate a client's right ear, in which direction should the nurse direct the irrigation stream?
[ ] **A.** 1 o'clock position
[ ] **B.** 5 o'clock position
[ ] **C.** 9 o'clock position
[ ] **D.** 11 o'clock position

54. Which of the following diagnoses is suspected in a client who presents with complaints of vertigo, tinnitus, ear fullness, and a fluctuation of hearing ability?
[ ] **A.** Labyrinthitis
[ ] **B.** Otitis media
[ ] **C.** Ménière's disease
[ ] **D.** Disequilibrium syndrome

55. What's a symptom of radial head dislocation (nursemaid's elbow) in a pediatric client?
[ ] **A.** Ligamentous instability
[ ] **B.** Excessive swelling
[ ] **C.** Refusal to use arm
[ ] **D.** Loss of arm length

56. A common metabolic oncologic emergency is hypercalcemia, when the total serum calcium concentration is greater than 10 mg/dL. Management for the client with hypercalcemia includes:
[ ] **A.** continuous cardiac monitoring.
[ ] **B.** maintaining slow I.V. rate.
[ ] **C.** I.V. mannitol.
[ ] **D.** I.V. calcitrol.

57. Which intervention would be appropriate for a client who suffers a seizure after receiving a lidocaine bolus and a lidocaine infusion?
[ ] **A.** Discontinue the lidocaine infusion, monitor the client closely, and notify the physician immediately.
[ ] **B.** Continue the lidocaine infusion, but obtain a specimen for repeat serum cardiac enzyme analysis.
[ ] **C.** Administer diuretics to decrease myocardial work.
[ ] **D.** Administer digoxin to help augment cardiac output.

58. Upper GI bleeding most commonly occurs as a result of:
[ ] **A.** neoplasms, gastritis, and duodenal ulcers.
[ ] **B.** Mallory-Weiss tears, peptic ulcers, and vascular anomalies.
[ ] **C.** peptic ulcers, acute mucosal lesions, and esophageal varices.
[ ] **D.** esophagitis, gastric ulcers, and hematologic disorders.

59. A repeat clean-catch urine specimen (or a catheterized specimen) may need to be collected if urinalysis shows the presence of:
[ ] **A.** bacteria.
[ ] **B.** increased epithelial cells.
[ ] **C.** increased white blood cells (WBCs).
[ ] **D.** pus.

60. Dietary restrictions the nurse will review at discharge with the client with a diagnosis of acute gout include avoiding or reducing the intake of:
[ ] **A.** dairy products.
[ ] **B.** whole grains.
[ ] **C.** red meat.
[ ] **D.** citrus fruits.

61. What's the earliest indicator of a change in a client's neurologic status?
[ ] **A.** Pupillary reaction
[ ] **B.** Motor response
[ ] **C.** Capillary refill
[ ] **D.** Level of consciousness (LOC)

62. A 14-month-old child with a sudden onset of colicky abdominal pain and vomiting is brought to the emergency department by his mother. His mother is unable to console him. A diagnosis of intussusception is suspected based on which physical finding?
[ ] **A.** Palpable olive-shaped mass in the upper abdomen
[ ] **B.** Tenderness over McBurney's point
[ ] **C.** Cullen's sign
[ ] **D.** Palpable sausage-shaped mass in the upper abdomen

63. Which finding indicates worsening pulmonary function in a client with flail chest?
[ ] **A.** Accessory muscle use
[ ] **B.** Increased pain with movement
[ ] **C.** Increased blood pressure
[ ] **D.** Shallow respirations

64. Which drug should be administered to a client who has taken an overdose of fentanyl (Sublimaze)?
[ ] **A.** Physostigmine
[ ] **B.** Flumazenil (Romazicon)
[ ] **C.** Atropine
[ ] **D.** Naloxone

65. About 16 hours after a fall, a client is transferred to the emergency department (ED) from a nursing home. The fall resulted in a comminuted fracture of the left hip. About 1 hour after arrival in the ED, the client begins to complain of chills and difficulty breathing. On auscultation of the client's chest, the ED nurse notes petechiae over the client's anterior chest and neck. What's the likely cause of the client's symptoms?
[ ] **A.** Compartment syndrome
[ ] **B.** Pulmonary embolus
[ ] **C.** Fat embolus
[ ] **D.** Myocardial infarction (MI)

66. A 4-year-old child presents with abrupt onset of high fever, stridor, drooling, tachypnea, and severe throat pain. What's the most likely diagnosis?
[ ] **A.** Epiglottiditis
[ ] **B.** Retropharyngeal abscess
[ ] **C.** Bacterial tracheitis
[ ] **D.** Viral croup syndrome

67. A 5-year-old client with a pea in his ear is admitted to the emergency department. What does the nurse need to remove the pea?
[ ] **A.** Alligator forceps
[ ] **B.** 30-mL syringe
[ ] **C.** Lidocaine
[ ] **D.** Triethanolamine polypeptide oleate-condensate

68. A young man comes to the emergency department complaining of a recurring tension headache. Which nursing intervention reflects an understanding of the causes of tension headaches?
[ ] **A.** Placing a warm towel on the client's neck
[ ] **B.** Performing rigorous, active range-of-motion (ROM) to the client's neck and jaw
[ ] **C.** Applying pressure over the contracted muscles
[ ] **D.** Administering ergotamine

69. On arrival in the emergency department, a multi-trauma client had a hematocrit (HCT) of 42%. After 1 L of fluid, the HCT was 35%; after 2 L, the HCT is 29.5%. The nurse notices that the urinary catheter drainage is now hematuric and the client is bleeding from the nasogastric and endotracheal tube sites. The physician makes a diagnosis of disseminated intravascular coagulation (DIC). Based on this diagnosis, the nurse can expect to:
[ ] **A.** administer heparin and fresh frozen plasma.
[ ] **B.** administer streptokinase and packed red blood cells.
[ ] **C.** administer tissue plasminogen activator (tPa) and platelets.
[ ] **D.** administer urokinase and whole blood.

70. A 36-year-old male client presents to triage after being hit in the right eye by an object. The client is complaining of diplopia and distortion in his visual fields. On examination, his visual acuity is decreased and there's no response to light. Which diagnosis is anticipated?
[ ] **A.** Globe rupture
[ ] **B.** Lens displacement
[ ] **C.** Hyphema
[ ] **D.** Retinal detachment

71. Neutropenia is defined as a neutrophil count of less than 1,000/mm^3. Disorders associated with neutropenia include all of the following *except:*
[ ] **A.** hepatitis.
[ ] **B.** influenza
[ ] **C.** diverticulitis.
[ ] **D.** measles.

72. During examination of the mouth of a client with facial trauma, the emergency nurse notes ecchymosis on the floor of the mouth. Which of the following diagnoses is consistent with this finding?
[ ] **A.** Zygotic fracture
[ ] **B.** LeFort fracture
[ ] **C.** Mandibular fracture
[ ] **D.** Maxillary fracture

73. Which injury should result in radiographic assessment by arteriography?
[ ] **A.** An injury to a long bone
[ ] **B.** A penetrating injury with the possibility of a fracture
[ ] **C.** An open fracture
[ ] **D.** An injury with suspected vascular damage

74. What's the treatment of choice for a client with an esophageal rupture?
[ ] **A.** Immediate intubation
[ ] **B.** Insertion of a nasogastric (NG) tube
[ ] **C.** Antibiotic administration
[ ] **D.** Chest tube insertion

75. The client receiving I.V. immune globulin therapy suddenly develops chest tightness, dyspnea, back pain, and chills. Which intervention is a priority for this client?
[ ] **A.** Assess vital signs.
[ ] **B.** Stop the infusion.
[ ] **C.** Administer subcutaneous epinephrine 0.1 mg/kg.
[ ] **D.** Administer diphenhydramine (Benadryl).

76. What's the purpose of corticosteroids in a client diagnosed with a brain tumor?
[ ] **A.** To control absence seizures
[ ] **B.** To provide symptomatic relief of agitation
[ ] **C.** To reduce cerebral edema
[ ] **D.** To reduce pain

77. Abrupt withdrawal of corticosteroid therapy puts a client at risk for:
[ ] **A.** glaucoma.
[ ] **B.** adrenal crisis.
[ ] **C.** psychiatric disturbances.
[ ] **D.** tardive dyskinesia.

78. An elderly client is brought to the emergency department by his neighbor, who states that he found the client in his unheated home. The outdoor temperature is 27° F (–2.8° C). The client is lethargic and confused. Vital signs are blood pressure, 90/46 mm Hg; pulse, 50 beats/minute; respirations, 14 breaths/minute; and temperature, 89.6° F (32° C). Which statement about treatment of clients with severe hypothermia is true?

[ ] **A.** The application of warm blankets is sufficient to prevent further heat loss.
[ ] **B.** Active and rapid external warming is the treatment of choice for this client.
[ ] **C.** Complications of rewarming include metabolic acidosis and cardiac arrhythmias.
[ ] **D.** After the temperature returns to normal, the client may be safely discharged.

79. Which term is applied to the lowest level of electrical energy required to initiate consistent capture with a pacemaker?

[ ] **A.** Underdrive pacing
[ ] **B.** Pacing threshold
[ ] **C.** Sensing threshold
[ ] **D.** Demand pacing

80. Hyperosmolar hyperglycemic nonketotic syndrome (HHNS) can be identified by which laboratory value?

[ ] **A.** Blood glucose level between 300 and 500 mg/dL
[ ] **B.** Plasma osmolality greater than 350 mOsm/kg
[ ] **C.** Normal blood urea nitrogen (BUN) level
[ ] **D.** Arterial blood gas (ABG) values of pH 7.12; PaO_2, 94 mm Hg; $PaCO_2$, 38 mm Hg; and HCO_3^-, 18 mEq/L.

81. Which type of injury is characterized by a pulling or stressing of a muscle or tendon beyond normal limits, resulting in damage to the fibers without bleeding?

[ ] **A.** Sprain
[ ] **B.** Abrasion
[ ] **C.** Strain
[ ] **D.** Contusion

82. After a motor vehicle accident, a client arrives in the emergency department complaining of dyspnea and sharp shoulder pain. Objective data reveal decreased breath sounds on the left, heart sounds shifted to the right, and bowel sounds in the middle of the chest. What's the most likely diagnosis?

[ ] **A.** Hemothorax
[ ] **B.** Ruptured diaphragm
[ ] **C.** Aortic dissection
[ ] **D.** Tracheobronchial disruption

83. Which statement indicates that the client with hypercalcemia has a good understanding of his condition?

[ ] **A.** "Exercise will help release calcium from my bones."
[ ] **B.** "Decreasing my intake of milk will prevent excessive intake of calcium."
[ ] **C.** "By decreasing my fluid intake to 3 L a day, I will eliminate more calcium from my system."
[ ] **D.** "My kidneys don't play a role in balancing calcium in my body."

84. After ingesting a bottle of aspirin in a suicide attempt, a client with severe salicylate poisoning has been admitted to the emergency department. The nurse should prepare to add which medication to the client's I.V. fluids?

[ ] **A.** Calcium gluconate
[ ] **B.** Folic acid
[ ] **C.** Sodium bicarbonate
[ ] **D.** Magnesium

85. The nurse has administered nalbuphine, a known opioid antagonist, for pain control. The nurse knows that the client needs assessment for opioid dependence after which outcome?

[ ] **A.** Respiratory depression
[ ] **B.** Nausea and vomiting
[ ] **C.** Gooseflesh and diarrhea
[ ] **D.** Seizures

86. The charge nurse walks by two staff nurses in the hall arguing over the need to switch holiday assignments. What's the best response for the charge nurse at this time?

[ ] **A.** Speak to each nurse individually and negotiate an acceptable resolution.
[ ] **B.** Tell the staff nurses to stop arguing and act like professional nurses.
[ ] **C.** Write an incident report for unprofessional behavior.
[ ] **D.** Provide a private opportunity for the nurses to deal with it themselves.

87. Adenosine (Adenocard) is administered to a client with paroxysmal supraventricular tachycardia. The client complains of faintness and becomes pale. The monitor shows asystole. The emergency department nurse should:

[ ] **A.** begin cardiopulmonary resuscitation (CPR).
[ ] **B.** administer 1 mg of atropine by I.V. push.
[ ] **C.** observe the client for several seconds.
[ ] **D.** administer epinephrine by I.V. push.

88. What's the most appropriate disposition of a client presenting to the emergency department with shunt malfunction?
[ ] **A.** Home with self-care instructions
[ ] **B.** Hospitalization to neurosurgical services for shunt revision
[ ] **C.** Home with home health consultation
[ ] **D.** Hospice services

89. Arterial and venous structures are most commonly injured in penetrating vascular trauma. In which type of injury is penetrating vascular trauma most commonly seen?
[ ] **A.** Gunshot wound
[ ] **B.** Blunt trauma
[ ] **C.** Stab injury
[ ] **D.** Crushing injury

90. Autotransfusion can be performed on a client with major blood loss from the chest. How many hours after the loss can the transfusion occur?
[ ] **A.** 4 hours
[ ] **B.** 5 hours
[ ] **C.** 8 hours
[ ] **D.** 10 hours

91. An 18-year-old male comes to the emergency department with multiple abrasions to his chest after falling off his motorcycle and sliding on his chest down the road. If the foreign bodies aren't properly removed, what permanent skin damage can occur?
[ ] **A.** Liposuction
[ ] **B.** Augmentation
[ ] **C.** Tattooing
[ ] **D.** Granulation

92. A new nurse on the unit is very upset and crying because the child that they were trying to resuscitate died. What's the best response for the charge nurse at this time?
[ ] **A.** Remind the nurse to control her feelings so that she can meet her client's needs.
[ ] **B.** Have the chaplain speak to the nurse.
[ ] **C.** Tell the nurse it's okay to cry and take her to a private area to talk.
[ ] **D.** Say nothing and walk away to allow her the privacy she needs.

93. The local TV station calls and asks about the condition of a police officer injured in an altercation with a robber. What's the best response by the staff answering the phone?
[ ] **A.** Refer the caller to the nursing supervisor.
[ ] **B.** Confirm the client's presence, but not the events or current condition.
[ ] **C.** Transfer the call to his wife and let her decide what to tell them.
[ ] **D.** Refer the caller to the legal department.

94. What's the best way for the charge nurse to handle the staff's reactions to a local police officer's fatal injuries at the end of the shift?
[ ] **A.** Encourage people to deal with it privately to prevent compromising client confidentiality.
[ ] **B.** Hold a group discussion session so that staff can share their thoughts and feelings.
[ ] **C.** Invite the staff out for drinks to help distract them from the disturbing event.
[ ] **D.** Ask pastoral care to have prayer for the individual's recovery next week.

95. A client is being treated with I.V. epinephrine and antihistamines after an anaphylactic reaction. Which evaluation finding suggests effective treatment?
[ ] **A.** Blood pressure, 86/62 mm Hg
[ ] **B.** pH, 7.45; PaO_2, 86 mm Hg; $PaCO_2$, 30 mm Hg
[ ] **C.** Patent airway, no pulmonary basilar wheezes
[ ] **D.** Pulmonary basilar wheezes

96. What's indicated for posterior epistaxis?
[ ] **A.** Nasal tampon
[ ] **B.** 16G indwelling urinary catheter
[ ] **C.** Nasal balloon
[ ] **D.** Gelfoam hemostatic agent

97. When evaluating the electrocardiogram (ECG) of a client with a potassium deficit, the nurse should expect which change?
[ ] **A.** Shortened QT interval
[ ] **B.** Tall, peaked T waves
[ ] **C.** Widened QRS complex
[ ] **D.** Inverted or flattened T waves

98. The emergency department clinical nurse educator provided an in-service on a new I.V. pump to the staff. What's the best indicator that the required information has been attained?
[ ] **A.** All staff score 100% on the follow-up written test.
[ ] **B.** Staff members indicate that they understand the machine and have no questions.
[ ] **C.** Any randomly picked staff member can state the step-by-step directions for operation.
[ ] **D.** Any randomly chosen staff member can accurately demonstrate operation of the pump by the end of the in-service.

99. When treating a client involved in a radiation accident, the emergency department (ED) nurse should:
[ ] **A.** treat life-threatening problems only after decontaminating the victim.
[ ] **B.** wear protective clothing.
[ ] **C.** wear a radiation meter.
[ ] **D.** contact the Department of Health.

100. A scuba diver presents with an avulsion or degloving injury of his hand from being attacked by a shark. Which solution should the hand be soaked in to prepare the tissue for debridement?
[ ] **A.** Hydrogen peroxide
[ ] **B.** Povidone-iodine preparations
[ ] **C.** Acetic acid
[ ] **D.** Normal saline

101. Objective assessment findings in the client with severe anemia include:
[ ] **A.** impaired thought processes.
[ ] **B.** weight gain.
[ ] **C.** bradycardia.
[ ] **D.** narrowed pulse pressure.

102. A workup for osteomyelitis would include all of the following *except*:
[ ] **A.** complete blood count (CBC) with differential.
[ ] **B.** joint aspiration.
[ ] **C.** blood cultures.
[ ] **D.** magnetic resonance imaging (MRI).

103. A 66-year-old client has marked dyspnea at rest, is thin, and uses accessory muscles to breathe. He's tachypneic, with a prolonged expiratory phase. He has no cough. He leans forward with his arms braced on his knees to support his chest and shoulders during breathing. This client has symptoms of which respiratory disorder?
[ ] **A.** Asthma
[ ] **B.** Emphysema
[ ] **C.** Acute respiratory distress syndrome (ARDS)
[ ] **D.** Chronic obstructive bronchitis

104. What should be the initial intervention to manage a severe laceration of the leg?
[ ] **A.** Apply a tourniquet and elevate the leg.
[ ] **B.** Obtain X-rays to assess for foreign bodies.
[ ] **C.** Control the bleeding, and assess the neurovascular function of the leg.
[ ] **D.** Pack the leg in ice to stabilize the wound.

105. When checking a client who states that her water just broke, the nurse notes a loop of umbilical cord in the vagina. The nurse applies pressure upward against the baby's head. Which of the following would indicate that this intervention was effective?
[ ] **A.** The umbilical cord retracts back into the uterus.
[ ] **B.** The umbilical cord changes from blue to pink.
[ ] **C.** The umbilical cord begins to pulsate.
[ ] **D.** The woman has the urge to push.

106. What's the least effective intervention for a client with flail chest?
[ ] **A.** Apply a sandbag to the flail area of the chest.
[ ] **B.** Intubate and ventilate the client.
[ ] **C.** Control pain to allow full lung expansion.
[ ] **D.** Limit fluids unless hypovolemic shock is present.

107. Which component must the nurse evaluate when assessing a client's labor contractions?
[ ] **A.** Pelvic type and contraction duration and frequency
[ ] **B.** Contraction duration, frequency, and intensity
[ ] **C.** Pelvic type and contraction frequency and intensity
[ ] **D.** Contraction type, duration, and intensity

108. A client comes to the emergency department with acute shortness of breath and a cough that produces pink, frothy sputum. Admission assessment reveals crackles and wheezes, a blood pressure of 82/45 mm Hg, a heart rate of 120 beats/minute, and a respiratory rate of 39 breaths/minute. The client's medical history includes diabetes mellitus, hypertension, and heart failure. Which disorder should the nurse suspect?
[ ] **A.** Pulmonary edema
[ ] **B.** Pneumothorax
[ ] **C.** Cardiac tamponade
[ ] **D.** Pulmonary embolus

109. A 42-year-old female arrives in the emergency department, gravida 5, para 4, with a history of hypertension in pregnancy. She complains of severe right upper quadrant abdominal pain. Based on clinical facts, the client is being evaluated for HELLP syndrome. The most serious complication of HELLP syndrome is:
[ ] **A.** abruptio placentae.
[ ] **B.** disseminated intravascular coagulation (DIC).
[ ] **C.** premature labor.
[ ] **D.** elevated liver enzymes.

110. Which statement indicates that a client with Ménière's disease understands his discharge instructions?
[ ] **A.** "I'll put these eye drops in my right eye every 6 hours."
[ ] **B.** "I'm going to send my daughter home tonight; she doesn't need to stay with me."
[ ] **C.** "I need to sit up slowly when I get out of bed."
[ ] **D.** "I'll put an ice pack on my ear to help the pain."

111. A 17-year-old female arrives at the emergency department via local emergency medical services (EMS) unconscious and intubated. She was last seen approximately 3 hours ago after a verbal fight with a family member. EMS workers report finding several empty pill bottles, including hydrocodone (Vicodin), lorazepam (Ativan), and phenytoin (Dilantin). They also report that there was vomitus on the floor near where she was found. Her underlying respiratory rate is approximately 3 breaths/minute. What's the most appropriate medication for improving her respiratory rate?
[ ] **A.** Albuterol
[ ] **B.** Dextrose 50% in water ($D_{50}W$)
[ ] **C.** Flumazenil (Romazicon)
[ ] **D.** Naloxone

112. A 53-year-old male comes to the emergency department with a 3-day history of left hip pain. He states that the pain began suddenly, is worsening, and that he's experiencing redness and swelling. When questioned about any recent trauma, he states that he fell while riding his bike a few days ago but didn't sustain any injury at that time. He states that he had a left hip fracture with open reduction with internal fixation (ORIF) 2 years ago, accompanied by a "bad infection" that required antibiotics. Physical examination reveals a warm, tender left hip and restriction in movement of this hip. What's the likely diagnosis for this client?
[ ] **A.** Joint effusion
[ ] **B.** Septic joint
[ ] **C.** Chronic osteomyelitis
[ ] **D.** Compartment syndrome

113. A 3-year-old child in respiratory distress is admitted to the emergency department. Vital signs are respiratory rate, 44 breaths/minute; pulse, 160 beats/minute; and temperature, 99.8° F (38° C). Nasal mucous membranes are pale, bluish gray, and boggy with clear mucoid discharge. The child has a high-pitched wheeze on expiration throughout the chest. Chest X-ray shows overdistended lungs. What's the most likely diagnosis for this client?
[ ] **A.** Bronchiolitis
[ ] **B.** Foreign-body obstruction
[ ] **C.** Asthma
[ ] **D.** Hypersensitivity pneumonitis

114. During assessment of a client with facial trauma, it's noted that the client has trouble closing his eyes. This indicates probable damage to which cranial nerve?
[ ] **A.** Oculomotor (III)
[ ] **B.** Trochlear (IV)
[ ] **C.** Trigeminal (V)
[ ] **D.** Facial (VII)

115. A 28-year-old female comes to the emergency department with hypertension in pregnancy. After establishing cardiac monitoring, vital signs, and fetal monitoring, the nurse is ready to start a magnesium drip. Magnesium sulfate is administered by I.V. infusion to clients to:
[ ] **A.** decrease uterine contractions.
[ ] **B.** rapidly lower the blood pressure.
[ ] **C.** reduce activity at the neuromuscular junction.
[ ] **D.** decrease pulmonary edema.

116. Which client has the highest risk for developing cardiogenic shock?

[ ] **A.** An elderly nursing home client with pneumonia
[ ] **B.** A client with acute anterolateral wall infarction
[ ] **C.** A restrained front-seat automobile passenger involved in a rear-end crash
[ ] **D.** A client who underwent cardiac surgery 4 weeks ago and who now presents with abdominal pain

117. A woman who's 12 weeks pregnant comes to the emergency department stating she thinks she's having a miscarriage. Symptoms present in the client experiencing a threatened abortion include:

[ ] **A.** mild vaginal bleeding and a closed cervical os.
[ ] **B.** malodorous vaginal bleeding and a closed cervical os.
[ ] **C.** moderate vaginal bleeding and an open cervical os.
[ ] **D.** heavy vaginal bleeding and an open cervical os.

118. Exposure to ammonia or chlorine gases are especially dangerous because:

[ ] **A.** ammonia and chlorine gases react with water in the lungs to produce acids that cause a secondary chemical burn.
[ ] **B.** ammonia and chlorine gases bind with hemoglobin competitively for oxygen.
[ ] **C.** ammonia and chlorine gases cause a hypotonic fluid to accumulate in the lungs, causing a volume overload in the circulatory system.
[ ] **D.** ammonia and chlorine gases cause paralyzation of the cilia of the airway, leading to decreased airway clearance.

119. A 22-year-old female involved in a motor vehicle crash is brought to the emergency department. She has sustained multiple injuries, including a C6 fracture, pelvis and limb fractures, internal injuries, and an altered level of consciousness (LOC). Spinal precautions are being maintained. Secondary assessment indicates abdominal tenderness, bleeding from the meatus, and multiple abrasions on limbs. Vital signs are blood pressure, 92/50 mm Hg; pulse, 118 beats/minute; respiratory rate, 10 breaths/minute. It's determined that the client should be transferred to the trauma center 50 miles away. Which intervention is most essential to complete before transfer?

[ ] **A.** Urinary catheterization
[ ] **B.** Intubation
[ ] **C.** Peritoneal lavage
[ ] **D.** Tetanus prophylaxis

120. A client is admitted to the emergency department after sustaining injuries in an explosion. The client was near the area of explosion and was thrown to the ground. The client has a fractured right humerus, a concussion, tinnitus, and a sanguineous discharge from a painful right ear. What's an appropriate intervention for this client regarding his painful right ear?

[ ] **A.** Instruct the client on the importance of following the prescribed antibiotic regimen.
[ ] **B.** Irrigate the right ear with warm normal saline.
[ ] **C.** Instill Auralgan eardrops for pain relief.
[ ] **D.** Investigate for evidence of cerebrospinal fluid (CSF).

121. A client comes to the emergency department after exposure to cold temperatures, complaining about severe pain in the tip of his nose. The nurse observes that the tip of his nose is a waxy white color. What type of injury does the client have to his nose?

[ ] **A.** Frost nip
[ ] **B.** Chilblains
[ ] **C.** Frostbite
[ ] **D.** Raynaud's disease

122. Which intervention is important when preventing infection in the client with neutropenia?

[ ] **A.** Providing perineal care after bowel movements
[ ] **B.** Following transmission-based precautions
[ ] **C.** Catheterizing the client as necessary for residual urine
[ ] **D.** Encouraging family to bring in favorite foods for the client

123. A client is admitted to the emergency department complaining of right ear pain. A diagnosis of acute external otitis or swimmer's ear is made. All of the following are signs and symptoms *except*:

[ ] **A.** tender ear.
[ ] **B.** swollen canal.
[ ] **C.** bulging tympanic membrane.
[ ] **D.** redness to pinna.

124. Which fracture has the highest potential for hemorrhage leading to hypovolemia?

[ ] **A.** Femur fracture
[ ] **B.** Forearm fracture
[ ] **C.** Pelvic fracture
[ ] **D.** Ankle fracture

125. A 5-year-old male has been complaining of a severe sore throat and dysphagia for 3 hours. His fever is 103° F (39.4° C). Dyspnea and drooling are observed. Based on this clinical presentation, which diagnosis best supports these symptoms?
[ ] **A.** Epiglottiditis
[ ] **B.** Croup
[ ] **C.** Diphtheria
[ ] **D.** Mononucleosis

126. Recurrent shoulder dislocations typically occur in clients:
[ ] **A.** younger than age 25.
[ ] **B.** ages 30 to 40.
[ ] **C.** ages 40 to 60.
[ ] **D.** older than age 60.

127. The emergency department nurse suspects a client has developed Rocky Mountain spotted fever after a recent tick bite. What's the typical rash pattern that develops?
[ ] **A.** The rash begins on the legs and spreads rapidly to other parts of the body.
[ ] **B.** A rash begins on the face, arms, and legs.
[ ] **C.** Lesions begin on the abdomen and back.
[ ] **D.** The rash begins on the wrists and ankles, spreads to the face, and then to the palms and soles.

128. A client with a hemothorax from blunt chest trauma is admitted to the emergency department. Three hours after receiving a blood transfusion, the client begins to lose 200 mL of blood each hour from the chest tube. What's the most likely explanation for this finding?
[ ] **A.** A vessel has been disrupted and requires surgical repair.
[ ] **B.** This is the expected rate of chest tube drainage.
[ ] **C.** The client is having a transfusion reaction.
[ ] **D.** A second chest tube should have been inserted to manage the loss.

129. Which medical diagnosis indicates a high risk for thrombotic stroke?
[ ] **A.** Hypotension
[ ] **B.** Diabetes insipidus
[ ] **C.** Myocardial infarction (MI) 20 years ago
[ ] **D.** Atrial fibrillation

130. A 35-year-old female comes to the emergency department complaining of right shoulder pain for the last week, with a history of right shoulder pain. The pain is worse at night and with activity. She reports a decrease in range of motion and mentions that she has just returned from vacation, during which she played tennis every day. She's right-handed and has no known history of shoulder or neck problems. A possible diagnosis for this client includes:
[ ] **A.** carpal tunnel syndrome.
[ ] **B.** rheumatoid arthritis.
[ ] **C.** bursitis.
[ ] **D.** Raynaud's disease.

131. Syndrome of inappropriate antidiuretic hormone (SIADH) is a metabolic complication that may occur most frequently in cancer of the lung but may also be seen in a variety of other cancers. Clinical manifestations of SIADH include:
[ ] **A.** weight loss.
[ ] **B.** increased appetite.
[ ] **C.** decreased bowel sounds.
[ ] **D.** seizures.

132. In which of the following diagnoses would you expect to find symptoms of spontaneous bleeding from swollen gums, fetid breath, and dirty gray ulcers on the bases of the tonsil?
[ ] **A.** Acute necrotizing ulcerative gingivitis
[ ] **B.** Ludwig angina
[ ] **C.** Gingivitis
[ ] **D.** Pericoronitis

133. The treatment for gonococcal arthritis is usually in-patient parenteral antibiotics. The current recommendations are:
[ ] **A.** ceftriaxone.
[ ] **B.** ampicillin.
[ ] **B.** erythromycin.
[ ] **D.** doxycycline.

134. When does intussusception occur in an infant?
[ ] **A.** The proximal bowel invaginates into the distal bowel.
[ ] **B.** Hypertrophy and hyperplasia of the circular antral and pyloric musculature result in gastric outlet obstruction.
[ ] **C.** A section of intestine twists on its own axis.
[ ] **D.** Solidified feces cause a mechanical obstruction.

135. What's the definitive therapy for a client with pneumothorax?
[ ] **A.** Administer analgesics.
[ ] **B.** Insert two I.V. lines with large-bore needles.
[ ] **C.** Administer supplemental oxygen.
[ ] **D.** Perform tube thoracotomy.

136. What's the appropriate disposition from the emergency department for a 50-year-old female who's provisionally diagnosed with temporal arteritis?
[ ] **A.** Send home with opioid pain medication.
[ ] **B.** Admit to intensive care to monitor arrhythmias.
[ ] **C.** Hospitalize for biopsy of temporal artery.
[ ] **D.** Refer to psychology services for stress management.

137. A gunshot wound to the right upper quadrant of the abdomen may cause injury to the:
[ ] **A.** appendix.
[ ] **B.** bladder.
[ ] **C.** transverse colon.
[ ] **D.** cecum.

138. During the oliguric phase of acute renal failure, which clinical manifestation would the nurse *not* expect to see?
[ ] **A.** An elevated blood urea nitrogen (BUN)
[ ] **B.** Red blood cells (RBCs) in the urine
[ ] **C.** A decreased serum creatinine level
[ ] **D.** High serum sodium level

139. A woman with pregnancy-induced hypertension is being evaluated in the emergency department. The nurse assists the client on to her left side. This intervention has been effective if the client experiences:
[ ] **A.** a decreased respiratory rate.
[ ] **B.** a decreased pulse rate.
[ ] **C.** a decreased headache.
[ ] **D.** a decrease in the diastolic blood pressure.

140. When assessing a client with moderate to severe anxiety, the emergency department nurse should expect to observe:
[ ] **A.** rapid, pressured speech; restlessness; and tachycardia.
[ ] **B.** exaggerated startle response, hyperactivity, and warm, dry skin.
[ ] **C.** dry mouth, clammy skin, and constricted pupils.
[ ] **D.** irritability, bradycardia, and dilated pupils.

141. Which isn't considered a possible treatment for the client experiencing acute renal failure?
[ ] **A.** Total parenteral nutrition (TPN)
[ ] **B.** Hemodialysis
[ ] **C.** Fluid challenge
[ ] **D.** Renal transplant

142. Five days after a colon resection, a client with diabetes comes to the emergency department (ED). This morning during a bout of coughing he felt a "pop." Now the incision is open, and intestines are protruding from the wound. Which intervention is most appropriate for the ED nurse?
[ ] **A.** Gently push the intestines back into the abdomen.
[ ] **B.** Cover the intestines with saline-moistened gauze.
[ ] **C.** Apply and inflate all sections of a pneumatic antishock garment.
[ ] **D.** Allow the intestines to be exposed to air.

143. What's the best example of a delegation given by a staff registered nurse to an unlicensed assistive personnel (UAP) or nurse's aide?
[ ] **A.** "Obtain a fingerstick glucose specimen on Mr. Green in 15 minutes and tell me the result."
[ ] **B.** "Can you please keep an eye on Mr. White next door while I go to lunch?"
[ ] **C.** "Check and let me know if Mrs. Black is feeling better after that pain shot. Thank you."
[ ] **D.** "Did Mrs. Brown in 913a have adequate output after that Lasix I gave her?"

144. A 54-year-old male with chest pain is brought to the emergency department. An electrocardiogram indicates the client is having an anterior myocardium infarction. Vital signs are blood pressure, 100/52 mm Hg; pulse, 80 beats/minute; respiratory rate, 20 breaths/minute; oxygen saturation, 100% on 2 L/nasal cannula. The decision is made to transfer to the nearby hospital 10 miles away for cardiac catheterization. Based on the initial assessment of the client, which intervention is most important before transfer?
[ ] **A.** Intubation
[ ] **B.** I.V. access
[ ] **C.** Thrombolytic therapy
[ ] **D.** Chest X-ray

145. Septic shock commonly causes which condition in children?
[ ] **A.** Hyperglycemia
[ ] **B.** Metabolic alkalosis
[ ] **C.** Hypoglycemia
[ ] **D.** Hypercalcemia

146. In a client with smoke inhalation, the nurse would expect to hear which breath sound?
[ ] **A.** Crackles
[ ] **B.** Decreased breath sounds
[ ] **C.** Inspiratory and expiratory wheezing
[ ] **D.** Upper airway rhonchi

147. Which intervention usually isn't performed before an interfacility transfer?
[ ] **A.** Report to the receiving hospital
[ ] **B.** Psychological support to the client and his family
[ ] **C.** Preparation for suturing lacerations
[ ] **D.** Copies prepared of the medical record

148. Which statement indicates that the nurse understands the requirements of the Emergency Medical Treatment and Active Labor Act (EMTALA)?
[ ] **A.** "The client has no insurance and must be transferred to another facility."
[ ] **B.** "We must stabilize the client within our capability before we transfer."
[ ] **C.** "We only have to provide an emergency screening examination."
[ ] **D.** "The physician isn't taking new clients."

149. What's the immediate priority in treating the child with asthma?
[ ] **A.** Starting an I.V. and administering corticosteroids
[ ] **B.** Intubation
[ ] **C.** Positioning the child and administering humidified air
[ ] **D.** Having the child cough and deep-breathe to get rid of excessive secretions

150. After a motor vehicle accident, a client comes to the emergency department with an injury to the right leg. On physical assessment, the nurse notices that the client can't raise his leg when it's straightened and lacks sensation to the anterior thigh. Assessment of the left leg is normal. What's the possible cause of this finding?
[ ] **A.** Damage to the median nerve
[ ] **B.** Damage to the femoral nerve
[ ] **C.** Damage to the tibial nerve
[ ] **D.** Damage to the peroneal nerve

151. A colleague expresses concern about copying the medical record of a client who has been unable to sign consent to release his confidential medical information, and then sending it to the hospital that will be receiving the client transfer. You discuss this concern with your colleague and advise her that:
[ ] **A.** she's correct to be vigilant about sharing medical information, but that in this case there's no concern over a HIPAA violation because the information is needed to continue safe care of the client.
[ ] **B.** she's correct to be concerned about this breach of confidentiality, and so no medical records will accompany the client to the receiving facility.
[ ] **C.** she's correct to be concerned, so you will obtain a consent from a family member whenever the family is located and can arrive; then you will send the medical records along to the receiving facility.
[ ] **D.** she's correct to be concerned, so you will send only partial and general information, such as demographics but no medical or nursing documentation.

152. The results from scientific investigation form the basis for which of the following?
[ ] **A.** The Internal Review Board (IRB)
[ ] **B.** Evidence-based practice
[ ] **C.** Interdisciplinary research
[ ] **D.** Performance appraisal

153. Migraine headache and acute angle-closure glaucoma may be difficult to distinguish because many of the symptoms are the same, including:
[ ] **A.** sudden loss of vision in one eye.
[ ] **B.** yellow-green discharge from the eye.
[ ] **C.** syncope.
[ ] **D.** severe unilateral headache, nausea, vomiting, and vision disturbances.

154. The distribution of lesions on the skin can help determine which of the following factors?
[ ] **A.** Type of lesion
[ ] **B.** Arrangement of the lesion
[ ] **C.** Color of the lesion
[ ] **D.** Disease

155. A client comes to the emergency department complaining of a maculopapular rash on his trunk, which follows skin cleavage lines in a Christmas tree pattern. He reports that the rash started as a small lesion 4 days ago. What's the most likely cause of the rash?
[ ] **A.** *Tinea corporis*
[ ] **B.** *Pityriasis rosea*
[ ] **C.** Allergic reaction to a drug
[ ] **D.** Eczema

156. Factors to consider when determining safe, high-quality, cost-efficient emergency staffing and productivity include which of the following?
[ ] **A.** Acuity, budget, and hospital policy
[ ] **B.** Acuity, length of stay, and emergency department (ED) skills mix
[ ] **C.** Nurse–client ratio, hospital census, and budget
[ ] **D.** Core measure metrics, nurse education, and length of ED stay

157. In developing a disaster plan for a hospital, all of the following are primary goals *except*:
[ ] **A.** to continue to care for clients.
[ ] **B.** to educate staff and test the plans.
[ ] **C.** to do a risk assessment of potential disasters.
[ ] **D.** to develop a plan of care for clients at the scene of the disaster.

158. During a mass casualty incident, the triage nurse evaluates a 54-year-old female with third-degree burns over 95% of her body. What disaster priority should the nurse assign to this client?
[ ] **A.** Priority 1—rush client to the resuscitation room immediately.
[ ] **B.** Priority 2—send her to the main emergency department for debridement and pain control.
[ ] **C.** Priority 3—delayed treatment, minor injuries.
[ ] **D.** Priority 4—expectant death; send her to the hospice area for pain control only.

159. If a child is suspected of ingesting poisonous hydrocarbons, an important nursing intervention would include which action?
[ ] **A.** Induce vomiting.
[ ] **B.** Keep the child calm and relaxed.
[ ] **C.** Scold the child for wrongdoing.
[ ] **D.** Keep the parents away from the child.

160. Which of the following descriptions refers to a puerperal infection?
[ ] **A.** Infection of the neonate's umbilicus
[ ] **B.** Infection of the maternal genital tract postpartum
[ ] **C.** Infection of the breast-feeding mother's nipples
[ ] **D.** Infection of maternal blood

161. Which fracture is commonly seen in the upper extremities and is related to physical abuse?
[ ] **A.** Longitudinal
[ ] **B.** Oblique
[ ] **C.** Spiral
[ ] **D.** Transverse

162. Which group of laboratory results, along with the clinical manifestations, establishes a diagnosis of Reye's syndrome?
[ ] **A.** Increased serum glucose and insulin levels
[ ] **B.** Increased bilirubin and alkaline phosphatase
[ ] **C.** Decreased serum glucose and ammonia levels
[ ] **D.** Elevated liver enzymes and prolonged prothrombin and partial thromboplastin times

163. A client comes to the triage desk with blurred vision, slurred speech, dry mouth, and bilateral arm paralysis. He is suspected to have which diagnosis?
[ ] **A.** Hypoglycemia
[ ] **B.** Stroke
[ ] **C.** Botulism
[ ] **D.** Brain tumor

164. Treating the condition from the previous question, identified as causing blurred vision, slurred speech, dry mouth, and bilateral arm paralysis, involves:
[ ] **A.** supportive care.
[ ] **B.** antibiotics given in high doses I.V.
[ ] **C.** oral antibiotics given over 60 days.
[ ] **D.** antitoxin and supportive care.

165. When preparing a client with suspected herniated nucleus pulposus for myelography, which nursing intervention should be done before the test?
[ ] **A.** Question the client about allergy to iodine.
[ ] **B.** Mark distal pulses on the foot in indelible ink.
[ ] **C.** Assess and document pain along the sciatic nerve.
[ ] **D.** Tell the client he may be asked to cough or pant to clear the dye.

166. A client comes to the emergency department with complaints of substernal chest pain, nausea, and weakness for the past hour. He's placed on oxygen, given sublingual nitroglycerin, has an I.V. started, and then receives morphine. His electrocardiogram shows ST-segment elevation in leads II, III, and aV_F. ST-segment elevation in these leads may indicate:
[ ] **A.** anterior myocardial ischemia.
[ ] **B.** inferior myocardial infarction.
[ ] **C.** unstable angina.
[ ] **D.** cardiac tamponade.

167. A 74-year-old woman comes to the emergency department complaining of shortness of breath, dyspnea on exertion, fatigue, and ankle edema. She has a history of hypertension but hasn't taken her medication for 2 months. Her blood pressure is 110/60 mm Hg, and her heart rate is 110 beats/minute and irregular. What's a likely cause for her symptoms?
[ ] **A.** Hypertensive crisis
[ ] **B.** Acute myocardial infarction (MI)
[ ] **C.** Diabetes mellitus
[ ] **D.** Heart failure

168. What's the immediate treatment of choice for acute angle-closure glaucoma?
[ ] **A.** Instillation of a topical anesthetic
[ ] **B.** Bed rest
[ ] **C.** Lowering intraocular pressure (IOP) by the administration of I.V. acetazolamide (Diamox) and mannitol (Osmitrol), and topical drugs, timolol (Timoptic) and pilocarpine (Carpine)
[ ] **D.** Irrigation of normal saline

169. Which finding wouldn't be present in a client with renal colic?
[ ] **A.** Severe, intermittent flank pain
[ ] **B.** Microscopic hematuria
[ ] **C.** Rebound tenderness
[ ] **D.** Restlessness, pallor, and diaphoresis

170. A client with recurrent renal calculi indicates understanding of her discharge instructions when she states all of the following *except:*
[ ] **A.** "I'll save all my urine for stone analysis."
[ ] **B.** "I'll urinate before and after sexual intercourse."
[ ] **C.** "I'll drink at least 1 quart of fluid per day to prevent dehydration."
[ ] **D.** "I'll reduce my intake of iced tea and dairy products."

171. Which symptom occurs early in multiple sclerosis (MS)?
[ ] **A.** Diplopia
[ ] **B.** Grief
[ ] **C.** Hemiparesis
[ ] **D.** Dementia

172. Disposition from the emergency department for a 55-year-old female who's provisionally diagnosed with temporal arteritis would be to:
[ ] **A.** send her home with opioid pain medication.
[ ] **B.** admit her to intensive care to monitor arrhythmias.
[ ] **C.** hospitalize her for biopsy of temporal artery.
[ ] **D.** refer her to psychology services for stress management.

173. A 20-year-old female comes to the emergency department complaining of cramping, abdominal pain, and mild vaginal bleeding. Pelvic examination shows a left adnexal mass that's tender when palpated. Culdocentesis shows blood in the cul-de-sac. The client probably has:
[ ] **A.** abruptio placentae.
[ ] **B.** ectopic pregnancy.
[ ] **C.** hydatidiform mole.
[ ] **D.** pelvic inflammatory disease (PID).

174. When approaching a family for organ or tissue donation, the nurse should keep in mind which guidelines?
[ ] **A.** Approaching a family is done only with a physician's written order.
[ ] **B.** The requester doesn't have to believe in the benefits of the organ donation but should support the process with a positive attitude.
[ ] **C.** The requester is knowledgeable about the basics of organ and tissue donation and is capable of educating the family members about brain death early in the organ donation process.
[ ] **D.** The family is offered the opportunity to speak with an organ procurement coordinator.

175. A 46-year-old female has a perforated eardrum as a result of aggressive cleaning with a hairpin. Which statement by the client would indicate the need for additional teaching?
[ ] **A.** "The hearing loss I am experiencing shouldn't be permanent."
[ ] **B.** "When healed, I should only clean my ears with a cotton-tipped applicator."
[ ] **C.** "I shouldn't use packing in my ear."
[ ] **D.** "My eardrum should heal without surgery."

Answer sheet

	A	B	C	D		A	B	C	D		A	B	C	D		A	B	C	D
1.	○	○	○	○	25.	○	○	○	○	49.	○	○	○	○	73.	○	○	○	○
2.	○	○	○	○	26.	○	○	○	○	50.	○	○	○	○	74.	○	○	○	○
3.	○	○	○	○	27.	○	○	○	○	51.	○	○	○	○	75.	○	○	○	○
4.	○	○	○	○	28.	○	○	○	○	52.	○	○	○	○	76.	○	○	○	○
5.	○	○	○	○	29.	○	○	○	○	53.	○	○	○	○	77.	○	○	○	○
6.	○	○	○	○	30.	○	○	○	○	54.	○	○	○	○	78.	○	○	○	○
7.	○	○	○	○	31.	○	○	○	○	55.	○	○	○	○	79.	○	○	○	○
8.	○	○	○	○	32.	○	○	○	○	56.	○	○	○	○	80.	○	○	○	○
9.	○	○	○	○	33.	○	○	○	○	57.	○	○	○	○	81.	○	○	○	○
10.	○	○	○	○	34.	○	○	○	○	58.	○	○	○	○	82.	○	○	○	○
11.	○	○	○	○	35.	○	○	○	○	59.	○	○	○	○	83.	○	○	○	○
12.	○	○	○	○	36.	○	○	○	○	60.	○	○	○	○	84.	○	○	○	○
13.	○	○	○	○	37.	○	○	○	○	61.	○	○	○	○	85.	○	○	○	○
14.	○	○	○	○	38.	○	○	○	○	62.	○	○	○	○	86.	○	○	○	○
15.	○	○	○	○	39.	○	○	○	○	63.	○	○	○	○	87.	○	○	○	○
16.	○	○	○	○	40.	○	○	○	○	64.	○	○	○	○	88.	○	○	○	○
17.	○	○	○	○	41.	○	○	○	○	65.	○	○	○	○	89.	○	○	○	○
18.	○	○	○	○	42.	○	○	○	○	66.	○	○	○	○	90.	○	○	○	○
19.	○	○	○	○	43.	○	○	○	○	67.	○	○	○	○	91.	○	○	○	○
20.	○	○	○	○	44.	○	○	○	○	68.	○	○	○	○	92.	○	○	○	○
21.	○	○	○	○	45.	○	○	○	○	69.	○	○	○	○	93.	○	○	○	○
22.	○	○	○	○	46.	○	○	○	○	70.	○	○	○	○	94.	○	○	○	○
23.	○	○	○	○	47.	○	○	○	○	71.	○	○	○	○	95.	○	○	○	○
24.	○	○	○	○	48.	○	○	○	○	72.	○	○	○	○	96.	○	○	○	○

	A	B	C	D		A	B	C	D		A	B	C	D
97.	○	○	○	○	126.	○	○	○	○	155.	○	○	○	○
98.	○	○	○	○	127.	○	○	○	○	156.	○	○	○	○
99.	○	○	○	○	128.	○	○	○	○	157.	○	○	○	○
100.	○	○	○	○	129.	○	○	○	○	158.	○	○	○	○
101.	○	○	○	○	130.	○	○	○	○	159.	○	○	○	○
102.	○	○	○	○	131.	○	○	○	○	160.	○	○	○	○
103.	○	○	○	○	132.	○	○	○	○	161.	○	○	○	○
104.	○	○	○	○	133.	○	○	○	○	162.	○	○	○	○
105.	○	○	○	○	134.	○	○	○	○	163.	○	○	○	○
106.	○	○	○	○	135.	○	○	○	○	164.	○	○	○	○
107.	○	○	○	○	136.	○	○	○	○	165.	○	○	○	○
108.	○	○	○	○	137.	○	○	○	○	166.	○	○	○	○
109.	○	○	○	○	138.	○	○	○	○	167.	○	○	○	○
110.	○	○	○	○	139.	○	○	○	○	168.	○	○	○	○
111.	○	○	○	○	140.	○	○	○	○	169.	○	○	○	○
112.	○	○	○	○	141.	○	○	○	○	170.	○	○	○	○
113.	○	○	○	○	142.	○	○	○	○	171.	○	○	○	○
114.	○	○	○	○	143.	○	○	○	○	172.	○	○	○	○
115.	○	○	○	○	144.	○	○	○	○	173.	○	○	○	○
116.	○	○	○	○	145.	○	○	○	○	174.	○	○	○	○
117.	○	○	○	○	146.	○	○	○	○	175.	○	○	○	○
118.	○	○	○	○	147.	○	○	○	○					
119.	○	○	○	○	148.	○	○	○	○					
120.	○	○	○	○	149.	○	○	○	○					
121.	○	○	○	○	150.	○	○	○	○					
122.	○	○	○	○	151.	○	○	○	○					
123.	○	○	○	○	152.	○	○	○	○					
124.	○	○	○	○	153.	○	○	○	○					
125.	○	○	○	○	154.	○	○	○	○					

Sample test 2

Answers and rationales

1. Correct answer—B.

Rationales: Bleeding is the primary adverse effect of thrombolytic therapy. The nurse should establish three I.V. sites before administering therapy and should avoid giving the client I.M. injections and drawing arterial blood gases. The client should be monitored for bleeding. Reperfusion arrhythmias and hypotension may occur with thrombolytic therapy and are treated symptomatically.

Nursing process step: Evaluation

2. Correct answer—B.

Rationales: Organic reasons for delusional behavior must be ruled out before the client is considered a psychiatric emergency. A psychiatric consult can be obtained once the client is cleared medically. Lithium isn't the drug of choice for this client because lithium is used for bipolar disease, not schizophrenia. Insisting that the delusions aren't real will only antagonize the client.

Nursing process step: Analysis

3. Correct answer—C.

Rationales: A change in the client's behavior or mental status may indicate increased intracranial pressure (ICP). The family should be advised to return with the client immediately if his behavior becomes abnormal. Aspirin should be avoided by a client with a head injury because it may increase bleeding. The use of opioids isn't recommended because these drugs may mask signs associated with increased ICP (increased drowsiness, confusion, and lack of coordination). Symptoms of a concussion should subside within 48 hours, and the client should be reevaluated if the symptoms exceed this length of time.

Nursing process step: Intervention

4. Correct answer—C.

Rationales: The advance directive is a legal document outlining a client's wishes regarding health care. If the client can't speak for himself or make decisions for himself, the durable power of attorney for health care gives another person the power to make health care decisions for him. The last will and testament and instructions for care after death aren't read until after the client's death.

5. Correct answer—B.

Rationales: Precipitating factors that can cause an attack of acute gout include excessive caloric intake or overindulgence in purine-containing foods, stress, alcohol intake, and excessive vitamin A intake.

Nursing process step: Analysis

6. Correct answer—C.

Rationales: Hypoxemia is the most common underlying cause of pediatric cardiopulmonary arrest. It leads to marked bradycardia and eventually asystole in the pediatric client. Ensuring optimum oxygenation is the most important intervention in this client population. The other options may lead to cardiopulmonary arrest in the pediatric client, but they're much less common.

Nursing process step: Analysis

7. Correct answer—B.

Rationales: Irrigation can cause the bean to swell and occlude the ear canal. Alligator forceps, a right-angled hook, and an ear curette can all be used to remove a vegetative foreign body.

Nursing process step: Intervention

8. Correct answer—A.

Rationales: Most insecticides are carbamates or organophosphates and are highly lipid-soluble and easily absorbed through the skin. If protection isn't worn, the insecticide may be absorbed through the skin of the nurse. The type and amount of insecticide spilled can be determined during the assessment. Respiratory protection is necessary if the insecticide is in a vapor or aerosol form.

Nursing process step: Analysis

9. Correct answer–B.

Rationales: Excretory urography is the test of choice for renal pedicle repair. Dye injected into the venous system should enter the kidney and provide visualization if the renovascular system is intact. Cystography is a diagnostic tool for the bladder, and retrograde urethrography is performed for a urethral injury. A KUB X-ray shows the shape, location, and size of these organs and helps to identify masses or radiopaque calculi.
Nursing process step: Evaluation

10. Correct answer–B.

Rationales: With an acute anterior MI, there will be ST elevation in leads V_2 through V_4, and ST depression in the inferior leads II, III, and aV_F. The ST elevations won't be found in the other leads.
Nursing process step: Evaluation

11. Correct answer–A.

Rationales: Common findings in a client with an open pneumothorax are sucking sounds from the wound on inspiration. A penetrating wound to the chest presents with diminished or absent breath sounds over the affected area and hyperresonance on the affected side along with dyspnea, chest pain, and tachypnea. Hemoptysis occurs most commonly with pulmonary contusion or tracheobronchial injury.
Nursing process step: Assessment

12. Correct answer–C.

Rationales: The priority for an intubated trauma client is to assess patency of airway. Tubes can become displaced during transport from the emergency medical service unit to the trauma room. To confirm nasotracheal tube placement, the nurse should first listen for air sounds over the epigastric area. If none are present, she should then listen over both lung bases during ventilation. All other interventions may be implemented after airway, breathing, and circulation have been assessed.
Nursing process step: Intervention

13. Correct answer–A.

Rationales: After being diagnosed with acute otitis externa, the client should be instructed to wear earplugs to keep the infected ear dry. Acute otitis externa is an inflammatory condition of the auricle and external auditory canal usually caused by gram-negative organisms. Keeping the ear dry makes it more difficult for these organisms to grow. Because of risks associated with vertigo, a client with Ménière's disease would be instructed to change position slowly and keep his home uncluttered. A client with otitis media would be instructed to notify the physician if ear pain increases when lying down since this may indicate that antibiotic therapy is ineffective.
Nursing process step: Evaluation

14. Correct answer–D.

Rationales: The treatment plan for a client in cardiogenic shock includes administering medications that decrease preload and afterload and increase contractility. As a result of this therapy, LVED pressure as well as demands on the heart should be reduced. Vasodilators reduce total peripheral resistance and decrease LVED pressure. Catecholamines increase heart rate, heart contractility, and vasodilatation in the postcapillary sphincters and pulmonary system. All other options are clinical manifestations of cardiogenic shock.
Nursing process step: Evaluation

15. Correct answer–B.

Rationales: A LeFort II fracture involves a pyramidal fracture that includes the central portion of the maxilla across the superior nasal area. It may also involve the orbit. This produces a free-floating nose and dental arch. Free-floating movement of the unilateral periorbital area doesn't describe a clinical situation. However, free-floating movement of the teeth and maxilla describes a LeFort I, and free-floating movement of all the facial bones describes a LeFort III fracture.
Nursing process step: Assessment

16. Correct answer–B.

Rationales: It's rare for a child to contract epididymitis, so the possibility of child molestation should be investigated. Causes of epididymitis include prostatitis, cystitis, and urethral instrumentation. Common causative organisms include *Escherichia coli, Neisseria gonorrhoeae, Mycobacterium tuberculosis,* and *Chlamydia.* Elevation of the testes sometimes relieves the pain. A client with epididymitis should be cautioned that all sexual partners should be examined and treated. Infertility can be a problem if epididymitis is untreated or partially treated because it can cause vas deferens scars or antisperm antibody production.

Nursing process step: Assessment

17. Correct answer–B.

Rationales: An injury to the left lower ribs would be more likely to cause a splenic injury. Heart failure, sickle cell anemia, and cirrhosis are chronic disease processes that have a direct effect on the liver, making it more susceptible to injury.

Nursing process step: Evaluation

18. Correct answer–B.

Rationales: Contracting with the client for safety is the primary focus. Although family notification, sedation, and involuntary commitment may be needed, they aren't the priority.

Nursing process step: Assessment

19. Correct answer–B.

Rationales: Because the client is both hypothermic and hypotensive, the priority treatment would focus on warming the client and fluid resuscitation. Although a CT scan may be indicated, the blood pressure must be addressed. Transfer to the ICU and blood transfusion may be needed following the initial treatment.

Nursing process step: Intervention

20. Correct answer–B.

Rationales: Code #1 in the code of ethics for ED nurses states that, "The emergency nurse provides services with respect for human dignity and the uniqueness of the client, unrestricted by considerations of social or economic status, personal attributes, or the nature of health problems." Personal beliefs can't compel the behavior of an entire profession. ED nurses may have many different personal or religious beliefs regarding human dignity, and the development of clinical expertise should coincide with a deeper understanding of ethical behavior. Clinical expertise can't guarantee ethical behavior because ethics deals with values, actions, and choices of right and wrong. Laws are binding rules of conduct enforced by authority. In many situations, laws and ethics may overlap; however, the ethical precept of treating other human beings with dignity and law can't mandate respect for their unique individuality.

21. Correct answer–C.

Rationale: MAP = systolic blood pressure + (diastolic blood pressure × 2) ÷ 3. So, in this case:
MAP = 126 + (70 × 2) ÷ 3; MAP = 126 + 140 ÷ 3;
MAP = 88.

Nursing process step: Assessment

22. Correct answer–A.

Rationales: The antigen-antibody reaction in anaphylactic shock induces the release of histamine, which causes massive vasodilation, a reduction in arterial pressure by dilating the arterioles, and an increase in vascular permeability. This creates a rapid shift of fluids into the interstitial spaces, and myocardial contractility is decreased because of inadequate venous return, resulting in decreased preload.

Nursing process step: Assessment

23. Correct answer–A.

Rationales: Labile emotions, hyperactivity, hypoactivity, poor social judgment, and grandiose context to speech are classic signs of bipolar disease. Vital signs are usually normal unless other contributing factors are present. A client with bipolar disease may have impaired thinking related to rapid progression of thoughts, flight of ideas, and grandiosity. A flat or inappropriate affect is usually associated with schizophrenia.

Nursing process step: Assessment

24. Correct answer–D.

Rationales: Nitroprusside is the first-line choice in a hypertensive crisis because it's a mixed arterial and venous vasodilator. This makes it more effective than the other medications.

Nursing process step: Intervention

25. Correct answer–B.

Rationales: Carbon dioxide is an acidic compound that's normally excreted by the respiratory system. A client with COPD presents with an elevated $PaCO_2$, resulting in the development of respiratory acidosis and hypoxemia. Metabolic acidosis is a common finding in renal failure, dehydration, and shock. Respiratory alkalosis commonly occurs with anxiety and other states that lead to hyperventilation. Metabolic alkalosis occurs in situations with increased loss of GI fluids.

Nursing process step: Assessment

26. Correct answer–D.

Rationales: Injuries at multiple levels on the same extremity make it unlikely that reimplantation will be successful. Loss of several digits seriously compromises hand function, so reimplantation should be considered. Reimplantation of the thumb should also be considered because the thumb constitutes 40% to 50% of the functional value of the hand due to its role in opposition and grasp and because this procedure has a high success rate. Reimplantation is usually successful in children because they regenerate transected nerves well and readily adapt to using a reimplanted part.

Nursing process step: Evaluation

27. Correct answer–A.

Rationales: Acidosis decreases the myocardial cells, ability to respond to the countershock. Synchronized cardioversion is inappropriate in ventricular fibrillation, which should be treated with unsynchronized defibrillation. Auscultation won't differentiate between ventricular fibrillation and asystole. The appropriate initial shock in ventricular fibrillation is 200 joules.

Nursing process step: Assessment

28. Correct answer–A.

Rationales: Coronary vasoconstriction, abdominal cramping, water intoxication, and tissue damage from infiltration are all adverse effects of vasopressin therapy. The most serious adverse effect, however, is coronary vasoconstriction, which can cause arrhythmias, ischemia, and decreased cardiac output.

Nursing process step: Evaluation

29. Correct answer–B.

Rationales: These symptoms suggest air embolism, which is caused by failure to exhale on ascent. Decompression sickness is caused by nitrogen bubbles in the bloodstream and is manifested by rash, fatigue, and dizziness. Nitrogen narcosis results when the client breathes dissolved nitrogen under pressure. Symptoms include fatigue, weakness, and decreased consciousness; it may result in death.

Nursing process step: Assessment

30. Correct answer–C.

Rationales: Epigastric pain is a GI symptom associated with liver engorgement and ascites. Cardiovascular manifestations include a decrease in systolic blood pressure with an increase in diastolic blood pressure. Tachycardia, not bradycardia, may be the first clinical manifestation of heart failure as the body attempts to compensate for a failing ventricle.

Nursing process step: Assessment

31. Correct answer–D.

Rationales: Clients don't typically present with swelling of their hands with carpal tunnel syndrome. Weakness, paresthesia, and pain at night are all classic symptoms of carpal tunnel syndrome. Other symptoms include decreased range of motion, elbow and shoulder pain, and occasionally nail and skin involvement.

Nursing process step: Assessment

32. Correct answer–C.

Rationales: Cocaine-induced myocardial ischemia has been associated with coronary artery vasoconstriction, coronary thrombosis, and increased myocardial oxygen consumption. In addition, these clients typically suffer from tachyarrhythmias.

Nursing process step: Evaluation

33. Correct answer–B.

Rationales: Clients receiving beta-adrenergic blockers require large, repeated doses of epinephrine to counteract the effects of the beta-adrenergic blockers. Glucagon 5 to 15 mcg/minute I.V. may be beneficial for refractory hypotension associated with beta-adrenergic blockers. All other medications should be administered per recommended doses.

Nursing process step: Intervention

34. Correct answer–A.

Rationales: Changes in leads II, III, and aV_F are indicative of damage to the inferior wall of the heart. The lateral wall shows changes in leads I, II, III, aV_F, V_5, and V_6. Anterior changes are shown in leads V_1 through V_4, I, and aV_L. Apical damage is shown in leads II, aV_F, V_5, and V_6.
Nursing process step: Assessment

35. Correct answer–C.

Rationales: Clenched fists, pacing, and tense posture demonstrate escalation of violent behavior. The emergency department nurse needs to recognize this behavior early so that appropriate intervention can occur. The other options may indicate the potential for violence as well, but not to the extent that clenched fists, pacing, and tense posture do.
Nursing process step: Assessment

36. Correct answer–C.

Rationales: Psychosis is a severe state in which a person loses the ability to interact with reality. This is evidenced by bizarre thinking, loose association of ideas, illogical speech, egocentricity, and withdrawal from relationships into an internal world of fantasies. The person may exhibit perceptual disturbances, including visual and auditory hallucinations and delusions of grandeur or persecution. Psychosis involves the loss of ego boundaries, diminished volition, and psychomotor abnormalities that demonstrate a marked decrease in reactivity to the environment. Catatonic patterns, such as stupor, posturing, unusual mannerisms, or grimacing may be present.
Nursing process step: Assessment

37. Correct answer–A.

Rationales: The pumping ability of the heart depends on contractility (force of ventricular contraction), preload (ventricular filling and end-diastolic volume), heart rate, and afterload (pressure against which the ventricle pumps). Cardiac output and index are the result of the pumping ability of the heart.
Nursing process step: Evaluation

38. Correct answer–B.

Rationales: A urine specific gravity of 1.050 is elevated and indicates decreased renal perfusion, possibly resulting in dehydration. The most appropriate intervention for this client is a bolus of crystalloid at 40 mL/kg. If urine output is less than 30 mL/hour, and adequate volume replacement hasn't been achieved, the client in shock may need to have an indwelling urinary catheter inserted to monitor urine output. Furosemide 40 mg I.V. isn't recommended in a client who's already volume-depleted.
Nursing process step: Intervention

39. Correct answer–D.

Rationales: Instilling a few drops of mineral oil into the ear canal will kill the insect, after which the dead insect can be removed with direct instrumentation. A cotton ball soaked in ether or 2% lidocaine will also anesthetize the insect, facilitating its removal. Normal saline and tap water are commonly used for irrigation of inorganic objects. A mixture of water and alcohol can be used for removal of organic objects because it won't produce further swelling of the object. However, irrigation with normal saline, tap water, or alcohol diluted with water won't readily kill the insect.
Nursing process step: Intervention

40. Correct answer–D.

Rationales: Hydrocephalus is treated with ventricular shunts, which are surgically implanted to augment drainage of cerebrospinal fluid from the brain. Pneumocephalus is treated by evacuation of air through the use of subarachnoid screws. Encephalopathy is treated with drugs: anticonvulsants, steroids, and antibiotics. A subdural empyema is a collection of material between the dura and arachnoid layers and is treated with antimicrobial therapy and surgical drainage.
Nursing process step: Analysis

41. Correct answer–B.

Rationales: Classic signs of cardiac tamponade include three main symptoms known as Beck's triad. They include hypotension, muffled heart sounds, and distended neck veins. Tracheal deviation is a late sign of a tension pneumothorax.
Nursing process step: Analysis

42. Correct answer—B.

Rationales: Herpes zoster (shingles) is characterized by clusters of vesicles that form in a line along nerve pathways. Vesicles are fluid-filled lesions less than 1 cm in size. The fluid is clear. Papules are solid masses of cellular growth usually less than 5 mm in size. Bulla are fluid-filled lesions larger than 1 cm. Pustules are fluid-filled lesions, but unlike a vesicle, the fluid inside is yellowish.
Nursing process step: Assessment

43. Correct answer—D.

Rationales: Blood transfusions should be used judiciously to treat a crisis. They have little or no role in treatment between crises. Large doses of continuous opioid analgesics may be needed and are the mainstay of pain management during the acute phase. Oxygen is administered to treat hypoxia and control sickling. Fluids and electrolytes are given to reduce blood viscosity and maintain renal function.
Nursing process step: Intervention

44. Correct answer—D.

Rationales: The right coronary artery supplies the right ventricle and right atrium. The inferior leads II, III, and aV_F look at the right side of the heart on the 12-lead ECG. Therefore, an ST-segment elevation observed in leads II, III, and aV_F would indicate an occlusion in the right coronary artery.
Nursing process step: Assessment

45. Correct answer—D.

Rationales: Increased ICP is a contraindication to performing a lumbar puncture, unless the benefits outweigh the risks. Performing a lumbar puncture on a client with increased ICP may result in brain stem compression or herniation. Allergy to a local anesthetic, blood in the CSF, and the presence of a spinal cord lesion aren't contraindications for lumbar puncture.
Nursing process step: Assessment

46. Correct answer—B.

Rationales: A decreased platelet count may be present if a blood dyscrasia is the cause of bleeding after a bleeding episode. Decreased hemoglobin may not be immediately apparent because of hemoconcentration. Hence, more time or serial hemoglobin determinations may be necessary to detect a fall in hemoglobin readings. Prothrombin times may be elevated in bleeding clients because of bleeding disorders or anticoagulant therapy. Creatinine is a test of kidney function.
Nursing process step: Assessment

47. Correct answer—C.

Rationales: Unless the client is ready to accept new information, building on previous knowledge is useless. The readiness factor is critical to acceptance and integration of new information. Client guilt can't be alleviated until the client understands the intricacies of the condition and the physiologic response to the disease.
Nursing process step: Assessment

48. Correct answer—A.

Rationales: Elevating the extremity and applying ice slow the swelling process and help relieve pain. Teaching the client how to walk with crutches isn't appropriate at this time because the pain distracts the client. If elevating the ankle and applying ice don't decrease the pain, then an order for medication is appropriate. A traction splint is contraindicated for this client; the traction splint is indicated for fractures of the femur and proximal tibia only.
Nursing process step: Analysis

49. Correct answer—B.

Rationales: A client presenting with heart failure is classified as acute, which means that the client must be seen within 30 to 60 minutes of arrival at the emergency department. A client classified as urgent must be seen immediately. A nonacute client can wait in turn to be seen, and a referable client can be seen at the physician's discretion and may be referred to another physician at another time.
Nursing process step: Evaluation

50. Correct answer—C.

Rationales: The two causes of intrapulmonary shunt seen in the client with ARDS are pulmonary edema and atelectasis. Common treatments for hydrostatic pulmonary edema include diuretics, inotropes, and decreased fluid intake. They aren't effective treatments for the early stages of ARDS. A key finding in ARDS is refractory hypoxemia that isn't improved by increasing the FIO_2. In fact, FIO_2 levels greater than 60% for prolonged periods result in atelectasis, worsening ARDS, and hypoxemia. Adding low levels of PEEP (5 to 10 cm H_2O) will assist in reopening the alveoli and improving tissue oxygenation.
Nursing process step: Intervention

51. Correct answer—D.

Rationales: Psychomotor learning requires the coordination of the brain and extremities to complete a task. Cognitive learning is a mental process that doesn't involve the extremities. Affective learning involves feelings and attitudes rather than cognitive or psychomotor skills. Social isn't a type of learning.
Nursing process step: Analysis

52. Correct answer—C.

Rationales: All NSAIDs should be taken with food or on a full stomach. The client shouldn't take NSAIDs on an empty stomach because of the possibility of gastritis or GI bleeding. Melena (dark, tarry stools) and hematochezia (bloody stools) are both symptoms of upper and lower GI bleeding. The use of NSAIDs with aspirin should be avoided. Also, it may take 1 to 2 weeks for full anti-inflammatory effects to take place.
Nursing process step: Intervention

53. Correct answer—D.

Rationales: When preparing to irrigate a client's right ear, the irrigation stream should be pointed toward the posterior superior aspect of the canal and not directly at the tympanic membrane. To irrigate the right ear, this would be toward the 11 o'clock position.
Nursing process step: Intervention

54. Correct answer—C.

Rationales: Ménière's disease is characterized by attacks of vertigo, tinnitus, a feeling of fullness in the ear, and a fluctuation of hearing ability. Labyrinthitis doesn't usually cause a feeling of ear fullness. Otitis media doesn't usually cause vertigo. Disequilibrium syndrome is characterized by headache and muscle cramps.
Nursing process step: Assessment

55. Correct answer—C.

Rationales: In a pediatric client, one of the hallmark signs of radial head dislocation is the client's refusal to use the affected arm. Other symptoms include limited supination and pain. No deformity may be obvious with this injury. Instability of the ligaments is associated with dislocations of the knee and doesn't frequently occur. Dislocations of the patella commonly present with excessive swelling in adults. Elbow dislocations present with a loss of arm length.
Nursing process step: Assessment

56. Correct answer—A.

Rationales: Severe hypercalcemia is a medical emergency. Continuous cardiac monitoring is necessary and emergency equipment should be readily available. Initial treatment includes vigorous hydration, possibly several hundred milliliters per hour for several hours. I.V. furosemide, not mannitol, may be given to promote diuresis. Calcitrol is a vitamin D analogue used to stimulate calcium absorption in the presence of hypocalcemia.
Nursing process step: Intervention

57. Correct answer—A.

Rationales: A seizure immediately after a lidocaine bolus is administered may indicate lidocaine toxicity and too-rapid administration of the drug. The infusion should be stopped and the client monitored while the physician is notified of this event. Neither diuretics nor digoxin is indicated in the immediate response to the seizure.
Nursing process step: Intervention

58. Correct answer—C.

Rationales: Peptic ulcers, acute mucosal lesions (resulting from gastritis, esophagitis, or Mallory-Weiss tears), and esophageal or gastric varices are the most common causes of upper GI bleeding. Upper GI bleeding is rarely caused by neoplasms, hematologic disorders, or vascular anomalies.
Nursing process step: Assessment

59. Correct answer—B.

Rationales: The presence of an increased number of epithelial cells, especially when they exceed the number of WBCs, is indicative of a contaminated specimen. Proper cleaning and retrieval of the specimen may not have taken place. The presence of bacteria, WBCs, and pus suggests pyelonephritis or a urinary tract infection.
Nursing process step: Evaluation

60. Correct answer—C.

Rationales: The client with gout should avoid high-purine foods, such as anchovies, liver, sardines, most meat, and alcoholic beverages. Dairy products, whole grains, and citrus fruits have low-purine content and won't precipitate an attack of gout.
Nursing process step: Analysis

61. Correct answer—D.

Rationales: The earliest indicator of a change in neurologic status is the LOC. A client who exhibits altered mental status or decreased LOC should be reevaluated by a nurse and a physician. A change in the reaction or shape of pupils is a late indicator of a neurologic problem. Motor response appears as a delayed sign of neurologic status changes. Capillary refill is an indicator of circulatory status.
Nursing process step: Assessment

62. Correct answer—D.

Rationales: Intussusception occurs most often in infants and toddlers aged 3 months to 2 years. They may present with a triad of crampy abdominal pain, vomiting, and bloody (currant jelly) stools. A sausage-shaped mass may be palpable in the right upper quadrant. Right lower quadrant tenderness at McBurney's point is associated with appendicitis. Cullen's sign, periumbilical ecchymosis, is consistent with a traumatic injury causing peritoneal bleeding. An olive-shaped mass in the upper abdomen is associated with pyloric stenosis, a narrowing of the outflow tract of the stomach.
Nursing process step: Assessment

63. Correct answer—A.

Rationales: The use of accessory muscles indicates worsening respiratory function. The client also has increased pain when moving. Increased pain leads to increased blood pressure and a tendency to breath shallowly. For these reasons, it's important to provide adequate pain medication to decrease the complications of immobility.
Nursing process step: Evaluation

64. Correct answer—D.

Rationales: Fentanyl is an opioid, and the antidote for opioids is naloxone. Physostigmine is the antidote for anticholinergics except cyclic antidepressants. Flumazenil is the antidote for benzodiazepines, and atropine is the antidote for organophosphates.
Nursing process step: Intervention

65. Correct answer—C.

Rationales: A fat embolism occurs after a bone fracture or surgical manipulation of bone. A fat embolus is a small fat globule that has been displaced into the blood. The origin, although largely unknown, is believed to be either from the fracture site or from altered lipid solubility brought on by the stress of the traumatic event. The fat globules can occlude blood vessels in the brain, lungs, heart, and other organs. Symptoms include a recent fracture or bone surgery, dyspnea, sudden onset of substernal chest pain, hemoptysis, cough, crackles, altered mental status, fever, and petechiae to the buccal membranes, conjunctiva, chest, neck, shoulders, or axillary folds. Because these symptoms closely mimic other syndromes, such as pulmonary embolus and MI, careful attention must be given to the circumstances surrounding the onset of symptoms and to the client's medical history.
Nursing process step: Analysis

66. Correct answer—A.

Rationales: A child with epiglottitis has a sudden high fever, marked drooling, stridor, and severe sore throat. A child with retropharyngeal abscess has abrupt onset of high fever, stridor, drooling, severe sore throat, hyperextension of the head, and stiff neck. In bacterial tracheitis, the fever is mild initially, followed by an acute increase; the child will also have a barking cough. Bacterial tracheitis doesn't cause drooling, and sore throat, if present at all, will be minimal. Viral croup syndrome causes a variable temperature (100° to 104° F [37.8° to 40° C]), barking cough, and mild (if any) sore throat; it doesn't cause drooling.
Nursing process step: Analysis

67. Correct answer—A.

Rationales: Alligator forceps are used to remove vegetable or other foreign bodies from the ear. The nurse also needs a good light source, large ear speculums, an ear curette, and ear suction. If the foreign body isn't a vegetable, a 30-mL syringe filled with water may be used to irrigate the ear—however, water shouldn't be used to remove vegetables because it causes them to swell, making removal more difficult. Lidocaine is useful in removing live bugs. Cerumenex is useful in removing earwax buildup only.
Nursing process step: Intervention

68. Correct answer—A.

Rationales: Muscular contraction or tension headache is an example of a nonvascular headache. Skeletal muscle contraction in the head or neck produces steady, pulsatile pain and limited motion of the head, neck, and jaw. Rigorous ROM causes increased pain. Pressure over contracted muscles worsens the pain, as do vasoconstrictor drugs such as ergotamine. A warm towel will induce vasodilatation and muscle relaxation.
Nursing process step: Intervention

69. Correct answer–A.

Rationales: DIC is a condition of excessive coagulation that eventually leads to inadequate homeostasis. The activation of the coagulation system leads to the formation of fibrin that binds with blood to form a clot. In DIC, the clots are deposited in the microvasculature of various organs. Excessive bleeding in DIC results from the consumption of all clotting factors. Fibrin degradation products further aggravate this situation because they act as powerful anticoagulants. Heparin is most effective when administered soon after recognition of symptoms. Fresh frozen plasma and cryoprecipitate are administered to replace clotting factors. Although the client is at risk for thrombus and emboli, thrombolytic agents, such as urokinase, streptokinase, and tPa, aren't used because they can cause excessive bleeding.
Nursing process step: Intervention

70. Correct answer–B.

Rationales: Lens displacement usually occurs as a result of direct trauma to the globe. Fibers around the iris break and the lens subluxes, causing diplopia, distortion, decreased visual acuity, and no response to light.
A globe rupture would cause severe pain and a complete loss of vision. Hyphema results in pain in the affected eye and blurred vision. A retinal detachment usually produces flashing and visible floaters in the eye.
Nursing process step: Assessment

71. Correct answer–C.

Rationales: Inflammatory processes, such as diverticulitis, cause an increase in neutrophils, or neutrophilia. Many viral diseases, such as hepatitis, influenza, and measles, as reflected in the other options, can cause a decreased neutrophil count, or neutropenia.
Nursing process step: Analysis

72. Correct answer–C.

Rationales: Signs of a mandibular fracture include malocclusion, ecchymosis of the floor of the mouth, and sublingual edema. A zygotic, LeFort, or maxillary fracture wouldn't cause ecchymosis of the floor of the mouth.
Nursing process step: Assessment

73. Correct answer–D.

Rationales: Arteriography is helpful if diminished or absent pulses indicate that there may be vascular damage. It isn't clinically indicated for long bone injuries if the vascular status is unaffected. Arteriography isn't usually indicated in open injuries (including penetrating injury) unless the wound is near major vascular structures or the wounding force was high-velocity.
Nursing process step: Assessment

74. Correct answer–C.

Rationales: The risk for infection is high in this client; therefore, administration of antibiotics is a priority. If other severe injuries are present and they compromise respiratory function, immediate intubation or chest tube insertion may be necessary. Insertion of an NG tube is contraindicated.
Nursing process step: Intervention

75. Correct answer–B.

Rationales: This client is having a hemolytic reaction to transfusion therapy. Therefore, the transfusion should be stopped immediately. The nurse should then initiate infusion of normal saline solution at a keep-vein-open rate. After contacting a physician, the nurse should be prepared to administer antihistamines and epinephrine. The client's vital signs should be reassessed frequently, as indicated by facility policy.
Nursing process step: Intervention

76. Correct answer–C.

Rationales: Corticosteroids reduce inflammation and cerebral edema and help prevent increased intracranial pressure. Anticonvulsants are used to control absence seizures. Antipsychotics and antianxiety drugs may be used sparingly to control agitation. Preferably, nonopioids are used to relieve pain. Opioids may make it difficult to assess the client's level of consciousness.
Nursing process step: Intervention

77. Correct answer–B.

Rationales: Adrenal crisis may occur as the result of sudden withdrawal from corticosteroid therapy. Symptoms of adrenal crisis include fever, myalgia, arthralgia, and malaise. An increased risk of developing glaucoma and subcapsular cataracts can be the result of prolonged use of corticosteroids. Psychiatric disturbances may present as an adverse effect during use, and they may include euphoria, insomnia, mood swings, and extreme depression. Tardive dyskinesia consists of irreversible, involuntary movements that may develop in people being treated with neuroleptics such as chlorpromazine.
Nursing process step: Analysis

78. Correct answer—C.

Rationales: Complications of rewarming include metabolic acidosis, cardiac arrhythmias, pneumonia, renal failure, pancreatitis, sepsis, and acute respiratory distress syndrome. The application of warm blankets isn't sufficient with such severe hypothermia. More active rewarming (peritoneal dialysis, warmed fluids, heated humidified oxygen, extracorporeal blood rewarming) may be needed. Rapid rewarming isn't advised because such a client is vulnerable to cardiac arrhythmias. External rewarming causes peripheral vasodilation. This action may divert blood flow to the skin and shunt cooled blood to the central circulation, thereby causing a brief drop in core temperature. It may also predispose the client to hypovolemia and ventricular fibrillation. Debilitated and elderly clients with core temperatures under 95° F (35° C) should be hospitalized.
Nursing process step: Intervention

79. Correct answer—B.

Rationales: The lowest level of electrical energy required to initiate consistent capture with a pacemaker is referred to as pacing threshold. It's determined by achieving pacing at a high level and then gradually decreasing the energy level until capture ceases. For successful capture, the energy is then set a few milliamperes above the threshold. Underdrive pacing is used to interrupt tachyarrhythmias. Demand pacers fire only when the heart rate drops below a set rate.
Nursing process step: Evaluation

80. Correct answer—B.

Rationales: Hyperosmolality is the result of accompanying hyperglycemia and hypernatremia. Hyperosmolality causes insulin levels to be reduced, preventing the movement of glucose into the cells and allowing glucose to accumulate in the plasma. HHNS is characterized by extremely elevated blood glucose levels, which range from 600 mg/dL to 2,800 mg/dL. The BUN level is normally elevated from severe dehydration. Fluid volume deficit is more severe than in diabetic ketoacidosis—up to 12 L of fluid must be replaced. Mild metabolic acidosis is reflected in ABG results from poor perfusion and anaerobic metabolism.
Nursing process step: Assessment

81. Correct answer—C.

Rationales: A sprain is the tearing of ligaments that results in inflammation and ecchymotic discoloration. An abrasion is a partial-thickness scraping away of the skin. A contusion is a closed wound in which ruptured blood vessels have hemorrhaged into the surrounding tissue and are self-contained.
Nursing process step: Assessment

82. Correct answer—B.

Rationales: The key diagnostic finding suggesting a ruptured diaphragm is the presence of bowel sounds in the middle of the chest. The left side of the diaphragm is more likely to be injured than the right side because it isn't as well protected. The abdominal contents herniate into the chest, causing compression of the lungs and great vessels. Hemothorax would produce diminished breath sounds but not shoulder pain or bowel sounds in the chest. Aortic dissection may cause a shift of heart sounds; however, the client decompensates quickly. A tracheobronchial disruption produces signs consistent with pneumothorax.
Nursing process step: Assessment

83. Correct answer—B.

Rationales: Increased fluid intake facilitates increased kidney excretion of calcium. Immobility, especially for extended periods, rather than exercise, causes calcium to leave the bones and become concentrated in the extracellular fluid. From there, it passes through the kidneys and precipitates to form calculi. Milk is high in calcium and should be restricted in a client with hypercalcemia.
Nursing process step: Evaluation

84. Correct answer—C.

Rationales: Sodium bicarbonate is used in severe salicylate toxicity to alkalinize the urine to a pH of 7.5 and to enhance excretion of salicylates. Calcium gluconate is the antidote for hydrofluoric acid. Folic acid is given in methanol poisoning. Magnesium is used in hydrofluoric acid exposure.
Nursing process step: Analysis

85. Correct answer—C.

Rationales: Administering a drug with opioid antagonist properties may precipitate drug withdrawal. In an opioid-dependent client, signs of opioid withdrawal include chills, diaphoresis, gooseflesh, abdominal pain, muscle cramps, diarrhea, tearfulness, and irritability. Respiratory depression, nausea, and vomiting are adverse effects of opioids. Seizures can occur as a result of sedative, hypnotic, or anxiolytic withdrawal.
Nursing process step: Evaluation

86. Correct answer—D.

Rationales: It's best to let adults attempt to work out their differences before an authoritative intervention, especially since the charge nurse wasn't asked to intervene. However, the nurses should relocate to a more secluded area so clients and their families don't overhear. Generic, judgmental advice-giving won't be effective. It isn't unprofessional to have a disagreement, so long as it's resolved and doesn't affect work.

Nursing process step: Intervention

87. Correct answer—C.

Rationales: Adenosine may cause momentary, but rapidly resolving, high-grade blocks and asystole. If they don't resolve rapidly, the nurse should begin CPR. No cases of asystole lasting longer than 30 seconds have been documented.

Nursing process step: Intervention

88. Correct answer—B.

Rationales: Hospitalization is required as well as neurosurgical services for shunt revision after the etiology of the shunt dysfunction has been established. Disposition home isn't appropriate until the shunt is once again functioning properly. Hospice and home health services wouldn't be indicated unless the underlying illness indicated such a referral.

Nursing process step: Analysis

89. Correct answer—A.

Rationales: Gunshot wounds cause more trauma to the tissues related to the bullet fragments. There's less exposure to tissues with stabbing injury, blunt trauma, and crushing injury.

Nursing process step: Analysis

90. Correct answer—A.

Rationales: Autotransfusion should be completed within 4 hours of the injury. Autologous blood is collected from the pleural cavity or mediastinal area and transfused to the client.

Nursing process step: Analysis

91. Correct answer—C.

Rationales: If the foreign bodies aren't removed, they will cause permanent scars or "tattooing." Liposuction is surgical fat removal. Augmentation is surgical enhancement. Granulation is filling in of a healing wound.

Nursing process step: Analysis

92. Correct answer—C.

Rationales: The charge nurse should at least offer support; nurses' emotions deserve a therapeutic response. Telling the nurse to control herself is denying her needs, and she probably wouldn't be as effective in client care until she can deal with her overpowering feelings. The nurse may not want to see the chaplain. Walking away is ignoring the need unless the nurse specifically asks to be left alone.

Nursing process step: Intervention

93. Correct answer—A.

Rationales: Public relations should be handled through a designated spokesperson, or the nursing supervisor if that spokesperson isn't available. Under the Health Insurance Portability Accountability Act (HIPAA) regulations for client confidentiality, even the presence of the client shouldn't be acknowledged without the client's consent. In addition, the client's wife should be asked before automatically transferring the call. It isn't necessary to contact the legal department with regards to client information.

Nursing process step: Analysis

94. Correct answer—B.

Rationales: To avoid post-traumatic stress syndrome, it's advised to have a critical incident stress debriefing (CSI). This involves expression of personal feelings, discussion, and working on unresolved emotional issues. Private discussions among caregiver staff don't breech client confidentiality. Denying and blunting emotions through avoidance, or numbing them with alcohol, only leads to delayed reactions. A prayer service is an option but shouldn't be the only action because it may not be consistent with some of the staff's personal values.

Nursing process step: Intervention

95. Correct answer—C.

Rationales: A patent airway without pulmonary basilar wheezes is an indicator that the treatment plan for this client is correct and that the client's condition is stabilizing. The other options don't indicate that this client's condition is improving.

Nursing process step: Evaluation

96. Correct answer—B.

Rationales: A 16G indwelling urinary catheter can be used to control bleeding and provide hemostasis for a posterior nosebleed. It's inserted into the nares and into the posterior nasal passage; it's then inflated and pulled against the nasopharynx. Other choices include gauze packs connected to a string, a posterior pack, and a double-balloon catheter. Gelfoam is an absorbable hemostatic agent that stimulates coagulation. The nasal tampon, the nasal balloon, and the Gelfoam hemostatic agent are for anterior bleeds.

Nursing process step: Intervention

97. Correct answer—D.

Rationales: In addition to flattened or inverted T waves, the ECG may show a prolonged QT interval and a prominent U wave. A client with hypokalemia is also more predisposed to developing ventricular ectopy. A shortened QT interval may be evidenced in hypercalcemia. Tall, peaked T waves with a short QT interval are indicative of hyperkalemia. A widened QRS complex may be observed with hyperkalemia.

Nursing process step: Evaluation

98. Correct answer—D.

Rationales: The best evaluation of learning is to be able to perform the necessary skills in a "return demonstration." A test, lack of questions, or statement of facts indicate that some level of theory-learning has taken place, which is essential; however, none demonstrates an ability to apply that knowledge.

Nursing process step: Evaluation

99. Correct answer—B.

Rationales: The ED nurse should wear protective clothing, such as boots, gloves, cap, and mask, to prevent contamination from radiation. A radiation meter isn't indicated in this situation. Life-threatening problems may be handled after the nurse has donned protective clothing and before the client is decontaminated. The Department of Health doesn't need to be contacted in a radiation accident.

Nursing process step: Intervention

100. Correct answer—D.

Rationales: Normal saline is noncytotoxic. Hydrogen peroxide is toxic to fibroblasts in normal dilutions. Povidone-iodine preparations are also toxic and may cause iodine toxicity. Acetic acid is used against pseudomonas and is also toxic to fibroblasts.

Nursing process step: Intervention

101. Correct answer—A.

Rationales: Severe anemia is defined as a hemoglobin level less than 6 g/dL. Impaired thought processes are a clinical manifestation. Weight loss, rather than weight gain, is observed, along with tachycardia and an increased pulse pressure.

Nursing process step: Assessment

102. Correct answer—B.

Rationales: CBC, sedimentation rate, blood culture, and MRI or computed tomography scan are the cornerstones of the evaluation. Joint aspiration isn't used in diagnosis of osteomyelitis.

Nursing process step: Analysis

103. Correct answer—B.

Rationales: These are classic signs and symptoms of a client with emphysema. A client with asthma is acutely short of breath during an attack and appears very frightened. A client with ARDS is acutely short of breath and requires emergency care. A client with chronic obstructive bronchitis is bloated and cyanotic in appearance.

Nursing process step: Assessment

104. Correct answer—C.

Rationales: The initial intervention would be control the bleeding and assess the neurovascular function of the leg to stabilize the client and determine the extent of injury. A tourniquet would be applied outside the hospital to a pulsating wound. X-rays and ice wouldn't be appropriate.

Nursing process step: Intervention

105. Correct answer—C.

Rationales: When the umbilical cord precedes the neonate, the cord may become compressed between the neonate's head and the pelvis, thus cutting off the blood supply to the neonate. When pressure is applied to the neonate's head, the nurse should be able to feel the cord pulsate, indicating blood flow. The nurse wouldn't want the umbilical cord to retract into the uterus, and probably wouldn't be able to see the color of the cord. The nurse wouldn't want the client to push at this time. A cesarean delivery is indicated in the case of cord prolapse.

Nursing process step: Evaluation

106. Correct answer—A.

Rationales: A sandbag applied to the injured chest area limits lung expansion and predisposes the client to atelectasis. Therefore, clients with flail chest should be immediately intubated and ventilated to manage the underlying pulmonary contusion. Pain must be controlled to facilitate adequate ventilation. Fluids should be limited to reduce the incidence of pulmonary edema.
Nursing process step: Intervention

107. Correct answer—B.

Rationales: The three components of a contraction that a nurse must evaluate are duration, frequency, and intensity of each contraction. Pelvic type has no bearing on contractions.
Nursing process step: Assessment

108. Correct answer—A.

Rationales: Shortness of breath, tachypnea, low blood pressure, tachycardia, diffuse crackles, and a cough producing pink, frothy sputum are late signs of pulmonary edema. Pneumothorax produces sudden, sharp pleuritic pain, exacerbated by chest movement; breathing and coughing; and absent breath sounds to the affected side. Cardiac tamponade produces muffled heart sounds, pulsus paradoxus, and jugular vein distention. Pulmonary embolus may cause fever, cough, hemoptysis, and a pleural friction rub.
Nursing process step: Assessment

109. Correct answer—B.

Rationales: HELLP syndrome is a life-threatening complication associated with hypertension in pregnancy. HELLP stands for hemolysis, elevated liver enzymes, and low platelets. Although all of the conditions listed may occur as a result of HELLP syndrome, DIC is the most serious.
Nursing process step: Analysis

110. Correct answer—C.

Rationales: Ménière's disease causes vertigo, a ringing or roaring noise in the ears, hearing loss, nausea, and vomiting. Slow positional changes can help the client control vertigo. Eye drops aren't useful, even if there's blurred vision. Because of the symptoms, the client may need help until the vertigo subsides; it would be in the client's best interest to have assistance at home. Hearing loss may not be permanent and hearing may return. No ear pain is associated with Ménière's disease; thus, an ice pack or other analgesic alternative for pain is unnecessary.
Nursing process step: Evaluation

111. Correct answer—D.

Rationales: Naloxone and flumazenil are both medications specifically for improvement of respiratory drive—naloxone for opioid overdose and flumazenil for benzodiazepines. Flumazenil is contraindicated for use in those with a history of seizures, a real possibility for this client. Albuterol is a bronchodilator that won't have any effect on her rate, and $D_{50}W$ is for the treatment of documented hypoglycemia.
Nursing process step: Intervention

112. Correct answer—C.

Rationales: Considering this client's history and presenting symptoms, he may have chronic osteomyelitis and should be fully evaluated. A joint effusion involves fluid in the joint. Septic arthritis presents more abruptly, causing intense pain, inflammation, and fever. Compartment syndrome occurs when perfusion to muscle and nerve tissue is decreased to a level inadequate to sustain the viability of the tissue. Symptoms involve intractable pain, paresthesia, and pallor.
Nursing process step: Analysis

113. Correct answer—C.

Rationales: Based on physical findings and chest X-rays, the correct diagnosis is asthma. Bronchiolitis occurs primarily in winter and spring during the first 2 years of life with a peak at age 2 to 6 months. It begins with a cough, rhinorrhea, and nasal congestion. The symptoms of foreign-body obstruction depend on the degree of obstruction; a sudden onset of coughing, choking, gagging, or wheezing is commonly seen. Bronchial foreign bodies usually cause wheezing or coughing and are commonly misdiagnosed as asthma. The client with a bronchial foreign body presents with hyperresonant percussion and diminished breath sounds distal to the foreign body. Hypersensitivity pneumonitis produces patchy infiltrates and atelectasis on chest X-rays.
Nursing process step: Analysis

114. Correct answer—D.

Rationales: Cranial nerve VII (facial) is responsible for motor facial muscles, closing of the eyes, and speech. The oculomotor nerve (III) controls most of the extraocular eye movements and the ability to raise the eyelids. The trochlear nerve (IV) controls the down and inward movement of the eye. The trigeminal nerve (V) controls the muscles of chewing and sensory taste.
Nursing process step: Assessment

115. Correct answer–C.

Rationales: Magnesium sulfate is administered to clients with hypertension in pregnancy to reduce the activity at the neuromuscular junction, thereby reducing the client's risk of seizures. Pregnant clients who are started on a magnesium drip must be closely monitored for respiratory depression and fetal distress.

Nursing process step: Evaluation

116. Correct answer–B.

Rationales: Cardiogenic shock is characterized by impaired ability of the heart to pump and decreased contractility of the myocardium. Stroke volume and cardiac output decline and result in increased left ventricular end-diastolic pressure. Myocardial infarction resulting in damage to greater than 40% of the left ventricular myocardium is the most common cause of cardiogenic shock. Other causes of cardiogenic shock are cardiomyopathies, valvular dysfunction, and rupture of papillary muscle, pericardial tamponade, tension pneumothorax, and pulmonary embolus resulting in obstructive or restrictive cardiogenic shock. Pneumonia is an inflammation of the lung parenchyma and is the leading cause of death in the geriatric population. Cardiogenic shock isn't a complication of pneumonia, and restrained passengers hit from the back are at low risk for developing cardiogenic shock unless they have sustained a myocardial contusion.

Nursing process step: Assessment

117. Correct answer–A.

Rationales: Symptoms of a threatened abortion include mild vaginal bleeding, cramping, and a closed cervical os. Malodorous vaginal bleeding may be indicative of infection. A client with an open cervical os would be experiencing an inevitable abortion.

Nursing process step: Assessment

118. Correct answer–A.

Rationales: Ammonia gas reacts with water to form nitric acid, and chlorine gas reacts with water to form hydrochloric acid and hypochlorous acid, which are irritants and can cause acid burns to susceptible tissues. Neither gas will bind with hemoglobin or cause paralyzation of the respiratory cilia. Any fluid accumulation in the lungs is hypertonic and will actually pull additional fluid from the vascular space and cause pulmonary edema.

Nursing process step: Assessment

119. Correct answer–B.

Rationales: The client's altered LOC, respiratory rate, and potential to aspirate in spinal immobilization dictate the need to establish a patent airway in a controlled environment before transfer. Urinary catheterization is contraindicated in this client given the possible urethra injury as indicated by bleeding at the meatus. Peritoneal lavage and tetanus prophylaxis aren't of the highest priority to perform before transfer. Peritoneal lavage is a diagnostic procedure that may delay the transfer.

Nursing process step: Analysis

120. Correct answer–D.

Rationales: When a significant traumatic event has occurred, the nurse should check for signs of a basilar skull fracture or other serious injuries. A ruptured tympanic membrane that has sanguineous discharge should be checked for the presence of CSF. When the ruptured tympanic membrane has been caused by a blast or other traumatic occurrence, antibiotics aren't usually indicated. Irrigating the ear is contraindicated in a ruptured tympanic membrane. Instead, gentle suctioning of any debris is recommended. Nothing should be instilled in the ear until other associated injuries have been ruled out and diagnosis is complete.

Nursing process step: Intervention

121. Correct answer–C.

Rationales: Frostbite looks waxy white because the skin is frozen. As the tissue thaws, there's severe pain from the injury, much like a burn. Frost nip is a stage of frostbite and presents as numb, white areas. Chilblains are superficial thermal injuries that are gradual in onset and aren't painful. Raynaud's disease, precipitated by exposure to cold or stress, usually affects the hands and feet and is more prevalent in women.

Nursing process step: Assessment

122. Correct answer–A.

Rationales: Providing perineal care after urination and bowel movements decreases the risk of infection. Option B is incorrect because transmission-based precautions are used for a client with suspected or documented transmissible or epidemiologically important pathogens for which additional precautions beyond standard precautions are needed to interrupt transmission in hospitals. The client should be placed in protective isolation from environmental sources of infection. Option C is incorrect because invasive procedures should be avoided to the greatest extent possible to decrease infection. Foods from outside sources should be discouraged to decrease the risk of exposure to bacteria.

Nursing process step: Intervention

123. Correct answer—C.

Rationales: Swimmer's ear refers to a bacterial or fungal infection in the external ear. Symptoms usually include an ear that's tender to the touch, a swollen ear canal, cellulitis of the pinna and surrounding structure, and possibly, purulent drainage. A bulging tympanic membrane is a symptom of acute otitis media.
Nursing process step: Assessment

124. Correct answer—C.

Rationales: Blood loss of 1,500 to 4,500 mL can occur with pelvic fracture. A closed femur fracture can result in 1,000 to 2,000 mL of blood loss into the surrounding tissue. Blood loss of 500 to 1,000 mL can occur with fractures of the elbow, forearm, tibia, or ankle.
Nursing process step: Assessment

125. Correct answer—A.

Rationales: The client's signs and symptoms, including the rapid onset, are supportive of epiglottiditis. Croup is usually seen in children up to age 3 and is preceded by several days of an upper respiratory infection. The classic clinical signs and symptoms of diphtheria are pharyngitis with a gray-green membrane, fever, and enlarged cervical lymph nodes. Mononucleosis is suspected with a prolonged illness that includes exudative tonsillitis, enlarged lymph nodes, and an enlarged spleen.
Nursing process step: Assessment

126. Correct answer—A.

Rationales: Shoulder dislocations typically occur in people under age 25. This is probably because such injuries occur as a result of severe trauma, such as a collision or a fall onto an outstretched arm. They commonly occur in such sports as football, basketball, and wrestling.
Nursing process step: Assessment

127. Correct answer—D.

Rationales: A rash on the wrist and ankles spreading to the palms and soles is specific to Rocky Mountain spotted fever. A rash beginning on the face, arms, and legs is typical of the rash pattern of smallpox. Lesions beginning on the abdomen and back are usually the rash pattern of chickenpox.
Nursing process step: Assessment

128. Correct answer—A.

Rationales: An ongoing blood loss of 100 to 200 mL/hour from a chest tube indicates a need for surgical repair. A transfusion reaction doesn't cause increased chest tube output. The most common transfusion reactions include hypotension, tachycardia, chest pain, dyspnea, nausea, vomiting, chills, flushing, hives, abdominal pain, flank pain, disseminated intravascular coagulation, fever, jaundice, increased serum bilirubin levels, hemoglobinuria, and decreased serum hemoglobin levels. If the client is thought to have a massive hemothorax, a second chest tube may be inserted to manage the blood loss.
Nursing process step: Evaluation

129. Correct answer—D.

Rationales: Recent MI, hypertension, diabetes mellitus, and atrial fibrillation are conditions related to a high risk of thrombotic or embolic stroke. A history of remote MI doesn't necessarily predispose the client to a thrombotic stroke. Hypotension isn't associated with an embolic stroke. Diabetes insipidus is a disorder of the posterior lobe of the pituitary gland due to a deficiency of anti-diuretic hormone.
Nursing process step: Assessment

130. Correct answer—C.

Rationales: Bursitis is caused by direct trauma to the area or strain due to repetitive motion such as sports activity. Carpal tunnel syndrome usually presents with pain and numbness in the hand. Rheumatic disorders usually manifest as gradual, bilateral joint inflammation with fever. Raynaud's disease causes pain and numbness of the hands and fingers.
Nursing process step: Analysis

131. Correct answer—D.

Rationales: Personality changes, seizures, and coma are manifestations seen in SIADH. Option A is incorrect because weight gain is seen. Option B is incorrect because anorexia, not increased appetite, is observed, and option C is incorrect because bowel sounds are hyperactive with vomiting.
Nursing process step: Assessment

132. Correct answer-A.

Rationales: Acute necrotizing ulcerative gingivitis is a noncontagious infection of the gums that occurs with the overgrowth of normal mouth bacteria resulting in spontaneous bleeding from swollen gums, fetid breath, and dirty gray ulcers on the bases of the tonsil. Ludwig angina, gingivitis, and pericoronitis wouldn't produce those symptoms.
Nursing process step: Assessment

133. Correct answer–A.

Rationales: Third-generation broad-spectrum cephalosporins are the drugs of choice because of the rapid rise in penicillin-resistant gonococci. After improvement from parenteral antibiotics has been achieved, a client can be switched to oral cefixime or ciprofloxacin.
Nursing process step: Intervention

134. Correct answer–A.

Rationales: Intussusception occurs in an infant when the proximal bowel invaginates into the distal bowel. The condition may lead to an infarction of the bowel. Hypertrophy of the pyloric musculature causes pyloric stenosis. Volvulus occurs when a section of intestine twists on its own axis. A mechanical obstruction is caused by an anatomic or "mechanical" problem in the bowel, not solidified feces.
Nursing process step: Assessment

135. Correct answer–D.

Rationales: The definitive therapy for a client with pneumothorax is tube thoracotomy. The first concerns are always airway, breathing, and circulation. Administering supplemental oxygen should occur while equipment is being gathered to insert the chest tube. The second intervention should be insertion of two I.V. lines with large-bore needles. The client with pneumothorax has severe chest pain, so analgesics should be administered.
Nursing process step: Intervention

136. Correct answer–C.

Rationales: Definitive diagnosis of temporal arteritis is biopsy of the temporal artery; therefore, the client would be hospitalized immediately. Because temporal arteritis can result in blindness, it's important to coordinate immediate definitive diagnoses at the time a provisional diagnosis is made. Unless other conditions require cardiac monitoring, it isn't required. Headaches caused by temporal arteritis don't have a stress-related etiology. Medication regimen is most likely a corticosteroid, not opioids.
Nursing process step: Evaluation

137. Correct answer–C.

Rationales: The direction a bullet takes after it enters the abdomen is impossible to predict. Damage may occur to the stomach, liver, or transverse colon. The appendix, bladder, and cecum are located in the lower quadrants of the abdomen.
Nursing process step: Assessment

138. Correct answer–C.

Rationales: In the oliguric phase of acute renal failure, both the BUN and serum creatinine levels are elevated, with the serum creatinine being the best indicator of renal failure because it isn't significantly altered by other factors. A urinalysis may show casts, RBCs, and white blood cells. Damaged tubules can't conserve sodium. Consequently, the urinary excretion of sodium may increase, resulting in normal or below normal levels of serum sodium.
Nursing process step: Analysis

139. Correct answer–D.

Rationales: The purpose of laying the client on her left side is to reduce the blood pressure by decreasing the venous pressure of the vena cava. Respiratory rate, pulse rate, and headache wouldn't be directly affected by this position.
Nursing process step: Evaluation

140. Correct answer–A.

Rationales: The sympathetic nervous system responds to a perceived threat by releasing epinephrine, which causes vasoconstriction. This vasoconstriction results in tachycardia, cold and clammy skin, dry mouth, and dilated pupils. Warm and dry skin, constricted pupils, and bradycardia wouldn't occur.
Nursing process step: Assessment

141. Correct answer–D.

Rationales: The challenge of nutritional management in renal failure is to provide adequate calories to prevent catabolism despite the restrictions that are required. If the client can't maintain adequate oral intake, TPN may be necessary for the provision of adequate nutrition. Hemodialysis may be required for such indications as volume overload, elevated potassium level, and blood urea nitrogen level greater than 120 mg/dL. A fluid challenge, typically administered in conjunction with diuretic therapy, may be initiated as the first step to determine whether there's adequate intravascular volume and cardiac output to ensure adequate perfusion of the kidneys.
Nursing process step: Analysis

142. Correct answer–B.

Rationales: The intestines should be covered with gauze moistened with sterile saline or water. Pushing them back into the abdomen may damage them further. If the intestines are allowed to dry, they may be irreversibly damaged. The abdominal portion of the pneumatic antishock garment shouldn't be inflated if viscera are protruding.
Nursing process step: Intervention

143. Correct answer—A.

Rationales: UAP delegation directions must be specific and shouldn't include the nursing processes of assessment and evaluation. "Keeping an eye" is too vague and involves assessment. A UAP can't cover registered nurse-level responsibilities. Judgments and interpretations, such as "feeling better" and "adequate," are evaluation.
Nursing process step: Analysis

144. Correct answer—B.

Rationales: The initial assessment of the client included airway, breathing, and circulation and confirmed that the client's airway and breathing aren't compromised. The next step would then be to evaluate his circulation and establish I.V. access. The chest X-ray is a diagnostic tool that can be obtained after the initial assessment and interventions are completed. Thrombolytic therapy may be ordered upon consultation with the cardiologist in the catheterization laboratory.
Nursing process step: Assessment

145. Correct answer—C.

Rationales: Septic shock commonly causes hypoglycemia in pediatric clients. Infants have limited glycogen stores that are rapidly depleted during stress. During the resuscitative stage, all pediatric clients should have serum glucose levels monitored. Hypoglycemia should be treated with 2 to 4 mL/kg of 25% dextrose solution I.V. Septic shock results in a metabolic acidosis state from decreased cellular perfusion. Hypercalcemia doesn't occur. Hypocalcemia results from impaired tissue perfusion during septic shock and should be treated with calcium chloride 10% solution 10 to 20 mg/kg I.V., administered slowly.
Nursing process step: Assessment

146. Correct answer—A.

Rationales: Smoke inhalation is related to acute respiratory distress syndrome (ARDS). In ARDS, the most commonly heard breath sounds are crackles through the lung fields. Decreased breath sounds or inspiratory and expiratory wheezing are associated with asthma, and rhonchi are heard when there's sputum in the airways.
Nursing process step: Assessment

147. Correct answer—C.

Rationales: Suturing lacerations can be time-consuming and can delay the transfer process for the seriously injured client. Wounds should be covered with sterile dressings for evaluation and intervention at the receiving hospital. Before transfer, the nurse should give a report to the receiving hospital and prepare copies of all documentation consent forms, laboratory results, and X-rays. The client and family will need emotional and psychological support throughout the transfer process.
Nursing process step: Intervention

148. Correct answer—B.

Rationales: EMTALA was enacted to prevent emergency departments participating in Medicaid from refusing to care for indigent clients. The hospital is obligated to provide an emergency medical screening examination to determine whether a medical emergency exists. In the event of a medical emergency, the hospital is required to stabilize the client within its skill and capability. Transfer to another facility may occur if additional medical resources are needed and the client or guardian consents.
Nursing process step: Analysis

149. Correct answer—C.

Rationales: The priority intervention starts with positioning the child to facilitate breathing and administering humidification oxygen by mask or face tent. The child may not need to be intubated if nebulizers are started to open airway passages. An I.V. line needs to be established and fluids given, but airway and breathing are the priority. Coughing and deep breathing at this time may cause the airways to close more. This intervention should be done later if needed.
Nursing process step: Intervention

150. Correct answer—B.

Rationales: Damage to the femoral nerve results in the client's inability to raise the affected leg when it's straight, to extend the knee, or to sense stimulus to the anterior thigh. Median nerve injuries are evidenced by inability to dorsiflex the affected wrist or extend the metacarpophalangeal joints. Sensory deviation with median nerve injury results in altered sensation to the dorsal web space between the thumb and index finger. Tibial nerve injuries result in altered plantar flexion of the foot and sensory changes to the sole. Peroneal nerve damage results in altered dorsiflexion of the foot and sensory changes to the web space between the great and second toes.
Nursing process step: Assessment

151. Correct answer–A.

Rationales: Caregivers need to be vigilant in protecting client confidentiality, but it's required that all pertinent medical records accompany the client, and it's in the client's interest so that care can continue. Failure to provide this information could result in an EMTALA violation being filed. Your colleague's concern isn't warranted in this case. It would be time-consuming and would potentially place the client in danger to wait for the possible later arrival of family members to sign a consent for the release of information. The client's consent can be assumed because of his serious injuries and unconsciousness. The complete medical record of the visit must be sent, not just demographics. If the records don't accompany the client, it's likely that tests and assessments will be unnecessarily duplicated and delays in care will result.

Nursing process step: Analysis

152. Correct answer–B.

Rationales: Research, from case studies to statistical results, guides evidence-based practice. The IRB precedes scientific investigation. Interdisciplinary research is a form of scientific investigation. Research may lead to tools used in performance appraisal, but it doesn't form the basis of the evaluation.

153. Correct answer–D.

Rationales: Migraine headaches and acute angle-closure glaucoma share the symptoms of severe unilateral headache, nausea, vomiting, and visual disturbances. Sudden loss of vision is a symptom of central retinal artery occlusion. Yellow-green discharge is a symptom of conjunctivitis, and syncope is a symptom of neither.

Nursing process step: Assessment

154. Correct answer–D.

Rationales: The distribution of lesions can help diagnose the illness, as with herpes zoster. The arrangement, type, and color are specific characteristics used along with the distribution in describing lesions.

Nursing process step: Analysis

155. Correct answer–B.

Rationales: Pityriasis rosea starts with a "herald patch" and then erupts in a Christmas tree pattern on the trunk. *Tinea corporis* is a skin infestation, usually seen as fine lines under the skin. Allergic reactions to drugs typically affect the entire body. Eczema is an erythematous papular rash typically affecting the antecubital and popliteal fossae.

Nursing process step: Assessment

156. Correct answer–B.

Rationales: Acuity, length of stay, and ED skills mix are essential components of safe staffing determination. Budget, policy, and ratios may be considered, but they don't have the same impact on safe, high-quality staffing. Metrics, education, and census haven't been shown to influence safe staffing and productivity.

157. Correct answer–D.

Rationales: When a major disaster occurs, the biggest mistake a hospital staff can make is to take all of the hospital's resources to the scene and deplete the hospital's staff and equipment. The primary goal of a hospital disaster plan is to maintain client care, provide for any possible disasters by planning and stocking adequate equipment and supplies, and provide care for the large numbers of clients from the disaster. Hospital personnel aren't trained to function at a disaster site. The hospital must also do a risk assessment to prepare for any local issues.

Nursing process step: Analysis

158. Correct answer–D.

Rationales: Rushing the client to the resuscitation room will tie up staff and supplies on this client, who has a high probability of mortality, thereby diverting resources that may be essential to save several clients whose chances for survival are greater. The client isn't a priority 3 because she does need immediate pain control.

Nursing process step: Assessment

159. Correct answer–B.

Rationales: Keeping the child calm and relaxed will help prevent vomiting. If vomiting occurs, there's a good chance that the esophagus will be damaged from regurgitation of the gastric poison. Additionally, the risk of chemical pneumonia exists if vomiting occurs. The parents should remain with the child to help keep him calm. Scolding the child may upset him and cause vomiting.

Nursing process step: Intervention

160. Correct answer–B.

Rationales: A puerperal infection is an infection of the maternal genital tract after delivery. Generally, it results from invasion by bacteria, such as group A beta-hemolytic streptococci, staphylococcus, coliform, and other organisms. Labor and delivery may reduce a woman's resistance to infection by bacteria usually found in the body. A puerperal infection isn't related to infection of the neonate's umbilicus or to a maternal nipple infection or blood infection.

Nursing process step: Analysis

161. Correct answer–C.

Rationales: Spiral fractures are commonly seen in the upper extremities and are related to physical abuse, usually when an extremity is grabbed and twisted. Longitudinal and oblique fractures generally occur with trauma. A transverse fracture commonly occurs with such bone diseases as osteomalacia and Paget's disease.
Nursing process step: Assessment

162. Correct answer–D.

Rationales: Reye's syndrome causes fatty degeneration of the liver, altering results of liver function studies. Serum bilirubin and alkaline phosphatase usually aren't affected. Decreased serum glucose levels, with reduced insulin levels, occur secondary to dehydration caused by intractable vomiting.
Nursing process step: Assessment

163. Correct answer–C.

Rationales: Early botulism is sometimes mistaken for a stroke because of the slurred speech and blurred vision, but the paralysis of botulism is an ascending bilateral paralysis that will progress and involve the arms, lungs, and legs. Hypoglycemia doesn't cause paralysis. A stroke or tumor doesn't normally affect both sides at the same time.
Nursing process step: Assessment

164. Correct answer–D.

Rationales: Providing supportive care only will assist the client's recovery but if used in conjunction with an antitoxin the client recovers faster. The antitoxin must be obtained from the Centers for Disease Control and Prevention. Since botulism's toxic effects are from the toxin formed by the bacteria, antibiotic therapy won't reduce or reverse the symptoms.
Nursing process step: Analysis

165. Correct answer–A.

Rationales: A radiopaque dye, usually iodine-based, is instilled into the spinal canal to outline structures during myelography. Pain may be expected along the sciatic nerve with a herniated nucleus pulposus, but this isn't as important as assessing a possible iodine allergy. During cardiac catheterization, the client is asked to cough or pant to clear the dye, and before cardiac catheterization or arteriogram, the nurse marks distal pulses in indelible ink.
Nursing process step: Intervention

166. Correct answer–B.

Rationales: ST-segment elevation in leads II, III, and aV_F is associated with inferior myocardial infarction. Anterior ischemia would be displayed as ST-segment depression in the anterior chest leads. Unstable angina and cardiac tamponade don't typically show isolated ST-segment elevation.
Nursing process step: Assessment

167. Correct answer–D.

Rationales: Dyspnea on exertion, ankle edema, and fatigue are all symptoms of heart failure. There are no symptoms of hypertensive crisis, and the client is normotensive. She hasn't described a history of diabetes, and she doesn't present with signs of diabetic ketoacidosis. She doesn't complain of chest pain or other signs of acute MI, though elderly women may have atypical presentations. The most likely cause of her symptoms is heart failure.
Nursing process step: Assessment

168. Correct answer–C.

Rationales: The treatment of choice is to lower the IOP to prevent damage to the optic nerve. This is done by immediate administration of I.V. acetazolamide and mannitol, and topical drugs, timolol and pilocarpine. Instillation of a topical anesthetic and bed rest wouldn't be the treatment of choice. Irrigation with normal saline is the treatment for foreign bodies or chemical burns.
Nursing process step: Intervention

169. Correct answer–C.

Rationales: Unlike appendicitis or ectopic pregnancy, there's no peritoneal irritation to cause rebound tenderness. Renal colic produces little or no abdominal tenderness. Intermittent sharp pain is caused by smooth-muscle contraction of the ureter. Microscopic hematuria is present in 80% of clients with renal colic. Clients are usually severely uncomfortable due to pain.
Nursing process step: Assessment

170. Correct answer–A.

Rationales: Tea and dairy products could contribute to the formation of calcium oxalate stone, the most common composition of renal lithasis. The client needs to save stone fragments, not collect her urine, for stone analysis. Instruct the client to drink at least 1 to 2 qt (1 to 2 L) per day to prevent dehydration. Due to migration of bacteria, voiding before and after sexual intercourse is a good practice to prevent urinary tract infection.
Nursing process step: Evaluation

171. Correct answer—A.

Rationales: Early symptoms of MS include diplopia and slurred speech. Paralysis is a late symptom of MS. Depression and a short attention span may also occur. Dementia is rarely associated with MS. Grief may occur as a result of the diagnosis, but it isn't a specific early symptom of MS.
Nursing process step: Assessment

172. Correct answer—C.

Rationales: Definitive diagnosis of temporal arteritis is biopsy of the temporal artery; therefore, the client would be hospitalized immediately. Because temporal arteritis can result in blindness, it's important to coordinate immediate definitive diagnoses at the time a provisional diagnosis is made. Unless other conditions require cardiac monitoring, it isn't required. Headaches caused by temporal arteritis don't have a stress-related etiology. Medication regimen is most likely a corticosteroid, not opioids.
Nursing process step: Evaluation

173. Correct answer—B.

Rationales: Most ectopic pregnancies don't appear as obvious life-threatening medical emergencies. Ectopic pregnancies must be considered in any sexually active woman of childbearing age who complains of menstrual irregularity, cramping abdominal pain, and mild vaginal bleeding. PID, abruptio placentae, and hydatidiform moles won't show blood in the cul-de-sac.
Nursing process step: Analysis

174. Correct answer—D.

Rationales: The family should be offered the opportunity to speak with an organ procurement coordinator. An organ procurement coordinator is knowledgeable about the organ donation process and should have exceptional interpersonal skills for dealing with grieving family members. Physician support in the process is desirable, but consent or written orders aren't necessary for a referral to the organ procurement organization. The requester must believe in the benefits of the organ donation and support the process with a positive attitude. The family should be approached about speaking to an organ procurement coordinator only after the family has been made aware of the client's condition and prognosis. Approaching a family member who believes that there's still hope for recovery will likely result in a negative outcome.
Nursing process step: Evaluation

175. Correct answer—C.

Rationales: The ear should be wiped clean with a cloth. Clients should be taught to avoid putting objects into the ear, including cotton-tipped applicators, to clean or scratch the ear canal. Hearing loss will be an initial sign of tympanic membrane rupture but shouldn't be permanent. The ear shouldn't be packed because this can lead to infection. Ruptured eardrums usually heal spontaneously within 1 to 3 months. Surgery is rarely required.
Nursing process step: Evaluation

Appendices

Types of cardiac arrhythmias

Use a standard electrocardiogram strip, if available, to compare normal cardiac rhythm configurations with the rhythm strips depicted here. (Note the various features, causes, and treatments of these common cardiac arrhythmias.) Characteristics of normal rhythm include:

- ventricular and atrial rates of 60 to 100 beats/minute.
- regular and uniform QRS complexes and P waves.
- PR interval of 0.12 to 0.20 seconds.
- QRS duration < 0.12 seconds.
- identical atrial and ventricular rates, with a constant PR interval.

Arrhythmia and features	Causes	Treatment
Sinus arrhythmia 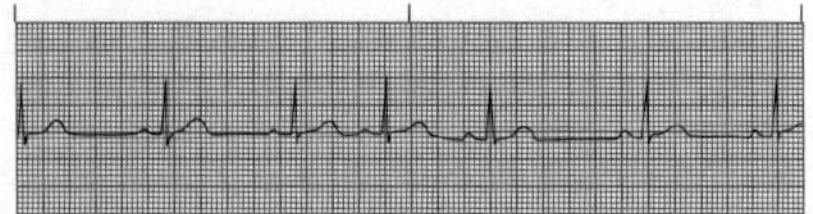 • Irregular atrial and ventricular rhythms • Normal P wave preceding each QRS complex	• Normal variation of normal sinus rhythm for athletes, children, and elderly people • Also seen in digoxin toxicity and inferior wall myocardial infarction (MI)	• No treatment necessary
Sinus tachycardia 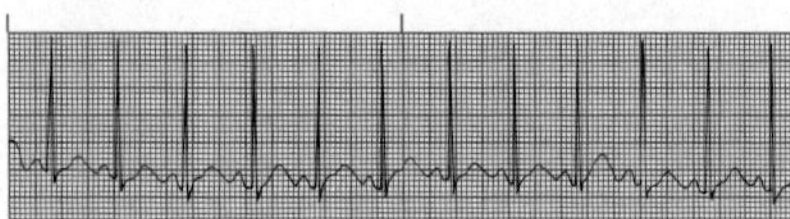 • Atrial and ventricular rhythms regular • Rate > 100 beats/minute; rarely, >160 beats/minute • Normal P wave preceding each QRS complex	• Normal physiologic response to fever, exercise, anxiety, pain, dehydration; may also accompany shock, left-sided heart failure, cardiac tamponade, hyperthyroidism, anemia, hypovolemia, pulmonary embolism, anterior wall MI • May also occur with atropine, epinephrine, isoproterenol, quinidine, caffeine, alcohol, and nicotine use	• Correction of underlying cause • Possible oxygen with or without normal saline infusion before Adult Cardiac Life Support (ACLS) protocol • Beta-adrenergic blockers or calcium channel blocker
Sinus bradycardia 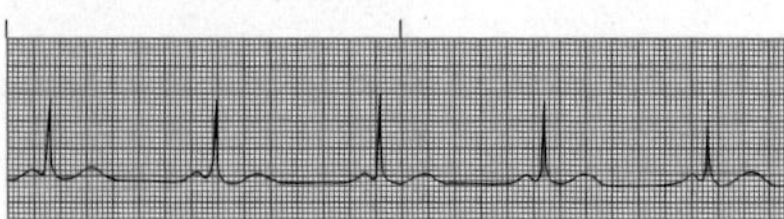 • Regular atrial and ventricular rhythms • Rate < 60 beats/minute • Normal P wave preceding each QRS complex	• Normal in a well-conditioned heart, as in an athlete • Increased intracranial pressure; increased vagal tone due to straining during defecation, vomiting, intubation, mechanical ventilation; sick sinus syndrome; hypothyroidism; inferior wall MI • May also occur with anticholinesterase, beta-adrenergic blocker, digoxin, or morphine use	• Correction of underlying cause • For low cardiac output, dizziness, weakness, altered level of consciousness (LOC), or low blood pressure: ACLS protocol for administration of atropine • Temporary or permanent pacemaker • Dopamine • Epinephrine

Arrhythmia and features	Causes	Treatment
Sinoatrial (SA) arrest or block *(sinus arrest)* 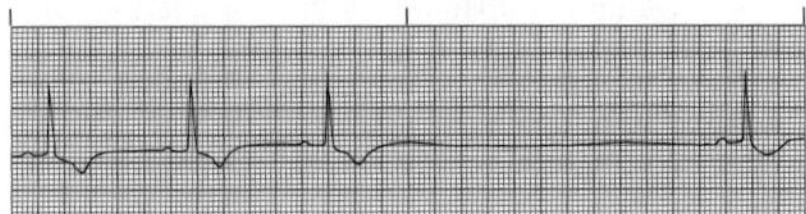 • Atrial and ventricular rhythms normal except for missing complex • Normal P wave preceding each QRS complex • Pause not equal to a multiple of the previous sinus rhythm	• Acute infection • Coronary artery disease (CAD), degenerative heart disease, acute inferior wall MI • Vagal stimulation, Valsalva's maneuver, carotid sinus massage • Digoxin, quinidine, or salicylate toxicity • Pesticide poisoning • Pharyngeal irritation caused by endotracheal (ET) intubation • Sick sinus syndrome	• No treatment if asymptomatic • For low cardiac output, dizziness, weakness, altered LOC, or low blood pressure: ACLS protocol for administration of atropine • Temporary or permanent pacemaker for repeated episodes
Premature atrial contraction *(PAC)* 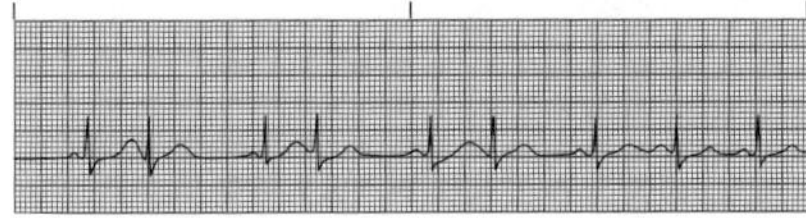 • Premature, abnormal-looking P waves that differ in configuration from normal P waves • QRS complexes after P waves, except in very early or blocked PACs • P wave often buried in the preceding T wave or identified in the preceding T wave	• Coronary or valvular heart disease, atrial ischemia, coronary atherosclerosis, heart failure, acute respiratory failure, chronic obstructive pulmonary disease (COPD), electrolyte imbalance, and hypoxia • Digoxin toxicity; use of aminophylline, beta-adrenergic blockers, or caffeine • Anxiety	• None (usually) • Treatment of underlying cause
Paroxysmal atrial tachycardia *(paroxysmal supraventricular tachycardia)* 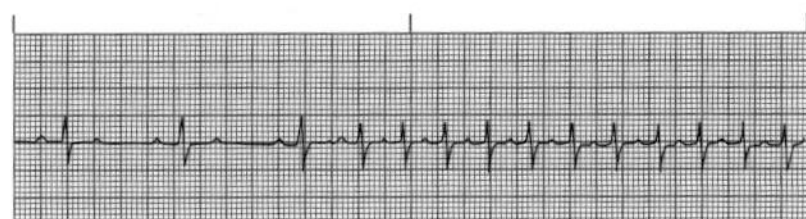 • Atrial and ventricular rhythms regular • Heart rate > 160 beats/minute; rarely exceeds 250 beats/minute • P waves regular but aberrant; difficult to differentiate from preceding T wave • P wave preceding each QRS complex • Sudden onset and termination of arrhythmia	• Intrinsic abnormality of AV conduction system • Physical or psychological stress, hypoxia, hypokalemia, cardiomyopathy, congenital heart disease, MI, valvular disease, Wolff-Parkinson-White syndrome, cor pulmonale, hyperthyroidism, systemic hypertension • Digoxin toxicity; use of caffeine, marijuana, or central nervous system stimulants	• If patient is unstable: immediate cardioversion • If patient is stable: vagal stimulation, Valsalva's maneuver, carotid sinus massage • If signs of good perfusion: ACLS priority—adenosine, calcium channel blockers, and cardioversion; if known heart failure or left ventricular failure: possible digoxin or beta-adrenergic blockers • If signs of poor perfusion: ACLS treatment priority—sedation then cardioversion; amiodarone or diltiazem if unresponsive to electrical therapy.
Atrial flutter 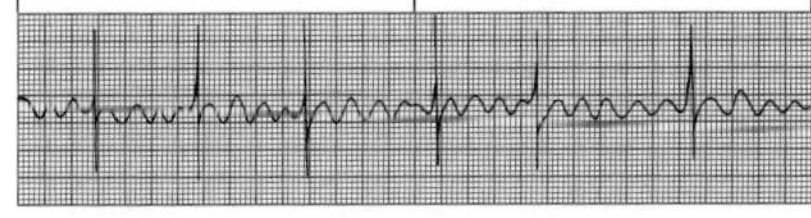 • Atrial rhythm regular; rate, 250 to 400 beats/minute • Ventricular rate variable, depending on degree of AV block (usually 60 to 100 beats/minute) • Sawtooth P-wave configuration possible (F waves) • QRS complexes uniform in shape but typically irregular in rate	• Heart failure, tricuspid or mitral valve disease, pulmonary embolism, cor pulmonale, inferior wall MI, carditis • Digoxin toxicity	• If patient is unstable with a ventricular rate >150 beats/minute or has signs of poor perfusion: immediate sedation and cardioversion starting at 50J and then ACLS medication therapy, which may include calcium channel blockers, beta-adrenergic blockers, or antiarrhythmics • If rate >150 beats/minute and no signs of poor perfusion: ACLS medication therapy is priority • Anticoagulation therapy, if necessary • Radiofrequency ablation to control rhythm

Arrhythmia and features	Causes	Treatment
Atrial fibrillation *(AFIB)* 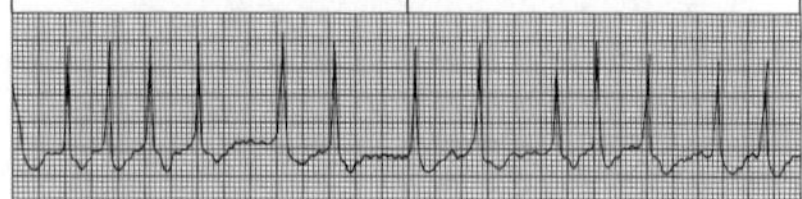 • Atrial rhythm grossly irregular; rate > 400 beats/minute • Ventricular rate grossly irregular • QRS complexes of uniform configuration and duration • PR interval indiscernible • No P waves, or P waves that appear as erratic, irregular, baseline fibrillary waves	• Heart failure, COPD, thyrotoxicosis, constrictive pericarditis, ischemic heart disease, sepsis, pulmonary embolus, rheumatic heart disease, hypertension, mitral stenosis, atrial irritation, complication of coronary bypass or valve replacement surgery	• If patient is unstable with a ventricular rate >150 beats/minute or signs of poor perfusion: immediate sedation and cardioversion starting at 120J biphasic or 200J monophasic then ACLS medication therapy, which may include calcium channel blockers, beta-adrenergic blockers, or antiarrhythmics • If rate >150 beats/minute and no signs of poor perfusion: ACLS medication therapy is priority • Anticoagulation therapy, if necessary • In some patients with refractory atrial fibrillation uncontrolled by drugs, radiofrequency catheter ablation
Junctional rhythm 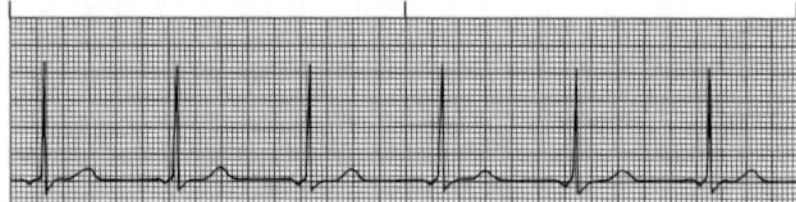 • Atrial and ventricular rhythms regular • Atrial rate 40 to 60 beats/minute • Ventricular rate usually 40 to 60 beats/minute (60 to 100 beats/minute is accelerated junctional rhythm) • P waves preceding, hidden within (absent), or after QRS complex; usually inverted if visible • PR interval (when present) < 0.12 seconds • QRS complex configuration and duration normal, except in aberrant conduction	• Inferior wall MI or ischemia, hypoxia, vagal stimulation, sick sinus syndrome • Acute rheumatic fever • Valve surgery • Digoxin toxicity	• Correction of underlying cause • Atropine for symptomatic slow rate • Pacemaker insertion if patient is refractory to drugs • Discontinuation of digoxin, if appropriate
Premature functional contraction 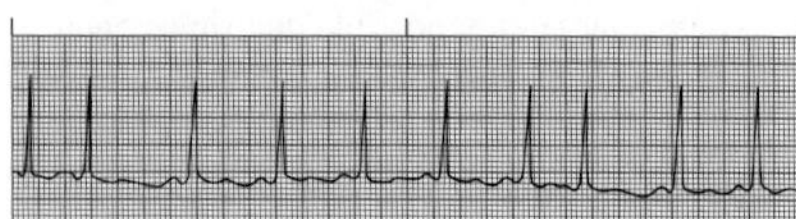 • Atrial and ventricular rhythms irregular • P waves inverted; may precede, be hidden within, or follow QRS complexes • PR interval < 0.12 seconds if P wave precedes QRS complex • QRS complex configuration and duration normal	• MI or ischemia • Digoxin toxicity and excessive caffeine or amphetamine use	• Correction of underlying cause • None (usually)

Arrhythmia and features	Causes	Treatment
Junctional tachycardia • Atrial rate > 100 beats/minute; however, P wave may be absent, hidden in QRS complex, or preceding T wave • Ventricular rate > 100 beats/minute • P wave inverted • QRS complex configuration and duration normal • Onset of rhythm typically sudden, occurring in bursts	• Myocarditis, cardiomyopathy, inferior wall MI or ischemia, acute rheumatic fever, complication of valve replacement surgery • Digoxin toxicity	• If stable without signs of poor perfusion: ACLS guidelines for amiodarone, calcium channel blocker, or beta-adrenergic blocker • If signs of poor perfusion or known history of heart failure: ACLS guidelines for amiodarone
First-degree AV block • Atrial and ventricular rhythms regular • PR interval > 0.20 seconds • P wave preceding each QRS complex • QRS complex normal	• May be seen in a healthy person • Inferior wall myocardial ischemia or MI, hypothyroidism, hypokalemia, hyperkalemia • Digoxin toxicity; use of quinidine, procainamide, beta-adrenergic blockers, calcium channel blockers, or amiodarone	• Correction of underlying cause • Possibly atropine if severe bradycardia develops • Cautious use of digoxin, calcium channel blockers, and beta-adrenergic blockers
Second-degree AV block Mobitz I *(Wenckebach)* • Atrial rhythm regular • Ventricular rhythm irregular • Atrial rate exceeds ventricular rate • PR interval progressively, but only slightly, longer with each cycle until QRS complex disappears (dropped beat); PR interval shorter after dropped beat	• Inferior wall MI, cardiac surgery, acute rheumatic fever, and vagal stimulation • Digoxin toxicity; use of propranolol, quinidine, or procainamide	• Treatment of underlying cause • Atropine or temporary pacemaker for symptomatic bradycardia • Discontinuation of digoxin, if appropriate
Second-degree AV block Mobitz II 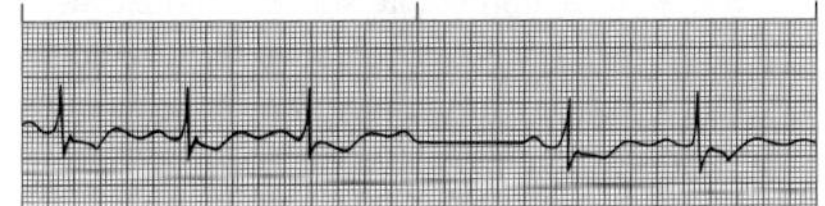 • Atrial rhythm regular • Ventricular rhythm regular or irregular, with varying degree of block • P-P interval constant • QRS complexes periodically absent	• Severe CAD, anterior wall MI, acute myocarditis • Digoxin toxicity	• Temporary or permanent pacemaker • Atropine, dopamine, or epinephrine for symptomatic bradycardia • Discontinuation of digoxin, if appropriate

Arrhythmia and features	Causes	Treatment
Third-degree AV block *(complete heart block)* 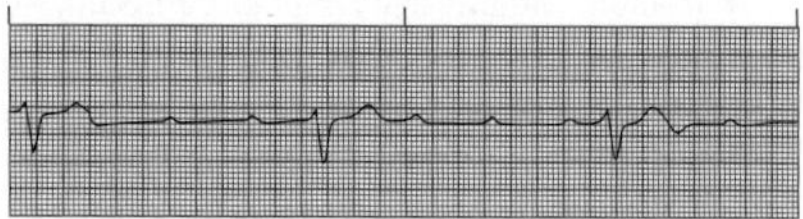 • Atrial rhythm regular • Ventricular rhythm slow and regular • No relation between P waves and QRS complexes • No constant PR interval • QRS interval normal (nodal pacemaker) or wide and bizarre (ventricular pacemaker)	• Inferior or anterior wall MI, congenital abnormality, rheumatic fever, hypoxia, postoperative complication of mitral valve replacement, Lev's disease (fibrosis and calcification that spreads from cardiac structures to the conductive tissue), Lenègre's disease (conductive tissue fibrosis) • Digoxin toxicity	• Temporary or permanent pacemaker • Atropine, dopamine, or epinephrine for symptomatic bradycardia
Premature ventricular contraction *(PVC)* 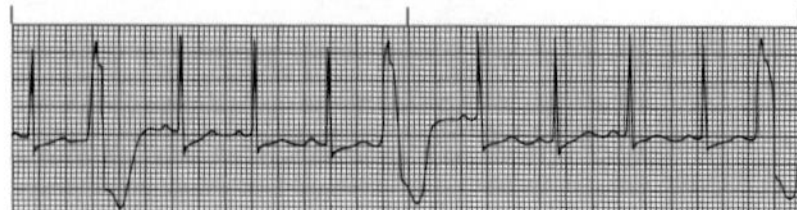 • Atrial rhythm regular • Ventricular rhythm possibly regular except for aberrant beats • QRS complex premature, usually followed by a complete compensatory pause • QRS complex wide and distorted, usually >0.12 seconds • Premature QRS complexes occurring singly, in pairs, or in threes; alternating with normal beats; focus from one or more sites • Ominous when clustered, multifocal, and with R wave on T pattern	• Heart failure; old or acute myocardial ischemia, MI, or contusion; myocardial irritation by ventricular catheter, such as a pacemaker; hypercapnia; hypokalemia; hypocalcemia • Drug toxicity (cardiac glycosides, aminophylline, tricyclic antidepressants, beta-adrenergic blockers [isoproterenol or dopamine]) • Caffeine, tobacco, or alcohol use • Psychological stress, anxiety, pain, exercise	• If symptomatic: procainamide, amiodarone, or lidocaine I.V. • Treatment of underlying cause: – Bicarbonate if known acidosis – Treatment for myocardial ischemia, as appropriate – Discontinuation of drugs causing toxicity – Potassium chloride I.V. if PVC induced by hypokalemia – Magnesium sulfate I.V. if PVC induced by hypomagnesemia • If symptomatic as a result of bradycardia: ACLS bradycardia algorithm
Ventricular tachycardia 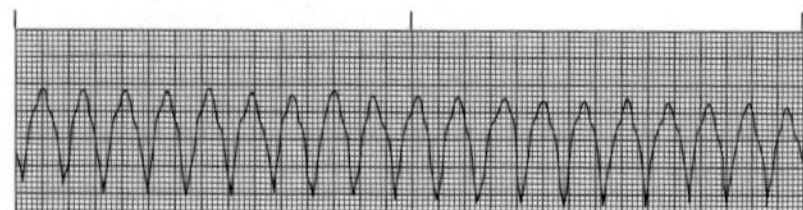 • Ventricular rate 140 to 220 beats/minute, regular or irregular • QRS complexes wide, bizarre, and independent of P waves • P waves not discernible • May start and stop suddenly	• Myocardial ischemia, MI, or aneurysm; CAD; rheumatic heart disease; mitral valve prolapse; heart failure; cardiomyopathy; ventricular catheters; hypokalemia; hypercalcemia; pulmonary embolism • Digoxin, procainamide, epinephrine, or quinidine toxicity • Anxiety	• With pulse with monomorphic wide-complex QRS complexes: administer adenosine (use adenosine cautiously in the presence of an irregular pulse); if unresponsive: amiodarone, procainamide, or sotalol; if persistent: possible cardioversion • If polymorphic and hemodynamically stable with a pulse: immediate shock, amiodarone, isoproterenol, over-drive pacing and cardioversion; if obvious Torsades or long baseline QT interval: possible magnesium sulfate • If with a pulse but unstable: sedation and cardioversion, then amiodarone • If pulseless: CPR, ACLS protocol for defibrillation STAT; then ACLS medication therapy, including epinephrine, vasopressin, amiodarone, lidocaine, bicarbonate, or magnesium sulfate as indicated; CO_2 monitor; advanced airway when available • If recurrent ventricular tachycardia: implantable cardioverter defibrillator

Arrhythmia and features	Causes	Treatment
Ventricular fibrillation • Ventricular rhythm rapid and chaotic • QRS complexes wide and irregular; no visible P waves	• Myocardial ischemia, MI, R-on-T phenomenon, untreated ventricular tachycardia, hypokalemia, hyperkalemia, hypercalcemia, alkalosis, electric shock, hypothermia • Digoxin, epinephrine, or quinidine toxicity	• If pulseless: CPR, ACLS protocol for defibrillation STAT; then ACLS medication therapy, including epinephrine, vasopressin, amiodarone, lidocaine, bicarbonate and magnesium sulfate as indicated; CO_2 monitor; advanced airway when available • If recurrent ventricular tachycardia: implantable cardioverter defibrillator
Asystole • No atrial or ventricular rate or rhythm • No discernible P waves, QRS complexes, or T waves	• Myocardial ischemia, MI, aortic valve disease, heart failure, hypoxemia, hypokalemia, severe acidosis, electric shock, ventricular arrhythmias, AV block, pulmonary embolism, heart rupture, cardiac tamponade, hyperkalemia, electromechanical dissociation • Cocaine overdose	• Cardiopulmonary resuscitation; ACLS protocol for ET intubation, transcutaneous pacing, and administration of epinephrine

Common life-support drugs

Drug	Indication
Adenosine (Adenocard)	*Paroxysmal supraventricular tachycardia (PSVT) involving atrioventricular (AV) node reentry* ▪ May cause flushing, dyspnea, chest pain, transient periods of sinus bradycardia, transient AV block, atrial fibrillation, and ventricular ectopy. ▪ Short half-life (less than 5 seconds). ▪ PSVT may recur. ▪ Theophylline decreases effectiveness. ▪ Dipyridamole potentiates effectiveness.
Aminophylline	*Acute bronchial asthma, bronchospasm associated with chronic bronchitis and emphysema* ▪ May cause palpitations, flushing, tachycardia or other arrhythmias, nervousness, irritability, headache, and hypotension.
Amiodarone	*Recurring ventricular fibrillation or unstable ventricular tachycardia; hemodynamically stable wide-complex tachycardia.* ▪ May cause hypotension and bradycardia. ▪ Reduces the clearance of warfarin (Coumadin) and digoxin.
Atropine (Atropen)	*Bradycardia, asystole* ▪ Lower dose (less than 0.5 mg) may sustain bradycardia. ▪ Higher dose (more than 3 mg) may cause full vagal blockage. ▪ Contraindicated for clients with glaucoma (use isoproterenol instead).
Beta-adrenergic blockers (atenolol [Tenormin], metoprolol tartrate [Lopressor], propranolol [Inderal], Esmolol [Brevibloc], labetolol)	*Reduce ventricular irritability in clients after myocardial infarction (MI); for emergency antihypertensive therapy in both hemorrhagic and ischemic stroke* ▪ Can cause bradycardia, AV conduction delays, and hypotension. ▪ Contraindicated in clients with symptomatic bradycardia, second- or third-degree block. ▪ Propranolol is contraindicated with cocaine-induced acute coronary syndrome.
Diltiazem	*Ventricular rate control in atrial fibrillation and atrial flutter; consider after adenosine for refractory supraventricular tachycardia* ▪ Blood pressure may drop from peripheral vasodilation. ▪ Use with caution with beta-adrenergic blockers and calcium channel blockers.
Diuretics (furosemide [Lasix])	*Acute pulmonary edema, cerebral edema after cardiac arrest* ▪ Venodilator effects occur within 5 minutes; can result in hypotension. ▪ Diuresis occurs within 60 minutes.
Dobutamine	*Acute heart failure, cardiopulmonary bypass surgery* ▪ Don't use with beta-adrenergic blockers such as propranolol. ▪ Clients with atrial fibrillation should receive digoxin first, or they can develop rapid ventricular response. ▪ Drug is incompatible with alkaline solutions. ▪ Infiltration may produce severe tissue damage.

Drug	Indication
Dopamine	*Shock, decreased renal function* ▪ Don't use for treating uncorrected tachyarrhythmias or ventricular fibrillation. ▪ May precipitate arrhythmias. ▪ Drug is incompatible with alkaline solutions. ▪ Infiltration may produce severe tissue damage. ▪ Solution deteriorates after 24 hours.
Epinephrine (Adrenaclick)	*Bronchospasm, anaphylaxis, severe allergic reactions, cardiac arrest, arrhythmias* ▪ Increases intraocular pressure. ▪ May exacerbate heart failure, arrhythmias, angina pectoris, hyperthyroidism, and emphysema. ▪ May cause headache, tremors, or palpitations. ▪ Monitor clients for signs of cerebral hemorrhage
Isoproterenol hydrochloride (Isuprel)	*Bronchospasm, heart block, cardiac arrest* ▪ Don't administer with epinephrine. ▪ Don't mix with barbiturates, sodium bicarbonate, any calcium preparation, or aminophylline. ▪ Contraindicated in heart blocks caused by digoxin toxicity.
Lidocaine (Xylocaine)	*Ventricular arrhythmias* ▪ Don't use if bradycardia is present or if client has high-grade sinoatrial or AV block. ▪ Don't mix with sodium bicarbonate. ▪ May lead to central nervous system toxicity. ▪ Light-headedness and dizziness are common.
Magnesium sulfate	*Hypomagnesemia, torsades de pointes* ▪ Serum magnesium and potassium levels should be determined. ▪ Can precipitate hypotension.
Nitroglycerin	*Angina, heart failure associated with MI* ▪ Angina not relieved with three sublingual tablets requires emergency medical services. ▪ May cause tachycardia, paradoxical bradycardia, and headache. ▪ Administration for more than 12 hours each day may produce tolerance. ▪ Hypovolemia decreases effectiveness and worsens hypotension.
Nitroprusside (Nitropress)	*Hypertension, increased systemic vascular resistance* ▪ Continuous blood pressure monitoring is required. ▪ Deteriorates when exposed to light; wrap in opaque container. ▪ May cause hypotension, headache, and vomiting. ▪ Cyanide toxicity may occur after 72 hours

Drug	**Indication**
Procainamide (Pronestyl)	*Ventricular arrhythmias including those associated with malignant hyperthermia* ▪ Can cause precipitous hypotension; don't use for treating second- or third-degree heart block unless a pacemaker has been inserted. ▪ Can cause AV block. ▪ Discontinue if PR interval or QRS complex widens or if arrhythmias worsen.
Sodium bicarbonate	*Metabolic acidosis, cardiac arrest* ▪ Don't mix with epinephrine; causes epinephrine degradation. ▪ Don't mix with calcium salts; forms insoluble precipitates.
Thrombolytic agents (activase [Alteplase], TNKase [Tenecteplase])	*Acute myocardial infarction, acute ischemic stroke* ▪ Alteplase is the only thrombolytic agent approved for acute ischemic stroke. ▪ Contraindicated in clients with a history of active internal bleeding within 2 days, history of stroke, or major surgery within 14 days.
Vasopressin	*Cardiopulmonary arrest as an alternative to epinephrine for clients without known cardiovascular disease* ▪ Potent vasoconstrictor. ▪ May cause hypotension or arrhythmias.
Verapamil	*Supraventricular tachyarrhythmias, angina, hypertension* ▪ Contraindicated in clients with aortic stenosis, hypotension, cardiogenic shock, severe heart failure, second- or third-degree AV block, or sick sinus syndrome. ▪ High doses or too-rapid administration can cause a significant drop in blood pressure. ▪ May increase serum digoxin levels.

Triage assessment principles

Triage involves gathering information about the client's presenting complaint and condition to determine acuity and priority of care. This acuity determination assists the triage nurse and the charge nurse to place clients appropriately so that the right client can be seen in the right place at the right time. Triage may also involve basic first aid and preliminary care. The Emergency Nurses Association recommends that, prior to performing triage activities, the emergency department nurse be experienced in emergency nursing care and trained in triage concepts.

Making triage decisions

To make triage decisions effectively, you must gather and interpret both subjective and objective data rapidly and accurately. Follow this rule: "When in doubt, triage up." That is, if you're uncertain as to the urgency of a client's condition, treat it as more, rather than less, urgent.

Triage activity consists of:

- obtaining a focused history of the client's chief complaint.
- performing a limited physical examination.
- classifying the client's problem for urgency.
- providing reassurance that the client will receive definitive medical care as soon as possible.

Obtaining a history

- Focus on the client's chief complaint.
- Document using the client's words; qualify his complaint as precisely as possible using the PQRST acronym (Provocate/Palliate, Quality/Quantity, Region/Radiation, Severity scale, Timing).
- Document the client's allergies and significant medical history.

Performing a physical examination

- Observe the client's general appearance, and assess his vital signs and level of consciousness (LOC).
- Take oral, axillary, tympanic, or temporal temperature as appropriate. Rectal temperature is the most accurate; take as indicated and ensure the client's privacy when possible.
- Check radial or apical pulse. Note rate, rhythm, and quality. While assessing pulse, check skin temperature and capillary refill time.
- Check blood pressure as quickly and accurately as possible.
- Note rate, depth, symmetry, and quality of respirations. Note skin color and turgor, facial expression, accessory muscle use, and any audible breath sounds.
- Assess LOC using a scale such as the Glasgow Coma Scale, or make a notation that the client is oriented to person, place, and time.

Classifying emergency conditions

Although triage acuity systems range from three to five levels, the Emergency Nurses Association, in collaboration with the American College of Emergency Physicians, released a position statement endorsing the use of a five-level triage.

Highest Triage Priority

Regardless of the system used, the highest triage priority includes those patients needing resuscitation or other immediate medical attention. Examples of highest priority conditions include respiratory or cardiac arrest, coma, or precipitous delivery.

Emergent conditions

The next level of priority, termed emergent, Level 2, or very urgent, includes those conditions needing medical and nursing attention as soon as possible. Start treatment using protocols or guidelines allowed by the facility, or notify the provider immediately if you triage a client complaining of:

- chest pain with dyspnea, cyanosis, diaphoresis, nausea, or vomiting.
- seizures.
- severe hemorrhage.
- severe head injury.
- poisoning or drug overdose.
- open chest or abdominal wounds.
- profound shock.

Triage responsibilities

Initial interventions, such as ice and elevation or wound care, typically need to be performed during triage. Client teaching can begin at triage with safety concepts, such as seat belts and car seat use, and hygiene concepts, such as proper hand washing.

Selected references

Briggs, J. K. (2011). Telephone triage protocols for nurses (4th ed.). Philadelphia, PA: Lippincott Williams & Wilkins.

Cavlovich, D. (2011). Ask an expert: Family presence at the bedside during resuscitation. *Nursing Made Incredibly Easy!, 9*(2), 56.

Emergency Nurse's Association. (2008). Emergency nursing core curriculum (6th ed.). Philadelphia, PA: W.B. Saunders.

Ernst, E. J., et al. (2011). Usefulness: Forensic photo documentation after sexual assault. *Advanced Emergency Nursing Journal, 33*(1), 29–38.

Foley, S. (2010). Short-term pharmaceutical management of the violent/aggressive patient in the emergency department. *Journal of Emergency Nursing, 36*(5), 504–506.

Fulde, G. (2009). Emergency medicine: The principles of practice (5th ed.). Philadelphia, PA: W.B. Saunders.

Gacki-Smith, J., et al. (2009). Violence against nurses working in US emergency departments. *Journal of Nursing Administration, 3*(7/8), 340–349.

Johnson, K. D., & Winkelman, C. (2011). The effect of emergency department crowding on patient outcomes: A literature review. *Advanced Emergency Nursing Journal, 33*(1), 39–54.

Mattu, M., et al. (2010). Avoiding common errors in the emergency department. Philadelphia, PA: Lippincott Williams & Wilkins.

Polly, D. M., et al. (2011). Applied pharmacology: Management of hypertensive emergency and urgency. *Advanced Emergency Nursing Journal, 33*(2), 127–136.

Proehl, J. (2008). Emergency nursing procedures (4th ed.). Philadelphia, PA: W.B. Saunders.

Shah, K. H., et al. (2010). Essential emergency trauma. Philadelphia, PA: Lippincott Williams & Wilkins.

Sheehy's emergency nursing: Principles and practice (6th ed.). (2010). St. Louis, MO: Mosby, Inc.

Stauber, M. A. (2011). Not all spinal cord injuries involve a fracture. *Advanced Emergency Nursing Journal, 33*(3), 226–231.

Index

t refers to a table.

t refers to a table.

E

t refers to a table.

I

t refers to a table.

N

t refers to a table.

Q

R

t refers to a table.

t refers to a table.